Sir Andrew Macphail

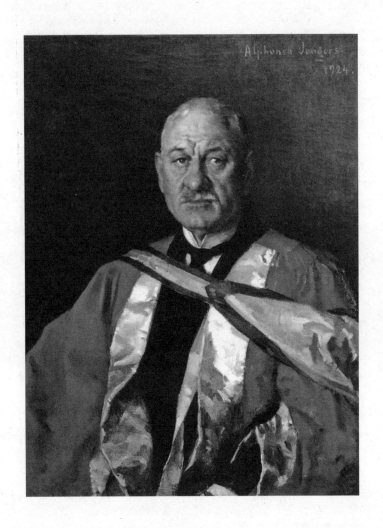

Sir Andrew Macphail

*The Life and Legacy of
a Canadian Man of Letters*

IAN ROSS ROBERTSON

McGill-Queen's University Press
Montreal & Kingston • London • Ithaca

© McGill-Queen's University Press 2008

ISBN 978-0-7735-3419-3

Legal deposit fourth quarter 2008
Bibliothèque nationale du Québec

Printed in Canada on acid-free paper that is 100% ancient forest free (100% post-consumer recycled), processed chlorine free

This book has been published with the help of a grant from the Canadian Federation for the Humanities and Social Sciences, through the Aid to Scholarly Publications Programme, using funds provided by the Social Sciences and Humanities Research Council of Canada.

McGill-Queen's University Press acknowledges the support of the Canada Council for the Arts for our publishing program. We also acknowledge the financial support of the Government of Canada through the Book Publishing Industry Development Program (BPIDP) for our publishing activities.

Library and Archives Canada Cataloguing in Publication

Robertson, Ian Ross, 1944-
   Sir Andrew Macphail : the life and legacy of a Canadian man of letters / Ian Ross Robertson.

Includes bibliographical references and index.
ISBN 978-0-7735-3419-3

1. Macphail, Andrew, Sir, 1864-1938. 2. Authors, Canadian (English) – 20th century – Biography. 3. Editors – Canada – Biography. 4. College teachers – Canada – Biography. I. Title.

PS8525.P42Z86 2008   C814'.52   C2008-902625-X

Typeset by Marvin Harder in Sabon Next LT Pro.

Frontispiece: Portrait of Sir Andrew Macphail, oil on canvas, by Alphonse Jongers, 1924. The painting hangs in the dining room of the Macphail Homestead, and this photograph was taken after professional restoration in 2007. A longtime member of the Pen and Pencil Club, Jongers lived at Macphail's home, 216 Peel Street, for some years as a result of financial reverses in the stock market crash and, while there, used 216 Peel as a studio. He subsequently moved to the Ritz-Carlton Hotel. As a portraitist he commanded fees of $5,000 or more.

Dedicated to the memory of Dorothy Macphail Lindsay

Contents

Contents

Introduction

At the end of the nineteenth century and the beginning of the twentieth, Canada seemed at last to be a "success." Industrialization was accelerating, cities were growing, and the West was being settled by immigrants from many countries. Yet with the achievements came a questioning of the costs, impact, and ultimate meaning of these changes for Canadian society. The foundation of the new prosperity was the National Policy of high tariffs, massive immigration, settlement of the West, and industrial expansion for the central provinces. This was not an unmixed blessing for all Canadians, since it entailed a drastic alteration in the regional balance of the country, encouragement of industry at the expense of agriculture, and increased specialization and reliance on machines for those who remained on the soil. The changes held profound implications for cultural patterns based on the older and more rural social order. Indeed, it seemed that a well-integrated and stable way of life was crumbling.

Andrew Macphail was the product of a region, the Maritimes, and a cultural heritage, that of the Scottish Highlands, which combined to make him acutely conscious of the social transformation underway. This study examines Macphail, his life, his world view, its roots, and the legacy of his life's work, but also attempts to convey the remarkable variety of fields to which he applied his energy. After receiving his early education in his native Prince Edward Island, he proceeded to McGill University where he graduated in both arts and medicine. In order to finance his studies, he developed into a prolific and highly skilled journalist, working for daily Montreal newspapers and at least one wire service. He became a practising physician and a professor in first the University of Bishop's College Faculty of Medicine and then McGill's Faculty of Medicine, where he spent thirty years as the first holder of its chair in the history of medicine.

An important editor of medical journals commencing in 1903, he was the driving force behind the foundation, eight years later, of Canada's first national medical periodical, the *Canadian Medical Association Journal*, and he served as its first editor. He was also outstanding for his independence of thought with respect to medical education, questioning the priority given to science, rather than direct contact with the sick, in the earliest stages of the curriculum.

But it was as a writer and as a non-medical editor that Macphail developed a truly national reputation among the literate public. He was founder, editor, and ultimate financial backer of the *University Magazine*, a markedly successful quarterly of broad focus, a publication that set new standards for Canada and flourished from 1907 to 1920. In establishing the magazine, which was published out of his home at 216 Peel Street, he built upon his experience and contacts as a member, since 1897, of the Pen and Pencil Club in Montreal. A remarkable group of artists and writers, it included the painters William Brymner, Maurice Cullen, Edmond Dyonnet, and Robert Harris, the humorist and political scientist Stephen Leacock, the physician and poet John McCrae, the architect and man of multiple talents Percy E. Nobbs, and the literature professor Paul T. Lafleur. They met fortnightly, usually about a dozen in number, on Saturdays, from autumn until spring, presenting original works for discussion and criticism in an atmosphere in which wine and spirits flowed copiously. The meetings were as much social as professional gatherings, in part because, as Macphail put it, "Artists would discourse upon writings, and ... writers would discourse upon pictures,"[1] a practice that militated against excessively competitive behaviour. He rapidly became an exceptionally frequent contributor to the programs of the club, delivering both poetry and prose.

Macphail's prose writing, much of it published in the *University Magazine*, quickly built for him a national name as a formidable political and social commentator in the years 1907–14. In this period Macphail was central to almost every aspect of English Canadian intellectual life, making his views forcefully known, and discovering and encouraging new talent. He articulated a philosophy of political and social conservatism whose pivotal components were imperialism and attachment to a traditional rural way of life. "Imperialism" in Canada as it was understood in the early twentieth century requires some explanation for readers in the twenty-first. The version that such figures as Macphail espoused was a form of Canadian nationalism that involved, especially after 1900, the assertion that a maturing Canada should do its full part in governing the British Empire. In other words, the entire emphasis was on assuming responsibilities, not on conquest or commerce. Macphail's friend Rudyard Kipling was delighted that his writing "dares to indicate that the new countries ... have duties."[2] Canadian imperialists such as Macphail envisioned a decentralized empire, with Canada playing an increasing role and exercising more power.

This sense of a maturing Canada, wanting to assert its equality within the British Empire, was evident in such enterprises as Macphail's quarterly. Before its first year was out, Earl Grey, the governor general of Canada, stated in private correspondence with the editor of the *Spectator* in London that "it compares not unfavourably with any of the home ... Monthlies."[3] One of the consistent themes in the *University Magazine*'s articles was the need for Canada to develop institutions and cultural bodies worthy of a mature country. In 1907 Lawrence J. Burpee, an Ottawa librarian, published a piece pleading for a much more systematic and coordinated approach to copying, storing, and making accessible historical documents related to Canada. He was highly critical of the status quo, which involved, according to him, much needless duplication of effort among institutions, and he pointed to positive counter-examples in such countries as Holland.[4] Three and one-half years later Burpee argued, again in the *University Magazine*, in favour of a national library, emphasizing that Canada lacked what small European countries and the republics of South America had. In this instance he scrutinized the practices of the Library of Congress in the United States for lessons that Canadians could learn.[5] In the next issue, John Edward Hoare of Montreal made a case for the development of local repertory theatre in Canada, to replace the overly commercial and lowest-common-denominator "sexology plays" that visiting companies brought to his city; he drew upon England, Germany, and Sweden for inspiration. Hoare believed that theatre based on the repertory model could travel, and he hoped the project would be a force unifying Canada.[6]

In summary, Macphail, the *University Magazine*, and its contributors frequently promoted what can be described as the self-improvement of Canada, and almost as frequently used non-Canadian examples as prods. They wanted to make Canadians understand that their country had passed the pioneering stage and the need to focus on immediate needs, and that consequently there should be a place for culture, the arts, and intelligent commentary. This drive was exactly analogous to Leacock's imperialist manifesto in political matters, "Greater Canada: An Appeal," which appeared in Macphail's quarterly and in which he exhorted Canadians to say, "The time has come; we know and realize our country. We will be ... [a] colony no longer."[7]

Macphail had burst upon the Canadian scene as an advocate of imperialism and as a singularly efficient and creative editor. He was also rapidly recognized as a master of the essay genre, publishing three volumes of his collected essays by 1910 and acquiring a reputation that has endured. When a major international project on the essay was being planned in the mid-1990s, an article on him was commissioned.[8] At the same time as Macphail was emerging as a leading Canadian essayist, he was becoming known as an outspoken critic of industrialization, tariff protection, American influences on Canadian life, and utilitarian education, among other modern trends; for example, he acquired fame – or notoriety, depending on the perspective – as an exceptionally emphatic antifeminist. More positively, he was a spokesman for a traditional way of life based on agriculture and, with it, the crafts that were being displaced by machine production. His ideals in these matters were modelled essentially, and sometimes explicitly, upon the sort of community in which he had grown up. This point of view was nourished by a continuing connection with his native district of Orwell, Prince Edward Island. Commencing in 1905, he returned there in the summers, and for several years he and a brother, a professor of engineering at Queen's University in Kingston, conducted agricultural experiments on the family property.

In order to explain why Macphail thought and advocated as he did, considerable attention must be given to the details of his early environment. His critical perspective and its significance can be fully understood only in the context of his social origins. Macphail was helpful to the investigator in this respect, for particularly in his later years he produced a considerable amount of self-revelatory writing. One result of this process of reflection and taking stock in the last twelve or more years of his life was *The Master's Wife*, a work that is now recognized as his creative masterpiece – a memoir of his early life in Prince Edward Island, presented through the mind of a child. That book, with its strikingly original technique, was published posthumously and eventually made him an iconic figure among those modern-day Prince Edward Islanders seeking to define a distinctive traditional local "way of life," with rural communities at the centre.[9] It is a development whose beginnings can be traced back to the 1970s[10] and which crystallized in the late 1980s with a successful popular, grassroots effort to save Macphail's birthplace – which had been donated to the province in 1961 – from falling into complete decay after many years of official neglect.

Acknowledgments

Many debts have been incurred over a long period, and it would be impossible to acknowledge all. Several persons have been mentioned at specific places in the notes, but in addition, certain individuals must be singled out. Carl Berger, professor emeritus, University of Toronto, has retained an interest in Macphail over several decades, offering insightful observations and asking many astute questions. Brook Taylor of Mount Saint Vincent University, my one-time student, former colleague, and present friend, has always encouraged this work, and it was he who suggested creation of the map of "Andrew Macphail's Montreal" for the benefit of those not familiar with Macphail's urban bailiwick. Paul Potter of the University of Western Ontario, once a fellow undergraduate at McGill and now an historian of medicine, has been aware for many years of Macphail's special combination of qualities, and has given me the benefit of his breadth of expertise.

Katherine Dewar's generosity was exceptional in allowing me to use the taped interviews she made in 1990 with persons who recalled Macphail from their youth. She was also one of the Friends of Macphail who, through their efforts, literally saved Macphail's home from falling down in the late 1980s. It is unfortunate that not all of those Friends are living to read this book. Harry Baglole's work in ensuring a proper reprinting of *The Master's Wife*, the result of years of persistent effort, deserves the gratitude of all students of Island history and of Canadian literature in general; he has been consistently sympathetic to efforts to preserve the Macphail Homestead as well as Macphail's memory on the Island. When it was time for me to seek images to support the written text, Jean Macphail Weber, a grandniece of the subject, was exceptionally helpful. My friend and former student David Carrington gave me the benefit of his technical expertise.

The map of Montreal was executed by Byron Moldofsky and Mariange Beaudry of the Cartography Office, Department of Geography, University of Toronto. With great generosity, Douglas Sobey, a research associate of the Institute of Island Studies, University of Prince Edward Island, created maps of Prince Edward Island that highlight areas of special importance for Macphail's life.

A grant from the Canada Council supported some of the research which made this book possible. Parts have appeared in different form in the following: "Andrew Macphail: A Holistic Approach," *Canadian Literature* 107 (Winter 1985): 179–86; and "Introduction" to a reprint of Sir Andrew Macphail, *The Master's Wife*, 3rd edition (Charlottetown: Institute of Island Studies, 1994). They appear here with permission.

In preparing the book for publication, Joan McGilvray of McGill-Queen's University Press, the coordinating editor, and Carlotta Lemieux, the copy editor, have performed with remarkable skill, attention to detail, and good judgment.

It bears repetition that many individuals helped this project in a variety of ways, and to all I am grateful. They are too numerous for me to hope to compile a list naming them without missing some. I am reminded of the text of an inscription on a plaque in the Baglio Anselmi Regional Archaelogical Museum in Marsala, Sicily, preceding a list of those who had assisted with their major find, a Phoenician ship sunk during the First Punic War, discovered in 1971: they were "too numerous to name individually," but those on the list could "be regarded as representative."

Early Years in Prince Edward Island

In an essay published in 1919, Andrew Macphail, by then knighted and a recognized leader in the field of Canadian letters, wrote, "The life of a Canadian is bound up with the history of his parish, of his town, of his province, of his country, and even with the history of that country in which his family had its birth."[1] Following Macphail's prescription, this study commences with his family, its migration from Scotland at least a generation before his birth, and a brief explanation of the context in which his grandparents left their homeland.

ANCESTRY

William Macphail,[2] an emigrating Scottish schoolmaster, was cast ashore with his family near the mouth of the River John in northeastern Nova Scotia on 1 September 1833. His intended destination was Napanee, Upper Canada, where a cousin was inspector of schools. Leaving his wife and two small children in Nova Scotia, the schoolmaster walked to Napanee. Apparently, he did not like Upper Canada, and after a short visit he returned on foot to Nova Scotia rather than sending for his family. The Macphails lived in several communities in Pictou County and on Cape Breton Island before moving to Prince Edward Island in September 1844. By this time, six more children had been born, one of whom had died.[3]

Macphail continued to teach in the New World and appears to have been highly successful in his profession, at least in pedagogical terms. In his surviving papers there is a statement by a parent whose children he had taught for several years at West River, Nova Scotia, where Dr Thomas McCulloch – the famed author and naturalist, principal of the Pictou

Academy, and founding president of Dalhousie College – had established a theological seminary and where standards were certain to be exacting. The writer praised Macphail in elaborate terms, stating that although he had encountered many schoolmasters, he had met none other who "produced either greater quantity, or quality of his pupils [*sic*] improvement, or progress in learning, or who devoted himself more entirely to the duties of his profession."[4] Macphail was a person of some learning and had attended King's College, Aberdeen, where he won a prize for Latin prose in 1820. But the scholarship fund that sponsored him became the object of factional strife within the Church of Scotland, and after four years of a seven-year course he was compelled to discontinue his studies and return to his native Nairn. He commenced teaching in the Highlands and in 1829, at the age of twenty-seven, married Mary McPherson of Inverness-shire.[5]

Teaching, never a lucrative profession, was also insecure in the Highlands of the 1830s. The progressive integration of the local ruling class with the commercially oriented English aristocracy throughout the eighteenth and early nineteenth centuries was uprooting the distinctive Highland society and culture. As historian Eric Hobsbawm has pointed out, the

> foundation of Highland society was the tribe (clan) of subsistence peasants or pastoralists settled in an ancestral area under the chieftain of their kin, whom the old Scottish kingdom had (wrongly) attempted to assimilate to a feudal noble, and English eighteenth-century society (even more wrongly) to an aristocratic landowner. This assimilation gave the chiefs the legal – but by clan standards immoral – right to do what they wanted with their "property," and entangled them in the expensive status-competition of British aristocratic life, for which they had neither the resources nor the financial sense. They could raise their income only by destroying their society. From the point of view of the clansmen the chief was not a landlord, but the head of their clan to whom they owed loyalty in peace and war and who in turn owed them largesse and support. Conversely the social standing of the chief in Highland society depended not upon the number of his acres of moorland and forest, but on that of the armed men he could raise. The chiefs were therefore in a double dilemma. As "old" chiefs their interests lay in multiplying

Sir Andrew Macphail

To date, among students of Canadian history (outside Prince Edward Island), Macphail has been known primarily as an imperialist. There is much more to be learned about this complex, multisided figure. As well as being devoted to rural life as he understood it, and critical of many modern trends, he actively supported the arts in Montreal long after his magazine had been wound up; and, more broadly, he was concerned to encourage Canadian writers, especially new ones such as Sinclair Ross, to write. A man of letters of a non-specialized type that has almost disappeared in the past century,[11] he was an unusually productive and wide-ranging author who attempted many genres in addition to the essay. Drama (including a play that has been identified as a Canadian adaptation of *The Taming of the Shrew*), the historical novel, and the short story are examples. Furthermore, an examination of Macphail delves into and reveals attitudes and preoccupations that have bedevilled Canadian thought for generations. Indeed, many of the tensions he explored – rural versus urban, centralist versus localist, specialism versus generalism, utilitarian versus humanistic education, to name but a few – continue to work themselves out today.

Macphail was also a man of action. When the First World War began, he insisted on participating as a medical officer with a field ambulance at the front, although in his fiftieth year and virtually blind in one eye as the result of an accident suffered in 1911. This volunteering has to be understood as a point of principle for him: he did not believe in theory without practice. One did not advocate going "back to the land" or "off to war" without being willing to get involved.

But with Macphail one must begin at the beginning.

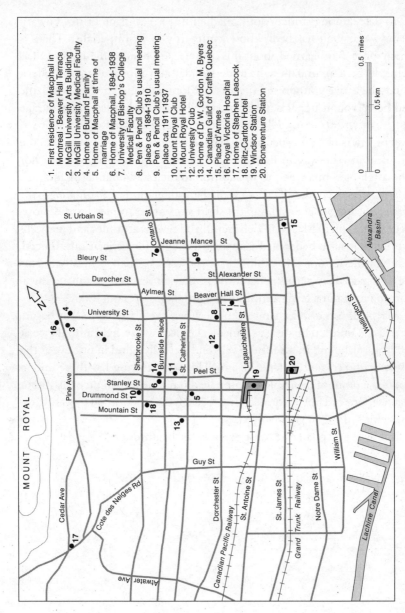

1. First residence of Macphail in Montreal : Beaver Hall Terrace
2. McGill University Arts Building
3. McGill University Medical Faculty
4. Home of Burland Family
5. Home of Macphail at time of marriage
6. Home of Macphail, 1894-1938
7. University of Bishop's College Medical Faculty
8. Pen & Pencil Club's usual meeting place ca. 1894-1910
9. Pen & Pencil Club's usual meeting place ca. 1911-1937
10. Mount Royal Club
11. Mount Royal Hotel
12. University Club
13. Home of Dr W. Gordon M. Byers
14. Canadian Guild of Crafts Quebec
15. Place d'Armes
16. Royal Victoria Hospital
17. Home of Stephen Leacock
18. Ritz-Carlton Hotel
19. Windsor Station
20. Bonaventure Station

Andrew Macphail's Montreal

Illustrations

Preface

This book is the product of several decades of interest in Sir Andrew Macphail, which began more than half a century ago when, as a small child, I had glimpses from a moving car of the stately pillars at the end of a lane that led to a deserted homestead located on a scenic clay road in southeastern Prince Edward Island. I came to know that the home and the pillars had belonged to someone called Sir Andrew Macphail and realized that – whoever he was – he had had a deep connection to the place. But it was only at university in the 1960s, first in Montreal and then Toronto, that I began to have a real idea of who he had been and what he had accomplished. Professor J.I. Cooper of McGill, now deceased, who remembered Macphail as a prominent person on campus in the 1930s, told me of Macphail's semi-autobiography, *The Master's Wife*, which he believed to be the best book of its kind, an account of the post-pioneering generation in rural Canada. When I was a graduate student at the University of Toronto in the first year of my doctoral studies, Professor Ramsay Cook suggested that I do my major research paper for the year on Macphail. Professor Carl Berger directed a subsequent PHD thesis on Macphail as a social critic. After completion of the thesis I moved on to other projects, but I noted that in Prince Edward Island there was a growing interest in Macphail and his legacy as the Island left its predominantly rural past behind. I did what I could to contribute to that consciousness, writing introductions to reprints of *The Master's Wife*, lecturing in Macphail's native district, and again lecturing when, in the late 1980s, it appeared that the provincial government was ready to allow his home, which had been given to the province in 1961, to deteriorate and fall into ruin. Thankfully, with the efforts of dedicated volunteers from across the Island, including summer residents, the house was saved and restored.

Also saved, after Macphail's death in 1938, was a susbtantial collection of his personal papers. I found these through the good offices of my mother, who had been taught by a niece of Macphail in a one-room school in Valleyfield, Prince Edward Island, early in the twentieth century. This niece, the native of a district adjacent to Valleyfield, provided me with an introduction to Macphail's sole surviving child, Mrs Dorothy Lindsay, who lived in Montreal and had custody of the papers. When I met Mrs Lindsay, she received me with exceptional hospitality and generosity of spirit. She gave me full and unfettered access to her father's papers; she made the space available for me to use them; she maximized my comfort and convenience; and she shared with me her recollections of him, his family, his associates, and his times. From our first meeting I had the sense that I was in her father's presence. To her memory this book is dedicated with a sense of gratitude and privilege.

When I used the papers they were in private hands, and that is how they are listed in the bibliography, as a private collection. Most of the material is no longer in private hands; anyone seeking additional clarification should contact me.

Ian Ross Robertson
March 2008

primitive subsistence peasants on increasingly congested territory; as "new" noble landlords, in exploiting their estates by modern methods, which almost certainly meant exchanging human tenants for livestock (which requires little labour), or the sale of their land, or both ... Most of them ... raised their incomes as best they could, exchanging the barbarous simplicities of their hills for the more sophisticated and expensive pleasures of the urban aristocratic life ... After the [Napoleonic] wars the times of horror began. Greedy or bankrupt landlords began to "clear" their uncomprehendingly loyal tribesmen from the land, scattering them as emigrants throughout the world from the slums of Glasgow to the forests of Canada.[6]

Between 1831 and 1841 the population of Nairnshire actually declined in absolute numbers. When, in the scramble for those jobs that remained, William Macphail was displaced from his school at Fort William, Inverness-shire, by a candidate with the backing of a local notable, William and Mary decided to emigrate. Three years later, his brother Hugh wrote from Inverness, "It is hard & difficult to live here, William. All that can be done is to 'Keep the Bones Green.'"[7] Within a few years, Hugh had emigrated to the United States.[8]

Even in the New World, the Macphails endured a precarious existence. A collection of papers deposited in the provincial archives of Prince Edward Island in 2004 provides an illustration. In 1840 a resident of Port Hood, Nova Scotia, apparently a merchant, wrote to William with a proposition. It seems that a son, William Jr, age 10, was with the merchant, who was writing to suggest that he keep the boy, "as you may not be *permanently* situated & having so young & helpless a family about you." Young William would be "*warm clothed* & well fed," the merchant stated. "If [he] was allowed to remain with me for some time I would make a smart, industrious man of him & in a year or two take him into the store & ultimately pay him as a clerk & do for him till he is old enough to look for himself – & take my word for it, it would be better for him in the end than to be at no steady employ, as he would be with you."[9] Notes on the paper regarding the address, one by a different hand, indicate that the father was moving about, most probably seeking work. The contents of the letter indicate that he was perceived as being in a vulnerable situation, perhaps not able to provide adequately for his family.

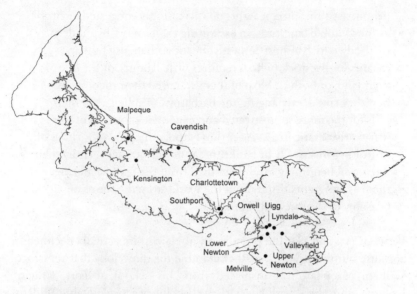

Prince Edward Island

PARENTAGE

In Prince Edward Island the Macphails eventually established a permanent residence at Upper Newton,[10] Lot 57, on the south shore of eastern
Queens County. The location of their home, virtually at the intersection
of the Selkirk Road and the Newton Road, can be identified on a map of
the colony dated 1863.[11] The two eldest children, William and Janet, aged
seventeen and sixteen, had schools of their own by 1847, and there is some
evidence that William had been doing at least some teaching in the Pictou
area of Nova Scotia in 1843 at age thirteen.[12] In Prince Edward Island he
taught in a number of districts and gained an enviable reputation as a progressive, capable, and strict though even-handed teacher in an era when
colonial schoolmasters were often unqualified, sadistic inebriates. In 1854
John Murdoch Stark, a Scottish school visitor who had recently arrived
on the Island, reported on the performance of scholars during his visit to
Macphail's school in Lower Newton: "I have much pleasure in stating that
they did their work in a most attentive and orderly manner, which is very
creditable to their indefatigable teacher."[13] This was significant praise from
a man whose outspoken intolerance of laziness and incompetence would

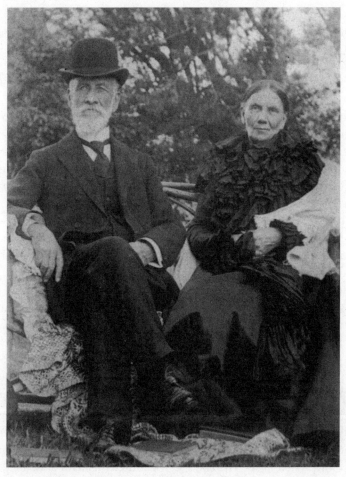

William and Catherine Macphail. This photograph of Andrew's parents is set in their garden at Orwell.

soon make him a target of anonymous abuse in the Island press from angry and ill-paid teachers.[14]

On 3 August 1858 William Macphail, whose father had died six years earlier, married Catherine Elizabeth Smith,[15] age twenty-three, a native of Lower Newton where he was still teaching. Her paternal grandparents had arrived on Prince Edward Island in 1802; the grandfather was a native of northern Perthshire.[16] One of their sons, the father of Catherine, was a spar-maker. In the words of Andrew, "To make a spar in the craft of ship-building is like making a sonnet in the craft of letters. He moved from place to place where a ship was being built and ready for her spars. A spar-maker works alone as a poet does. He would set up his benches in a retired grove apart from the yard; he would eat and sleep by himself. His work took him as far as the Miramichi." Andrew repeated a family story about his grandfather: "In that strange place his custom was not known, nor his reticence, as he thought, sufficiently respected. A sailor was incautious. He struck the man with his fist and killed him. The Smiths were a passionate people." But Andrew conceded that the Macphail family members were never able to extract from Catherine a categorical confirmation or denial of the story of the homicide on the Miramichi: "She wished her family to be well thought of. She did add, however, that … she had heard that his [her father's] forearm was as thick as another man's thigh. The utmost she would admit was that if he had struck the sailor he would have killed him, and 'it served him right.'"[17]

The first children of William and Catherine, twin brothers, were born in 1859; one died fifteen minutes after delivery.[18] Others soon arrived, and when Andrew was born on 24 November 1864 he was the fourth to survive birth; ten would do so by 1877.[19] With a growing family, William felt the need to supplement his annual salary of £50. For a time he considered leaving his profession to become a shopkeeper, but an experiment in buying tea and tobacco for resale led to a net loss of some £20. After this disappointment, William decided to attempt to provide for basic necessities through farming in addition to teaching. In March 1861 he accepted a new position paying £60 in the neighbouring school district of Uigg, and three years later he purchased, at a cost of £220, the residue of a 999-year lease (which had commenced in 1829) to the 100-acre farm on which the school stood. The actual location of the farmhouse was in the district of Orwell, in a part of it then known as Orwell Head. Like most Island land occupiers at the time, William was a tenant, and he would remain such until the legislated abolition of leasehold tenure in the late 1870s. The owners of the land on Lot 50 were two sisters, Maria Matilda Fanning and Louisa Augusta Wood, who resided at the prestigious address of No. 3 The Circus, Bath, England; they were daughters of a former lieutenant governor, the Loyalist Edmund Fanning (1739–1818).[20]

William had had a series of religious experiences between 1859 and 1861, commencing on the occasion of the death of his nineteen-year-old brother, John McPherson Macphail, who was beginning his fifth year as a teacher.

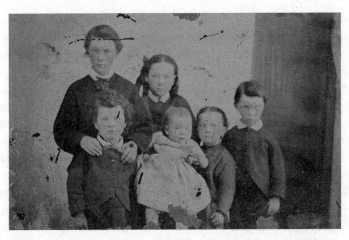

The Macphail children, 1869. These are the eldest six children of William and Catherine Macphail. *Back row, left to right:* William John James, Margaret Ann, Finlay Smith; *front row, left to right:* Andrew (John Andrew), Janetta Clark, Mary Isabella.

Although William's most frivolous activity as a young man had probably been the writing of verse, he worried about his lack of religious enthusiasm at a time when Protestant evangelism was sweeping the Island. By September 1861 he could write that at last "there is a progress of enlightenment going on in me."[21] An elder in the "McDonaldite" Church of Scotland[22] throughout his adult life, he did not fit the stereotype of the reformed sinner giving up a life of abandon. He had never been irreligious or blasphemous in his behaviour or speech, and had none of the conventional vices to put aside. Yet there is a discernible change of tone and emphasis in his correspondence after 1861: less concern is manifested for his own spiritual state and more for that of others. Although not a self-righteous or bigoted man, he was in many ways the archetypal mid-Victorian father: strictly sabbatarian, imbued with a strong sense of duty, personally fastidious, and, all in all, very much in earnest. His son Andrew later recalled:

> Everything the Master did was correct - his manner of eating, of drinking, of holding a pen or a book, of sitting in a chair or arising from it; and he did his best to instil a sense of correctness in his children. A child who was too tired or too indolent to sit erect was allowed the option of going to bed. To "sprawl in a chair" was to him the mark of a slovenly and undisciplined mind. He had words of

deadly directness. To stroll on a forest path with motive ulterior to
the purpose of passing through was "to lurk in the woods." For a boy
to proceed at any other pace than a run was to linger, loiter, dawdle,
meander, creep, saunter.[23]

Sixty-five years after his death a granddaughter remembered that nobody
was supposed to move a chair when sitting on it. "Each chair had a reason
for being where it was."[24]

In 1868 William Macphail was appointed school visitor for Queens
County. The inspection of schools had been a chronic problem following
Stark's departure eleven years earlier. Since the number of district schools
had greatly increased, the job was divided among three visitors, one for
each county. Although Macphail received the same salary of £150 as each of
his two colleagues, his responsibilities were almost as heavy as theirs combined. Nonetheless, his reports were a model of thoroughness, exhibiting
greater care and attention to detail than those of any school visitor since
Stark. With the exception of seven months in 1872–73, Macphail continued
to hold this position until the end of 1878, when he failed to meet a new
set of qualifications. It was the implementation of the reforming Public
Schools Act of 1877 that displaced him; ironically, he had been advocating
many of its features for years.[25] He returned to rural school teaching.

But at the beginning of 1882 Macphail was appointed supervisor of
the provincial Hospital for the Insane, located a short distance outside
Charlottetown, following a scandal over mistreatment of a patient the previous year. As recommended by a commission of inquiry, the duties of the
supervisor were redefined to permit closer oversight of subordinates, and
the major reason the government turned to Macphail was his exceptional
reputation for integrity. But there was another element to the outcry, for
the patient was a McDonaldite, and most of the five attendants implicated
were Roman Catholics. Indeed, Macphail had participated in organizing a
denominational protest; in the circumstances, the appointment of him, a
McDonaldite of undoubted rectitude, was a prudent measure on the part
of W.W. Sullivan, the first Roman Catholic premier of the Island and only
two years in office. Macphail served as supervisor until 1900 and appears
to have displayed the same diligence as he did when inspecting schools.
His responsibilities increased greatly in 1889 when there ceased to be a
medical superintendent residing on the premises; he became the chief officer present around the clock. This remained the situation until the turn
of the century, when a new medical superintendent was appointed, with

instructions to reside at the hospital and devote his entire time to the position. The former school visitor was relegated to the new office of bursar, responsible only for business matters, as distinct from ward work. He retired in 1903 at age seventy-three.[26]

Macphail's school visitorship during the years 1868–78 required that he spend much of his time travelling, and his appointment in 1882 to a full-time position in the Charlottetown area meant that his normal place of residence for more than twenty-one years was not in Orwell. Consequently, the influence of his wife Catherine came to be felt more strongly within the household than before. She took the religious side of life considerably less seriously than William did and indeed was disinclined to any display of emotion or enthusiasm; Andrew wrote that he had never seen her cry or laugh. A greater tolerance for the milder vices of this world accompanied her generally more bland disposition.

Catherine's family home, that of the Smiths of Lower Newton, provided, in Andrew's words, "a pagan refuge"[27] for the children. The Smith family included seafarers and shipbuilders, and all were supposedly immune from the negative effects of strong drink; one uncle had fathered a child out of wedlock, and there was no attempt to obscure the fact. "The boy's name, contrary to custom, appears on his father's tombstone, although with proper reticence the mother's name is not given."[28] Andrew later recalled that visits to his mother's uncles "gave entrance into a wholesome and real world … The mother never wavered in the belief that her own people required no special act of grace … their strength was increased by using the good things of this world; self-denial was for the weak and timorous. They even boasted that they were not afraid of the devil; he did not interest them. It was a secret pleasure to her that her own sons were disposed to follow the way of her own people."[29] Andrew also remembered having overheard her cautioning her husband not to follow the austere example of "a highly censorious Elder [who] found scriptural warrant against all pictures" and who demanded when staying overnight that the Macphails turn them to the wall. "It is fun they [the children] make of him; and they will end by making fun of you," she warned.[30]

This comparatively secular influence was reinforced by the presence of William's mother, who outlived her husband by thirty-six years. Mary McPherson Macphail was "an inveterate reader of newspapers, magazines, and other romances – everything but the Bible."[31] She also loved the brandy that Andrew Smith – one of Catherine's uncles who was a sea captain – brought into the house after every voyage; she "drank freely, and her

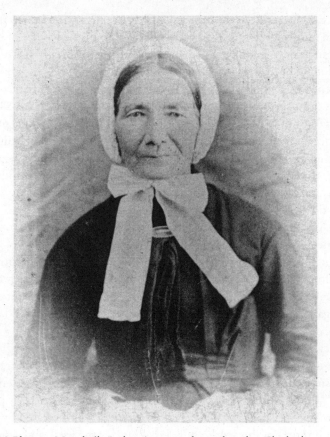

Mary McPherson Macphail, Andrew's paternal grandmother. She had a profoundly secular influence on the Macphail children. This photograph is probably the image that Edmond Dyonnet used when he painted her portrait several years after her death. A photograph of the Dyonnet portrait appears in the first and third editions of *The Master's Wife*; the portrait itself hangs in the Macphail Homestead in Orwell.

eyes shone."[32] A vivid character, she was "the one authority upon all matters that lay beyond our little Island world. She was of 'the old country'; she had crossed the sea, and all knowledge was imputed to her. What did a mountain look like? Did it rise up from the level ground? Or, was it approached by lesser mountains? How high were the waves of the sea? And how could they wreck a ship? The answers to these questions occupied many a winter evening, and created a profound unrest in young minds."[33] She purveyed information on witches and fairies, and was a source of songs, ballads, and traditional tales of "forays, robberies, and murders."[34]

An overwhelming proportion of the community in Orwell was Scottish by birth or of Scottish-immigrant parentage. The way of life, religious customs, and hierarchy of values were those of the old country. As in Scotland, agriculture was not overly specialized. The farmers grew oats, wheat, potatoes, barley, and turnips, and raised sheep, hogs, and cattle. Almost everyone was a Presbyterian of one variety or another; in addition to McDonaldites there were orthodox Kirkmen, Secessionists, and Free Churchmen. When in 1869 William Macphail and his fellow elders drafted a letter asking that they be allowed to retain their pastor, they stated that the great majority of their people were unilingually Gaelic Highlanders, requiring a Gaelic-speaking minister.[35]

The most prestigious member of the community was of course the minister, whose advice was sought on all subjects. Second came the *dominie*, or schoolmaster, for he held the key to "the escape" from manual labour. The transplanted Highlanders did not consider the latter degrading, but neither did they romanticize it. They wanted better for their children, and choosing a teacher was a serious matter. In mid-1878, for example, William Macphail pleaded with a young man (who went on to become a McGill gold medallist and the rector of Montreal High School) to come to Orwell: "Some of our boys here are now in the most critical period of their life ... I fear their prospects will be blighted, if we shall have the misfortune of a poor inexperienced teacher."[36]

The hoped-for "prospects" of these boys obviously did not lie on the farm. If they wanted to learn farming, home was the place for them. "Schooling" was for those suited by nature for it; those who were unfit were discouraged from continuing by being beaten when they failed to "learn" a lesson. The results were impressive: in Andrew Macphail's lifetime, 153 students from that two-room school, known as Uigg grammar school, servicing a district of never more than forty families, went forth to take one or more university degrees. But education in Orwell was clearly for a minority: "A boy must prove that he was one of the few capable of learning ... In any year not more than three boys were considered qualified to profit from books ... These three were set apart, and upon them the master lavished all his care. He offered two forms of education, his undivided attention and his undivided neglect ... At the age of 14, these three had read six books of Euclid, Algebra to quadratic equations, quite difficult Latin, and the new Testament in Greek."[37]

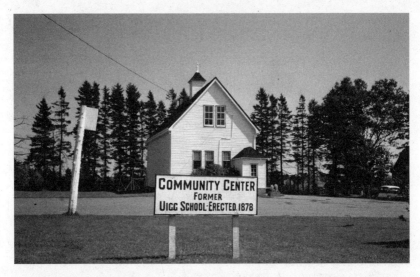

Uigg grammar school. This two-room school, built in the wake of the reforming
Public Schools Act of 1877, serviced a district of never more than forty families.
In Macphail's lifetime, 153 former students took one or more university degrees.

ANDREW MACPHAIL, SCHOLAR AND TEACHER

The system worked well for Andrew Macphail, and in 1880, at the age of fifteen, he was awarded an entrance scholarship into Prince of Wales College
in Charlottetown. There were only two granted for all of Queens County,
and he had faced a field of 150 applicants at a competitive examination held
over two days in the town: "When I returned home, the mother said nothing; the Master made some observations that seemed irrelevant; the grandmother said, 'Well, what else would you expect?' She remembered, part in
sorrow, part in pride, 'that none of your father's name ever worked.' The
long tradition of scholarship was unbroken."[38] This tradition had extended
some four hundred years, and seven of William Macphail's ten children
were to obtain at least one university degree.[39]

Prince of Wales College, an intermediate institution between a grammar school and a university, was under the sway of Alexander Anderson,
a Scot from Aberdeen who had been a gold medallist at the University
of Edinburgh.[40] Several decades later Macphail recalled, "Of the many
teachers I have since known he was the best. His authority was absolute;

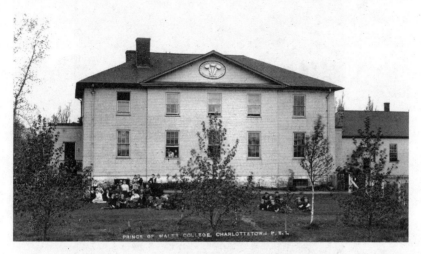

Prince of Wales College, 1894. Established in 1860, the college was renowned for its success in preparing students for further academic work, despite a building that was much less than adequate. Graduation from it was recognized as providing the first year of university work. Macphail attended on a scholarship and was admitted into second year at McGill University.

therefore he was never known to exercise it … He treated the crude boys as if they were grave young gentlemen determined to become scholars and win by their scholarship any highest place in the world … This teacher had the curious idea that boys came to school to learn; not to waste their time, or their parents' money."[41] Each year a small number went forth from Prince of Wales and won academic honours, whether they went to McGill, Queen's, Dalhousie, Edinburgh, or Princeton. In 1888 McGill University gave Anderson the recognition of an honorary degree.[42]

Macphail remained at Prince of Wales for two years and appears to have done well. By the latter part of his first year his father was writing to express the hope that the excellence of his essays would not cause suspicion of parental aid. There were, including Anderson, three masters, whose emphasis bore heavily on classics, mathematics, English literature, and history. Agriculture and the natural sciences were treated with a certain disdain and taught largely in terms of theory; for each science course the laboratory was used not more than once a year. French was taught as one

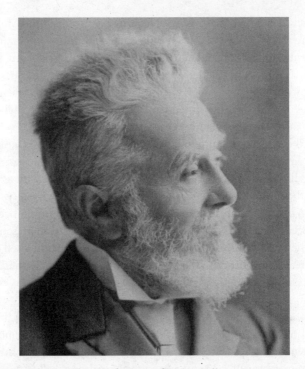

Alexander Anderson, principal of Prince of Wales College, 1868–1901. Anderson
won Macphail's lifelong admiration, and in the 1890s Macphail presented the
college with a medal, named after Anderson, to be awarded to the outstanding
graduating student.

would teach a dead language – the grammar constituted an interesting
intellectual exercise. There was no pretence at a utilitarian justification for
the curriculum.[43]

Despite the burden of his studies and some private tutorial work,
Macphail does not appear to have led a cloistered or narrowly academic
life in Charlottetown. He found time for playing cards and took an interest in the newly admitted female students at the college. With the encouragement of Thomas Le Page, a poet and staff member, he became seriously
interested in literature and was a regular participant in the activities of the
Shakespeare Club. That he was beginning to evolve a new scale of values is
evident from the fact that his father found occasion to admonish him for
travelling on the Sabbath, something to be avoided at all costs.[44]

Andrew Macphail took his first teaching position in rural Melville, Lot 60, where a new school had been built in 1878. Both his father and grand-father had taught there, and in 1853, in that district, his Aunt Janet had been the first female teacher to gain employment in the much broader area known as "Belfast," which encompassed approximately twenty school districts.[45] Situated about fifteen miles south of Orwell, Melville does not appear to have been a hive of activity.[46] In an early letter to his father, Macphail cryptically commented, "Living here is dull but interesting and novel from its very sameness. Though I have not very much of what one would call *pleasure* I do not feel that spirit of *ennui* with which one is apt to be inflicted [*sic*] when a break occurs in the round of gaiety."[47] He had hoped to obtain a grammar school, and from the beginning made it clear to the local trustees that he would leave if a better position presented itself. This restlessness no doubt increased after his school was closed owing to an outbreak of diphtheria. When in December a cousin notified him that he was resigning his grammar school position to continue his education, Macphail seized the opportunity.[48]

Fanning Grammar School – named for the same landholding family that had owned the farm where Andrew Macphail had been born – was in Malpeque on the north shore of eastern Prince County some fifty-five miles west of Orwell.[49] Macphail was principal of the two-room school, which had two storeys; he taught the higher grades in the upper storey, and a female teacher taught the lower grades on the ground level. He boarded in a stone house virtually adjacent to the school property. The settlement was older, more sophisticated, and more prosperous than his native district. Some inhabitants, probably those of Loyalist background, even had black servants. There was little place in the community for the evangelical intensity to which the young schoolmaster had been accus-tomed in Orwell. When the people of Malpeque went to church, they were – although Presbyterians – little troubled by questions of sin, repentance, and conversion:

An evangelist was regarded as a curiosity, as a diversion. One of these was much encouraged by the large attendance. He asked those who were "saved" to stand up. No one moved. Moderating his appeal, he asked those who "desired to be saved" to stand up. The result was no better. Then, with a touch of irony, he appealed to all who wished to lead a "better life." The only response was from a low

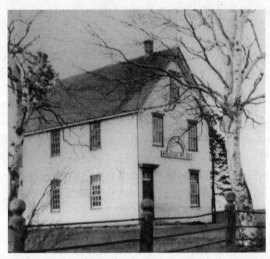

Malpeque grammar school, 1942. Macphail was principal here for two and one-half years. The position was prestigious, and he found the community of Malpeque, with its relative sophistication and worldliness, to be to his taste.

fellow who was known to be a fool and was suspected of being a thief. "Happy people," the evangelist exclaimed, and abandoned that cultivated field.[50]

To Macphail, barely eighteen years old, it was "a new world": "In Malpeque in winter there were parties of 30 or 40 persons every night, at which young and old, men as old as my father, danced with agility and laughter, with Joe McLellan to play the fiddle. Old and young lived together without hypocrisy on the one side, without fear on the other ... Until I went to college, I had never attended a party at which dancing was practised."[51]

Macphail took to the new way of life immediately. Within a few weeks of his arrival one of his friends was writing, "To read your letter one would almost be led to think you had fallen on a Paradise."[52] The correspondence Macphail sent and received in his two and one-half years at Malpeque indicates that the secularizing trend engendered during his studies at Prince of Wales continued to develop. He showed more interest in obtaining guest lecturers, such as Le Page on literary topics, than in organizing and teaching Sabbath schools, which his father would have preferred. On at least one occasion William Macphail expressed distress that his son should be writing to him on the Sabbath. When Macphail took his holidays in Orwell, "the Master was quick to notice a change, and between him and his wife there was veiled reference to the distinction between proper pride and false pride."[53] The latter was presumably pride related to the things of this world.

A highly successful teacher, Macphail became popular with both the students and their parents. He gained access to the family library of Dr William Keir, the son of the late Rev. John Keir, a longtime Secession minister who had studied at the University of Glasgow and had an impressive selection of theological works; 420 of his leather-bound books now form a collection at the National Presbyterian Museum in Toronto.[54] He was held in such regard as a scholar that, according to historian John Moir, in the year following Thomas McCulloch's death, the Synod of Nova Scotia had "begun the revival of Pictou Academy by appointing [Keir] as professor of theology."[55] His son, the physician, has also been identified as an author – one who in 1862, writing under the name Fabrius Cassius Funny Fellow, had published a thirty-five-page poem that was bitterly satiric with respect to a royal commission on the differences between landlords and tenants on the Island, but at the same time replete with Island patriotism and praise for his own community of Malpeque.[56] Macphail proceeded to read all the books in the Keir library, which were heavily weighted towards literature, theology, philosophy, and medicine. With the strong encouragement of his father, who had always regretted his own lack of time for "home study," the young schoolmaster furthered his intellectual development by wide reading. His correspondence shows a steady stream of requests for books to his friend James H. Good in Charlottetown and his eldest brother William John James Macphail in the United States. These letters and his correspondence with booksellers in other places indicate a marked interest in works by the greats of English literature. Among the more modern writers, he was drawn to the essayist and literary critic William Hazlitt and especially the novelist George Eliot. Possibly because of his heavy reading, he began to show the first signs of eye strain, and by 1885 he was wearing eyeglasses.[57]

These were unhurried years for Macphail, among the most joyful of his life, and marked by a clear and public blossoming of his talents. He took a prominent part in community activities and appears to have been the prime mover in the local literary society, or "institute," issuing invitations to speakers and giving lectures himself. As a teacher, in addition to his success and acceptance within the district, he attained recognition outside his own community. After a visit to Fanning Grammar School, the provincial superintendent of education praised Macphail's work and invited him to deliver a paper to the Teachers' Institute at their meeting

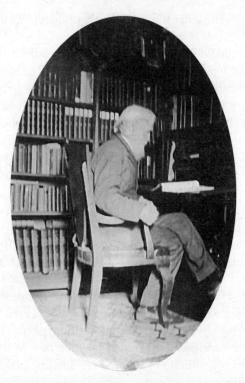

Dr William Keir in his study in Malpeque. This physician had a substantial library and granted complete access to the young school principal, who read everything in it. The influence of Keir's father, the Rev. John Keir, had been instrumental in establishing the reputation of the local grammar school. The desk and chair pictured here are still in use and are now located in Charlottetown. Much of the library is in a museum in Toronto.

in Charlottetown; the Prince of Wales faculty members would be present. He began to develop his journalistic abilities by contributing reports to the local press on Malpeque events. While a teacher, Macphail took his first trips off the Island at the urging of his brother in the United States. "Willie J" or "Will" was a highly skilled craftsman and worked in Boston and St Augustine, Florida. As soon as he arrived in the United States, Will began to invite his younger brother to visit him. Although in 1883 Andrew got only as far as Saint John, New Brunswick, he went to Boston the following October, visiting the city's educational institutions and taking the conventional tours.[58]

More than education and intellectual self-improvement engaged
Macphail in these years. His correspondence, with Good in particular, reveals a young man who had come a long way from the gravity and
self-denial of the Highlanders of Orwell. When inviting Macphail to visit
him in Charlottetown at Easter 1884, Good, a student at law, wrote:

> We'll raise a racket some how &
> With thee I'll drain the modest cup
> (Although the *Club* might think it odd)
> And we will drink well liquored up
> Success unto our darling m—d.[59]

In addition to partaking of liquor and tobacco (both of which his father
had renounced), Macphail appears to have been known as a humorous
raconteur. The young schoolmaster even indulged a romantic bent by
writing a sonnet on the absence of a ladyfriend. He also learned to shoot,
ride, swim, and sail; he bought a boat and developed a taste for rowing
out to sea "so far that the land was lost in the distance and the dark, medi-
tating upon strange things."[60] There were mishaps: "I learned to handle a
gun, to such good purpose that one morning before dawn at one shot I
killed three ducks, but unfortunately they were domestic ducks belonging
to Charles Taylor."[61]

Yet during his last year at Malpeque one aspect of his life weighed heavily on Macphail: his future. In the best Victorian manner, he gave the most
earnest consideration to the choice of a profession. It would appear that
the only two callings he seriously considered were medicine and the ministry. He listened to a sermon on "honesty in the discharge of one's duties
to his day & generation,"[62] and as secretary of the Malpeque literary society
arranged to have Neil McLeod, a Summerside teacher, lecture on that apos-
tle of the active life of duty, Thomas Carlyle. After the sermon, the lecture,
a lengthy conversation with McLeod, and much self-analysis, Macphail
made his decision in solitude: it would be medicine. His motives appear
to have been characteristic of his age. Good, in replying to a letter of early
1885, commended him upon being "so anxious about your duty to others."[63]
Compared with the decision on which profession to enter, the choice of a
university was easy. After inquiring about King's in Halifax and a college
in New York City, he settled upon McGill. He wrote to the principal, Sir
William Dawson, outlining his background, and received permission to
write examinations for entry into second year.[64]

When Andrew Macphail left for Montreal in September 1885, he felt in many ways much richer than when he had arrived in Malpeque. He was almost twenty-one and was experienced as a teacher, private tutor, and journalist; he had written poetry. He was now an adult, a fact attested to by his father's request for advice on the proper course concerning the education of the younger Macphail children. Not only did he have $300 ($230 of it saved from an annual salary of $380) with which to launch his university education, but he had been exposed to a wider range of experience in those two and one-half years than ever before: "For the first time I learned, what I had always suspected, that humanity is not one, but a congeries of families each with a unity of tradition, a similarity of interest, an equality of education, an identity of thought, manners, and morals; a 'society' in which the upper members could of their own free will penetrate to the bottom; in which the lower members could only by sheer merit and incredible difficulty rise to the top."[65] In short, they "were happy and to me important years ... In those years I learned more than I taught."[66]

Macphail was now ready for "a wider world."[67] He was leaving Prince Edward Island, but the Island and its spell never left him. The author Stephen Leacock, who would become one of his closest friends in Montreal and who shared a rural upbringing, thought he understood: "The Canadian countryside in those days was dark and solitary, and life there had little converse and less amenity. Yet it bred, unconsciously, a love of the open air, of early hours, of the remembered stillness of the woods and the unceasing breaking of the sea."[68] Lured by these attractions, Macphail returned at every opportunity, for he found that what he had known in his youth provided, in his mind, an alternative to the urban way of life to which he was migrating. Although he would adapt fully to the requirements he encountered and would within a decade be living a life almost unimaginably different from his earliest days, he retained a deep respect and affection for the people he had known in Orwell, Charlottetown, and Malpeque. Orwell had provided the foundation for his values, and Malpeque had supplied a partial bridging between the austerity of Orwell and the much more expansive and permissive society of Montreal. As for Charlottetown, for Macphail that really meant Prince of Wales College, and it – and particularly Anderson, its principal – had built on the sound education he had received in his native district and prepared him for the intellectual demands of his new environment.

Years later Macphail recalled, "On the way into the mysterious world to a great University, oppressed by a sense of inexperience and ignorance, I was striving even at that desperate moment to repair this unworthiness by reading Greek prose composition. A senior student also on his way discovered me at the task. 'Put that book away,' he said, 'and tell them you come from the Prince of Wales College.' I told them so, and they admitted me into the second year."[69]

Studies, Career, and Family Life in Montreal

Andrew Macphail made Montreal his principal place of residence for the remainder of his life. In 1894 he wrote to his mother that Orwell would always be home for him as long as she was there, yet in reality there was no turning back.[1] He probably never went as far as his eldest sibling William John James ("Will"), who in a letter written in 1892, when at home during a period of uncertain health and underemployment, stated, "Living here is a slow death"[2] – but Andrew did not return to live there. As well as choosing a career, he was in the process of settling permanently in Canada's largest city.

UNIVERSITY STUDENT AND JOURNALIST

Macphail adjusted quickly to Montreal and to McGill University. Within a week of his arrival he felt permanently established. "I like Montreal thoroughly – its broad clean streets, its fine trees, rows of fine houses and its hearty [?] cordial people," he told his mother. With the help of friends from Prince Edward Island, he had obtained lodging and board to his satisfaction: lodging on Beaver Hall Terrace (now Côte du Beaver Hall), board on University Street. "Both places," he assured her, "are quite above the average in culture and comfort."[3] When he presented himself at McGill, he was excused from all examinations for entry into second year except one, English, which he passed with ease. He was entirely capable of doing the work; in classics, at least, he was somewhat astonished at the lack of difficulty in the curriculum. "I found myself in a class of grown men who were reading the journalistic Xenophon as if he were a serious author. From this I sought refuge in the library."[4]

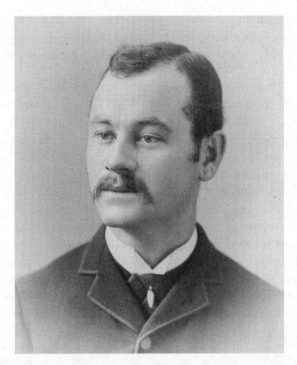

Andrew Macphail, November 1886, in Montreal. This would be one of the first photographs of Macphail taken in Montreal.

McGill University in 1885 was a small and intimate institution.[5] There were only 428 students, and among Macphail's teachers were the principal, Sir William Dawson, and the dean of arts, Alexander Johnson. The attacks by Dawson, an eminent geologist and paleontologist, on the Darwinian explanation for the origins of the human species had made him a celebrity among the non-university population. Indeed, in William Macphail's household, Dawson was "believed to be ... [one of] the two righteous men in Canada."[6] Now William's son was attending the great man's lectures and being invited to his home. The dean also was a scientist, but he could teach the classics equally well; like Alexander Anderson of Prince of Wales College, his emphasis was on underlying principles rather than practice of scientific method. But the teacher who stimulated Macphail most was Charles Moyse, a graduate of University College, London, and professor of English literature, who had administered the entrance examination in English. With his guidance, Macphail read through the entire McGill library, just as he had devoured the Keir library in Malpeque. He particularly enjoyed Matthew Arnold, John Ruskin, Walter Pater, Walter Bagehot, Ernest Renan, and Charles-Augustin Saint-Beuve.[7]

Macphail had greatly underestimated the cost of his education and maintenance in Montreal, and within two months of arrival was writing to his mother, "If I had known expenses were so great I doubt whether I should have come up and I am glad I did not [know], for the wisdom of the step I have taken is becoming more evident."[8] He could rely on his eldest brother and his father for temporary financial aid; but Will was paid only the wages of a skilled labourer, and his father, with an annual salary of between $600 and $800, had six children younger than Andrew. Any long-term solution to his financial problems would have to be of his own making. Thus he began to give private tuition, for which he received more per hour than he had received per day in Malpeque. In addition, he appears to have done some reporting for the *New York Tribune* and the *New York Times*. By early 1886 Macphail's relatives, friends, and acquaintances were expressing the fear that he might injure his health by overwork.[9]

Despite the demands of his studies and his journalistic and tutorial work, Macphail found time for extracurricular university activities. In January 1886 he participated in the entertainment at the Arts Undergraduate Dinner, where he distinguished himself by consuming a large number of toasts without noticeable ill effects - in the tradition of his mother's family. Two years later he was president of a committee presenting the arts undergraduates' musical program, "Conversazions." He became a popular campus orator and in 1890 spoke on behalf of his medical class at a dinner at which Governor General Stanley, Sir John A. Macdonald, Wilfrid Laurier, Sir Donald Smith, and many other notables were present; the Montreal *Gazette* reported that "his remarks were varied with a vein of refreshing humor and sarcasm."[10]

Macphail was also a prominent student journalist. In October 1887 he joined the editorial board of the *University Gazette*, a fortnightly whose function was "to mirror the intellectual and literary progress of the University, and also to act as a chronicle of College item and class report."[11] Twelve or fourteen numbers appeared throughout the academic year, each composed of between twelve and eighteen pages. After serving as assistant editor-in-chief and acting editor-in-chief in 1888, Macphail assumed the editorial chair with the 11 January 1889 number. He remained editor-in-chief through the 1889–90 session, after which the publication was discontinued because of financial problems and friction between the faculties over its control. The *University Gazette* was a somewhat bland publication, although contributors included such distinguished persons as Charles G.D. Roberts. The most notable aspect of Macphail's editorial policy was his advocacy of a place for Canadian history in the McGill curriculum.[12] He may have participated in an organized attempt by students, through petitioning, to introduce Canadian history. In this, the students were somewhat ahead of their time. It appears that the first such course at McGill was not presented until 1899 – taught by Dean F.P. Walton of the law school, and focusing on the history of Canadian constitutional law.[13]

The *University Gazette* did not absorb much of Macphail's time, for the editorial board met only once a week, on Saturday afternoon.[14] While still an undergraduate he joined the Montreal *Gazette* as a reporter. In addition, he held various summer jobs. He spent at least portions of two summers on the Island assisting at the provincial Hospital for the Insane, where his father had been supervisor since 1882, and he was in New York State, probably working as a journalist, for at least two summers.[15]

With precarious financial resources and no scholarship, Macphail was compelled to work exceptionally hard. From the beginning, he took a combined arts and premedical course in order to shorten the number of years he would require at university. When he received his Bachelor of Arts degree in 1888, he had completed in three years a curriculum normally covered in five. Despite his robust constitution, he felt considerable strain in his last year as an undergraduate. A week before the end of exams he wrote, "It was a long spring and an amount of work is gone through with that really was impossible and which nothing could induce me to undertake again. The Medical examinations are over … and for the past five weeks it has been one steady grind night and day at the Arts work."[16] By the time he received his degree fifteen days later, he "was not well … from the reaction of the year's hard work."[17] Macphail, who was never one to exaggerate his health problems or to solicit sympathy, told his father, "After the work was over I was afraid I had bent too far and would not recover my former tone."[18]

But Macphail recuperated within a few weeks, and that autumn he returned to McGill, where he applied his academic energies solely to medicine. About the time of his arts graduation he had been appointed to the editorial staff of the Montreal *Gazette*, a job that apparently paid more than reporting. In his new role he reviewed musical and dramatic productions, and wrote a column under the title "Olla Podrida."[19] Macphail's reviews and columns offer revealing glimpses of his intellectual development and assumptions. The breadth and depth of his artistic knowledge is impressive, especially in music. As a critic, he always gave reasons for praise or censure, and he showed particular appreciation for the qualities of economy, measure, and restraint.[20]

Macphail had an elevated and demanding conception of the artist's proper role: "It is not enough [for musicians] to be conscientious performers, filling well the places they have chosen. As musicians they have a duty in placing high ideals before the public, in living up to these themselves and urging a fuller appreciation of them." Thus they should foster the taste of their audiences and attempt to raise the level of general culture. The role of the audiences in cultivating the arts was to patronize the artists. He was quick to criticize small turnouts which, he warned, could lead to Montreal being bypassed by the best companies.[21]

Although Macphail praised "truth" in performances and distrusted "artificiality," he sharply distinguished between this sensibility and that of contemporary realism and naturalism. His aesthetic appreciation was linked to a sense of poetry and mystery, whereas the naturalists displayed "hideous skill ... [in] depicting the ugly and loathsome." The function of the arts was to provide spiritual comfort and a refuge from everyday life, not to confront the audience with reality in its starkest form.[22]

These inclinations were also evident in Macphail's assumptions about nationality. In true romantic fashion, he wrote that "painting, architecture, music and poetry are but the expression of national life and the striving after an individual ideal ... [which] has root far back in a nation's life, and each nation breathed forth its aspirations in its own note." Linked with this was his view that there was a need "to discourage the centralizing power that brings the members of one class or one sect together ... and to promote a community of interest which is the root of mutual justice and a community of sentiment upon which real loyalty is based."[23]

Thus the major elements in Macphail's position on nationality were a belief in the uniqueness of each nation's spirit and a belief in the necessity for fostering a community of interest and consciousness within the nation. Nonetheless, these assumptions did not lead him into a nationalist instrumentalism in the interpretation of artistic merit:

> For literary purposes the world is one community with the same
> experiences and aspirations, and if there is a difference in their
> expression it is but a passing phase arising from the pitch of culture

which marks the development of each. Literature ... is not confined
by geographical limits, and we are apt to confound local coloring
with the universal heart of it. The use of a national literary society is
chiefly for historical purposes, and the creative side falls in abeyance;
indeed there is a real danger of creating a narrowness that fails to see
any good thing outside of its own isolated Galilee.[24]

It is apparent from the preceding quotations that his romanticism coloured
his style on occasion. Precise in his critical writing, he was at this stage
in his development abstract and sometimes vague when setting down his
own ideas.

Macphail worked hard at his newspaper articles and enjoyed considerable success. He was soon appointed night editor of the *Gazette* but left
that position to join the *Montreal Star* as commercial editor. In the summer
of 1889 he gave up editorial work and became Montreal correspondent
for the Great North Western Telegraph Company of Canada, a wire service apparently affiliated with Associated Press. He established a reputation for promptness and accuracy, and his reports began to appear regularly in the Toronto *Globe* and a number of American papers, including
the *New York Times*. By late 1889 he was earning $2,000. This was a very
respectable income for the era and represented an immense improvement
in Macphail's fortunes. At Malpeque he had been paid $380 per year, and
as recently as 1887–88 his income for the academic year had been $209.
Macphail enjoyed this work and many years later recalled that almost all
his favourite authors during this period were journalists. He seriously considered giving up medicine for journalism, and consulted his father, who
advised him to continue his course for a number of reasons, the most telling of which was probably that if he gave it up he would eventually regret
not finishing what he had begun.[25]

Macphail's income from journalism, which his father estimated as
comparable to that of a practising physician, enabled him, while yet a student, to assist other members of his family in their education. There was
a remarkable sense of solidarity within the Macphail family, and while at
Malpeque saving for university, Andrew had provided aid to Alexander[26]
and Janetta ("Nettie"), who then attended Prince of Wales College. At a
difficult point in his first year at McGill, he had received money from his
younger sister Mary Isabella ("Belle"). Now he was sufficiently prosperous
to assist his eldest brother Will, who in the autumn of 1888 had entered a
medical course in Washington, DC; Andrew appears to have been Will's

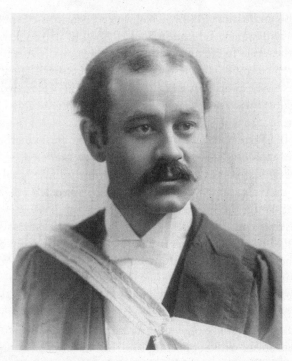

Andrew Macphail in academic dress, 25 March 1891. This photograph was taken shortly before his graduation in medicine.

closest friend and most regular correspondent within the family. A year later, when Nettie returned to Prince of Wales and Alexander wrote for advice on entering McGill, Andrew was able to help Nettie and pledge aid to Alexander.[27]

Despite working as a full-time journalist, Macphail experienced no great difficulty in his medical curriculum. Indeed, he appears to have been less fatigued at the time of his graduation in 1891 than he had been three years earlier. Part of the secret was that he "learned to sleep without appearing to be asleep, and by that gift was spared many a useless lecture."[28] But there was more to it than that; of sixty-seven important examinations during his university years he passed all but one. Although, according to his own account, he stood near the middle of his class in most courses, he may have been overly modest, for surviving evidence indicates that at least in his senior arts year, two-thirds of his grades were firsts.[29]

Before his graduation, Macphail had won an essay contest sponsored by the American Humane Education Society, open to the English-speaking world, on the topic "In the interests of humanity should vivisection be permitted, and if so, under what restrictions and limitations?" There were two prizes of $250 to be awarded for the best contributions of 8,000 words or less for and against vivisection; entering this competition afforded Macphail early experience in extended writing. He prepared a paper favouring vivisection, and a jury of Harvard medical professors chose it from among nineteen submissions. The essay was a straightforward defence of the practice as an essential means of increasing scientific knowledge that would ultimately decrease human suffering and prevent needless loss of life. He argued that taking the interests of humanity as the goal, only physiologists themselves could rationally decide whether each particular vivisection should or should not be performed. Even the requirement of "a probability of beneficient results must not be pushed too closely, for science must be untrammeled … One truth may be an unseen way to the germ of others. Science has only to do with the seeking of truth, utility will follow in its train."[30]

Macphail's essay was closely argued, the problem presented in rigorously logical form, with supporting evidence introduced at appropriate points. Only in a few instances did he resort to hyperbole, sarcasm, and the technique of *reductio ad absurdum* – and these exceptions seem to have been intended to add humour rather than to cover weaknesses in the essential argument. His assumption was that much of the opposition to vivisection was rooted in ignorance and misinformation, and that disclosure of the facts would clear the air, establishing common ground between the vivisectionists and their erstwhile opponents. This was not quite the case, and Macphail found himself "overwhelmed … with Anti-Vivisection literature often accompanied by bitter words and scoffs and taunts and jeers."[31] In fact, he did not hear the end of it for several years. The controversy stung him but did not change his mind; he remained convinced that defence of vivisection was not advocacy of cruelty. About the same time he wrote a pamphlet condemning the use of checkreins on horses, a tract which a leading American Anti-Vivisectionist praised as "splendid."[32] Whatever the merits of vivisection, his essay on the subject helped him to graduate in 1891 with $1,200 and no debts.

On 4 April 1891, three days after he received his MD, Macphail signed a contract in New York with a syndicate of news organizations that included the *New York Times*, the Montreal *Gazette*, the *Detroit Free Press*, the *Chicago*

Times, and Associated Press. The contract stipulated that he was to sail around the world, his fare being paid in exchange for the rights to a series of articles on the places he visited. Macphail embarked for Britain at the end of May and remained there a month before proceeding to Paris. While in England he visited Haslemere, the summer retreat of many British intellectuals; it was there that George Eliot had written *Adam Bede*. Macphail was enthralled with rural England, which met his every expectation. In London he was repelled by the congestion and noise, and his journalistic work reveals, as well as an aesthetic point of view, a certain suspicion of urban working-class mores:

> The omnibus strike … was not an unmixed evil in the quietness
> and safety of the streets, caused by the absence of a long and ugly
> procession of chameleon hued caravans. The men complained that
> they were worked for fifteen to twenty hours a day, that they were
> subject to obnoxious fines, that they were liable to instant dismissal,
> and that they were underpaid; but the truth of the matter seems to
> be that the recent introduction of the ticket system prevented the
> men from supplementing their wages by pilfering from the company.
> However, they have been granted such demands as were thought
> reasonable.[33]

All in all, he was well pleased with the mother country: "If there is any trace of effeteness it lies so well concealed that it has yet escaped a keen and well paid observation."[34]

After visiting a number of European cities in early July, Macphail boarded the Canadian Pacific Railway's ss *Empress of China* for Japan, where he spent a full month. En route he saw Port Said, Cairo, Colombo, Singapore, and Hong Kong. He liked the Orient. In a published article, he praised Japan for "its delicacy, its gentleness, its ingenuousness."[35] And among his papers is an unpublished diarylike manuscript, in which, when reflecting on the role of Christian missionaries in China, he acknowledged the complexity of the issues and commented, "I think upon the whole the native Chinese live lives as moral as our own." Further, in disputing the view that the Chinese were frequently opium smokers, he wrote, "The Chinese are probably more lied about than any other people." But despite the pleasures of discovering other cultures and customs, by the end of September he was glad to be back in Canada. His return to Montreal via the still new Canadian Pacific Railway line from British Columbia – a journey of seven days – gave him his first view of the Canadian West, and he was deeply impressed: "Until one has crossed the Continent he has no conception of the power of Canada."[36]

MARRIAGE, THE SQUARE MILE, PARENTHOOD, AND BEREAVEMENT

On Macphail's return to Montreal he became engaged to Georgina Nightingale Burland, age twenty-one, known as Georgie, the youngest daughter of George Bull Burland, a leading Montreal businessman. Burland *père* was president of the British North American Bank Note Company of Montreal and Ottawa, responsible for printing bank notes, postage stamps, and the like; according to Peter Keating, an historian writing in the *Dictionary of Canadian Biography*, the firm was "noted for the quality of its work."[37] Burland had also been publisher of several magazines, including the *Canadian Illustrated News*, an early attempt to reach a mass Canadian readership. A map of the Montreal printing industry as it stood in 1890, which an historical geographer published in 2000, suggests that Burland Lithography may have been the largest printing operation in the city.[38] In addition, Burland was engaged in a wide range of philanthropic endeavours. A story in *La Presse* in 1905 reported that he had recently given $25,000 to l'Hôpital Général, that on an annual basis he often donated $100,000 or more to charities, and that he, an anglophone in culture and a Congregationalist in religious affiliation, included French Canadian and Roman Catholic organizations among the recipients. The same story estimated his fortune as amounting to between $12 and $15 million.[39] Both he and his children, especially his son Jeffrey Hale, were later prominently involved in the struggle against tuberculosis. The prevalence of the disease in Montreal was especially great when compared with that in other large North American cities, and within their city the Burlands took the lead.[40]

Georgie's name first appears in Macphail's surviving correspondence in 1890, although he had known her elder brother Jeffrey for several years. (Shortly after Jeffrey's death in 1914, Macphail wrote that they had been "intimate friends for thirty years,"[41] a calculation which suggests that the two men had met soon after Macphail's arrival in Montreal in 1885.) Jeffrey was president of the board of directors of the *University Gazette* when Macphail joined its editorial board in 1887, and they appear to have been drinking companions.[42] They shared an interest in Canadian history and a commitment to disseminating knowledge of it. In October 1891 Jeffrey offered $2,500 to be used "to secure the production of a textbook of Canadian History, written from a Dominion standpoint and suitable for use in all the schools of Canada." Profits from sales would be used to fund lectures and libraries in Canadian history in various Canadian normal schools, the contemporary term for teachers' colleges.[43] The Burland family lived on University Street, bordering the McGill campus on the east, and it is possible that Macphail met Georgie in the first instance through his connection with her brother, and partially because of the proximity of the Burland home to McGill.

Letters from Andrew ("Jack" in at least some of them) to Georgie survived over the years, and the tone is affectionate.[44] There is a tenderness in his manner that makes them stand out from the hundreds upon hundreds of his other surviving letters. Andrew and Georgie seem to have planned their engagement before his departure for England, but decided not to announce it. The reason for the delay may have been related to the fact that she preceded him to England, and to the likelihood – based on a reading of two letters from Andrew to his brother Will in the United States – that they planned to meet in England. Even in October 1891, Andrew and Georgie did not set a definite date for the marriage; that decision was deferred for two years.[45]

The twin paths of Macphail's working life for the next decade – physician and medical professor – had been set in place by the time he interrupted his busy routine of teaching and practice to marry Georgie late in 1893. The wedding on 19 December was a grand occasion, reflecting the Burland family's wealth and social prominence. A Montreal newspaper reported that the father of the bride gave the newlyweds a cheque for $5,000 and that there were also several cheques for $100. Some five hundred guests attended the reception. Andrew and Georgie then proceeded on a five-month honeymoon tour of Britain, Germany, Italy, and the French Riviera. On 18 May 1894 Dr and Mrs Macphail announced their return to Montreal with a reception held in the Burland home at 287 University Street; flowers were everywhere, and an orchestra was in attendance.[46]

Later in the year Andrew and Georgie moved from 2430 St Catherine Street (at the corner of Stanley Street), Macphail's bachelor quarters, to a row house at 216 Peel Street, which was a present from George Burland – a further act of generosity on his part. The Peel Street house, which was to be Macphail's Montreal residence for the rest of his life, was near McGill University, between St Catherine and Sherbrooke Streets. A few doors

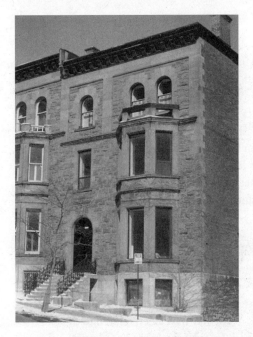

Peel Street row house. Built in 1894, this row house is similar in dimensions, and possibly in appearance, to 216 Peel Street, where Macphail lived from 1894 to 1938. His house, which no longer stands, was farther south on Peel and on the opposite side of the street. This house's present number is 3501.

north of the intersection with Burnside Place – which has since become part of de Maisonneuve Boulevard – it was also somewhat to the north of the midpoint between the two major east-west arteries. Although the area has long been composed exclusively of commercial establishments and large apartment buildings, an author in 1941 wrote that in the 1890s "there used to be many fine old houses and well-to-do families there."[47] A modern scholarly analysis of rents as a measure of affluence on Montreal streets and segments of streets in 1901 shows the section of Peel south of Sherbrooke as belonging to the highest category. In fact, Peel was one of the relatively few streets on which rents south of Sherbrooke attained that ranking.[48] The new residence, which was on the west side of the street, had a garden at the back and was sufficiently spacious to serve also as Macphail's medical office.

Both 216 Peel Street and the Burland home on University Street were situated within the area that became known as the Golden Square Mile. Roderick MacLeod, who has written a doctoral thesis on the area in the nineteenth century, has concluded that this "tightly-knit community," which had been forming since around 1840, was "mature" by the 1890s.[49] For decades it was regarded as Canada's most exclusive residential area, and MacLeod has defined it as being bordered by Mount Royal on the north, the Canadian Pacific Railway tracks on the south, Cote des Neiges

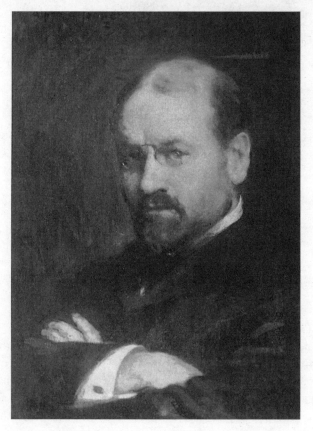

Portrait of Andrew Macphail, 1897. Copy of painting signed by Alphonse Jongers and dated 1897 by him. The present whereabouts of the original portrait is unknown.

Road on the west, and what are now Durocher, Aylmer, and St Alexander streets on the east.[50] In his words, "Its idyllic setting on the mountainside, overlooking the city and the St Lawrence River, was a natural magnet for wealthy nineteenth-century families."[51] Julia Gersovitz, the author of a superb master's thesis on the Square Mile (she did not use the word "Golden") from 1860 to 1914, has argued that there was a sharp differentiation between the areas north and south of Sherbrooke, one that ultimately can be attributed to the physical features of the landscape: those areas north of Sherbrooke, on an ascending land surface, had the best views and were home to "the grand mansions, isolated one from another by acres

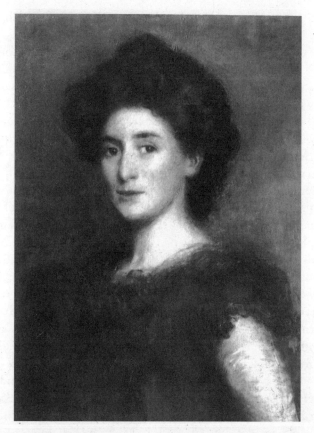

Portrait of Georgina Burland Macphail, *ca.* 1900. Copy of painting whose date
is not known; the photograph is dated 11 May 1900. The present location of the
original portrait is unknown, and although the identity of the portraitist
is uncertain, it may be Jongers.

of garden. The area had an immediate image of exclusiveness and exclu-
sion, of wealth and power."[52]

In October 1894 a son, Jeffrey Burland, was born to the Macphails.
They had one other child, a daughter, Dorothy Cochrane, in 1897.[53]
Fragmentary written evidence gives some indication of Georgie's activities
other than motherhood and household management. She reported to her
mother-in-law in 1896 that she was taking vocal and instrumental music lessons, "which means plenty of hard work."[54] In addition, she carried forward
the Burland family tradition of philanthropic activity. At her death she was

described as "an officer of the Montreal Foundling and Baby Hospital …
[and] also deeply interested in the work of the Industrial Rooms, and the
Day Nursery."[55] Living sources with first-hand knowledge of Georgie and
the marriage with Andrew are not available, since Georgie has been dead
for more than a century. Jeffrey, the older child, died without issue in 1947,
and his widow passed away in 1968. Dorothy, who lived until 1988, was less
than five years old when she lost her mother and, despite her superlative
memory, would not have been in a position to comment on the quality of
the marriage.

Given what is known of Macphail the parent and also the way his family
and neighbours took to Georgie when she went to Orwell in 1896, it is safe
to infer that she was traditional in her attitudes and in her sense of her role
– no "bluestocking." She appears to have charmed the Macphail family and
the people of Orwell, just as she had quickly become very close to Nettie
Macphail when the latter entered McGill in 1893. Andrew's elder sister
Maggie wrote enthusiastically, "How beautifully *we* & *Georgie* got along, &
how *highly* we esteem her & have learned to love *her* also for her own sake
…I find she has the same good *old fashioned* principles & beliefs that I have,
so it cannot be my '*bringing up* in an *out-of-the-way* place & never having
seen anything' that is the reason I am not 'progressive' enough … Even the
people around took to Georgie & know exactly just how fine & good &
sensible she is, as *Margaret Neil* said to me 'Och would John Andrew get
any other kind.'"[56] Maggie's husband remarked, "She is as good as a man –
to talk to."[57] As Andrew commented to Georgie, she had "bewitched them
all … down there."[58]

Macphail himself certainly conveyed to his children and grandchildren
that they were to behave much as he had been expected by his father to
behave: not to disturb the adults - in short, "to be born adult," as a grand-
child recalled in 2000.[59] His daughter remarked to the present author in
1969, "I wish I were young now," when children were not so constrained.[60]
There is no reason to suspect that Georgie held dramatically different views
from her husband on such matters as proper child rearing. Indeed, there
is evidence to suggest that she was less liberal than he in some of her attitudes. In a letter written during the summer of 1893, he comforted her and
counselled patience in dealing with the religious skeptics she encountered
at a summer retreat in Rockland, Maine; the issue appears to have been
the efficacy of churchgoing.[61] As for Macphail's spare time, starting early in
1897, for about six months of the year – from autumn to spring – he spent
alternate Saturday evenings at an all-male club where there was fellowship, intellectual stimulation, and plenty of drink. This pattern of taking

refuge in clubs was probably not anything out of the ordinary, especially in Canada's metropolis, Montreal, for husbands and fathers who had access to such amenities.

On 22 April 1902 Georgie, who had never been robust, died suddenly of diabetes. At the time of her death she was in a New York City hotel with Andrew and the children. They had come from Pinehurst, North Carolina, a famed winter resort, where they had apparently spent a lengthy period, and they were intending to proceed to Saratoga, known as an all-season health resort.[62] Macphail reported to his father, "I had a year's warning. ... [but] she did not even know the end was coming – though I did. I was with her constantly for two months."[63] Despite having known a year in advance, the trauma was intense for Macphail; over a full year after Georgie's death he used black-bordered envelopes to enclose his correspondence.[64] Prior to this, the greatest tragedy in his life had been the death of his brother Will in 1893, shortly after he had left him convalescing in Orwell. Now, at thirty-seven, Macphail was left alone with two small children. He largely withdrew from social life and let his medical practice dwindle, eventually confining it to the examination of applicants for life insurance.[65]

Georgie thus exited from the grand narrative of Macphail's life in 1902. He was an intensely private man; "reticence" is the noun he probably would have chosen to describe the quality, for in his mind it clearly connoted pro- priety in the way one exercised self-discipline in not speaking too much about oneself, particularly one's innermost thoughts. In keeping with this reserve, it appears that rarely if ever did he refer to his wife after her pass- ing. Stephen Leacock wrote in an obituary article following Macphail's death, "In the thirty-seven years I knew him I never heard him once refer to what I know had been the greatest sorrow of his life." He added, "Those of us of weaker temper carried our troubles to Andrew but never were asked to share his."[66] In Macphail's posthumously published memoir *The Master's Wife*, 246 pages in length, Georgie is not mentioned even in a veiled fash- ion, although both children are present. While the book focuses particu- larly on his youth in Prince Edward Island, from time to time it does flit forward and back between places and generations. Self-revelatory as it is in other respects, there is no clue regarding his marriage. His daughter recalled in 1970 that he had never mentioned her mother to her from the time of death until she reached the age of twenty or twenty-one, except when he wrote dedications to his children in his books.[67]

Macphail's reticence extended beyond the matter of referring or not referring to his dead wife. When his friend Archibald MacMechan extended his sympathy on the death of Macphail's brother-in-law Jeffrey Burland,

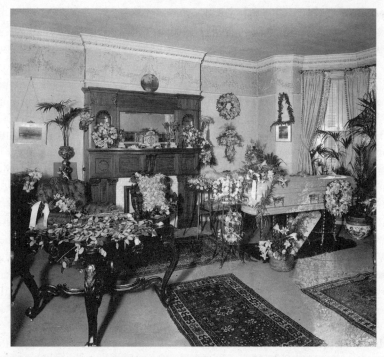

The drawing room at 216 Peel Street at the time of Georgina's death.
Note Georgina's casket on the right. This photograph was taken in May 1902.

he remarked that he assumed they were friends although "you have never
mentioned his name in my hearing."[68] In his reply Macphail praised the
dead man's character and revealed that he was going to New York to meet
his body, which was coming from England, where he had died – a fact
which suggests that he had remained close to his in-laws but simply was
disinclined to speak about this bond, even with someone with whom he
was on very friendly terms.[69]

    In 1903, the year following Georgie's death, an exceptionally important
dimension of Macphail's life began to emerge. He sent his two children,
in the company of a German governess, to Orwell to spend the summer
with his parents; his father retired in June. The following year, Dorothy
alone was sent. In late June of 1905 Macphail accompanied his children
to Orwell, the beginning of a long-term trend. He had perhaps signalled
his intent in 1904 by paying for the renovation of the family home. On 4
July 1905 his father died, but his mother remained in the house until her

passing in 1920.[70] After that, the house was occupied seasonally, when the family arrived from Montreal. Macphail was thus able to remain in frequent contact with his native province and his native district for the rest of his life.

PHYSICIAN AND MEDICAL PROFESSOR AT BISHOP'S

After returning to Canada from the Orient, Macphail had established himself in medical practice at 2446 St Catherine Street and bought a piece of land on which he hoped to build a house eventually – this, of course, was before George Burland gave him the row house at 216 Peel Street. On 1 December 1891 he wrote to his brother Will, who also had graduated in medicine that year, "Business is flourishing mildly at first but in time I hope to get my share of work in this town. I have very comfortable offices and knowing a lot of people practice will grow."[71] Yet he soon decided that he needed further study, and on 11 May 1892 he sailed for England. He was absent less than six months but during that time became a licentiate of the Royal College of Physicians (London) and a member of the Royal College of Surgeons (England). He also assisted some doctors in their private practice and appears to have done a bit of journalistic work on the side. As a result, as he recalled many years later, "I emerged a lean and broken wretch; it required the twelve days of the return voyage to restore me."[72]

For the following ten years the practice and teaching of medicine dominated Macphail's working life. His private practice appears to have grown steadily, and in December and January 1892–93 he signed contracts as medical examiner for three life insurance companies. On 31 May 1893 he was elected professor of the diseases of children at the University of Bishop's College Faculty of Medicine, which was located in Montreal, separate from the main campus at Lennoxville. Less than a year later he acquired an additional position at Bishop's, as professor of pathology and bacteriology.[73]

Macphail's medical practice continued to expand in the latter part of 1894. Over the next two years he was appointed pathologist to the Protestant Hospital for the Insane in Verdun and the Samaritan Free Hospital for Women; he was also appointed visiting physician at the Protestant House of Industry and Refuge. Along with the scholarly and innovative T.J.W. Burgess, medical superintendent at the Verdun institution, he undertook research into mental disease.[74] But a series of blood-poisoning attacks and a presumed connection between them and the conditions of surgical work compelled him to give up surgery about 1898. Through the 1890s a number of his articles appeared in professional journals, particularly the *British Medical Journal*. Not all his publications were of a clinical nature: in 1900 he wrote on "The After-History of Applicants Rejected for Life Insurance."[75]

In 1896 Macphail interrupted his medical work to do research for the dominion government on discolouration in canned Prince Edward Island lobsters. The lobster canning industry, which had scarcely existed when the Island entered Confederation in 1873, had commenced a boom period by the early 1880s but had been plagued with problems of spoilage, which in turn were rooted in lack of regulation.[76] After three months of work in Montreal, Macphail and Arthman Bruère, a professor of physiology in the Bishop's medical faculty, proceeded in mid-May to the Island, where they established a laboratory. It is not clear why the federal government selected the two medical professors for the project or what their relevant expertise was or was thought to be. But with a fisheries cruiser at their disposal, they made experiments throughout late May and June, working between ten and twenty hours a day. On 25 May Macphail wrote to Georgie that the work was "very hard and obscure and I sometimes think there is no end nor bottom nor track in it."[77] Nevertheless, within two weeks of this letter, he and Bruère discovered a probable explanation, which revolved around lack of cleanliness in the canning factories. After taking several samples tinned by an improved process back to Montreal for aging, they were able to confirm their hypothesis. The improvements they recommended were instrumental in retaining the British export market for Canadian lobster packers.[78] But the most recent writer on the subject has noted that not all canneries adopted their recommendations, with the result that consistency of quality remained an issue for decades after their report.[79]

Since Macphail was on the Island at the end of May, he was able to make the first presentation of a gold medal he had donated to Prince of Wales College. The prize, which Principal Anderson had originally wished to name the Macphail or Uigg Medal, eventually became known, at Macphail's insistence, as the Anderson Medal. Being a gold medal, it superseded the Governor General's silver medal as the highest scholastic honour at the college and remained so for seventy-odd years. Macphail had previously presented a gift to McGill University, and in both the Prince of Wales and the McGill cases he characteristically insisted on as little personal publicity as possible.[80] The lobster research had also provided Macphail with an opportunity to have Georgie and their small son visit the Island for the first time.

As already noted, following Georgie's death in 1902, Macphail had let his medical practice decline almost to the point of non-existence. Perhaps its main manifestation was the continuing presence of the "Doctor Macphail" nameplate on his door during his lifetime, with the occasional result that strangers (sometimes from out of town, because of the proximity to the major Montreal railway stations) arrived at his home seeking treatment – and sometimes, according to his daughter, seeking access to drugs.[81] But despite the personal loss and his apparent lack of interest in immersing himself in a conventional medical career, Macphail was not the man to become inactive. His energies were partially redirected. He continued to teach, and at the beginning of 1903 he became managing editor of the *Montreal Medical Journal*. His teaching was interrupted in 1905 when McGill University absorbed the Bishop's College medical faculty. Macphail played a leading role in the amalgamation, since he had been convinced for some time that Bishop's lacked the hospital facilities, financial resources, and staff necessary for an efficient and modern medical school. He had made no secret of his views in conversations with his colleagues and in 1904 had put his thoughts in writing; he explicitly stated "that there was no reasonable prospect of obtaining these essentials for teaching at Bishop's and that therefore the holding of classes should cease."[82] Certainly a reading of the minutes of the Bishop's medical faculty suggests that it was not a particularly happy place to be: there were problems in recruiting and retaining suitable professors, and there was the almost constant spectre of hostility from McGill.[83]

Early in 1905, with the forced retirement of the ailing medical dean of Bishop's, and in response to a sense of crisis within the Faculty of Medicine regarding the future, a three-member negotiating team, including Macphail and the poet-physician William Henry Drummond, opened discussions with a group from McGill. Macphail's appointment to the body was understandable, given the views he had already expressed, and he soon demonstrated a willingness to stand up to colleagues who were apparently inclined to drag their feet in pursuing the ostensible objective of amalgamation. A pivotal moment came when, in his absence from a meeting of the Bishop's Faculty of Medicine, the other two negotiators reported that the McGill side seemed to be averse to coming to terms and that there was no real point in continuing. Macphail obviously disagreed, and at the following meeting he contradicted his colleagues, setting the record straight, in his mind, so as to move the process forward. He had his opposing interpretation of the state of negotiations attached as an addendum to the main body of the minutes for the meeting from which he had been absent.[84]

Once matters had progressed further, it was Macphail who on 1 March 1905 read and explained the proposed terms of amalgamation to the faculty as a whole. At a meeting on the following day, he suggested that a committee be appointed to confer with the Bishop's medical students and to assure them that their interests were being protected; then he served as a member of that committee. In short, if anyone spearheaded the movement for amalgamation, Macphail was that person, and in pressing the case he had found himself in a minority on at least one important occasion but was not daunted. No one else emerges from the official records in the way Macphail does.[85]

The union was consummated on 9 May 1905, and in practical terms it proved to be the extinction of a rival of McGill rather than any sort of unification of equals - or even of two groups both of whose members deserved a modicum of respect. With the discontinuance of medical classes at Bishop's, Macphail was left without a teaching position. It was clearly understood at the time that McGill was under no obligation to hire the Bishop's staff. This had been underlined for Macphail personally on 6 May 1905 when a motion was presented to the McGill Faculty of Medicine for his appointment as the university's first professor of the history of medicine; the fourteen members present rejected the proposal. Macphail's leading advocate was probably pathologist J.G. Adami, one of the most eminent medical men of the era, who had moved his appointment and who on 16 March 1904 had unofficially proposed to him that he consider changing to McGill. Yet the sponsorship of Adami and Robert F. Ruttan, another medical professor of high stature, and the apparent sympathy of Principal William Peterson, who was in the chair on 6 May 1905, were insufficient to carry Macphail's case. The probable explanation is the long-standing enmity (the word is not too strong) between the rival medical schools and his identification with the losing side. In any event, when the question of Macphail and the new chair arose again at the medical faculty on 13 June 1907 and it was specified that the position would not entail a seat on the faculty, those present resolved to recommend the establishment of the chair and Macphail's appointment to it. Eight days later the board of governors confirmed the faculty's decision.[86]

Macphail was the only senior member of the Bishop's medical faculty at the time of amalgamation in 1905 to be appointed subsequently to McGill.[87] Many years later, in a published article, he wrote that the terms of the merger had "not been adequately fulfilled."[88] Since he did not specify, there can be no certainty, but it is probable that he was referring to the question of appointments. This had been a contentious point during negotiations. He and his fellow negotiators for Bishop's had informed colleagues in advance that McGill had said men would be appointed who would strengthen their medical faculty but that such appointments would not be automatic. The Bishop's negotiators do not appear to have expected them to be virtually non-existent.[89] There was, in addition, the associated issue of the prospects for Bishop's graduates, and there, too, there had been disappointment, according to Macphail. In a memorandum written in 1918, he stated that the "final arrangement" had been that all would be considered "on their merits without reference to their previous affiliations." Yet thirteen years after amalgamation, he was not aware of any Bishop's medical graduate who had been considered for appointment to McGill – "a real grievance," in his view.[90]

MCGILL'S FIRST PROFESSOR OF THE HISTORY OF MEDICINE

Macphail's duties as professor of the history of medicine at McGill involved ten or twelve lectures per annum. In the university calendar it was stated that "the intention [is] to examine the causes which produced the varying conceptions of medicine in times past, rather than burden the student with a narration of facts and a recital of biographies."[91] In other words, Macphail's aim was to move beyond the conventional and produce an intellectual or social history of medicine. The lectures were not restricted to students in any particular medical year, and attendance was voluntary.[92] According to H.E. MacDermot, a future historian of the Canadian medical profession who took the course in 1909–10, Macphail's lecturing style was very deliberate, and the material was delivered in a droning monotone. No questions were ever asked in those days, MacDermot reported, not even at the end of lectures; thus, the lack of any sort of dynamic interaction between professor and students in the formal classroom setting was not unusual at the time. Most who enrolled attended regularly, though there was no examination. Macphail himself was a considerable attraction, and there were opportunities outside the classroom for students to watch him at work, to make his acquaintance, and to make themselves, as individuals, known to him.[93]

Although Macphail's formal responsibilities were not onerous, he made the position into more than a sinecure and took considerable interest in those who showed any enthusiasm for the work. One night a week he met with a small group of students at the medical building to discuss style in medical writing, a subject on which he held passionate views. MacDermot remembered that Macphail used case reports as illustrative material, and that he was the only one of his lecturers to take any interest at all in writing.[94] One of his aphorisms was, "If a writer of prose takes care of the sound the sense will take care of itself."[95] MacDermot later reported, "It is one of the first things he impressed upon his students, and I have heard him repeat it over and over."[96] Macphail was not a harsh critic – especially not to his juniors, MacDermot emphasized – but there was an air of finality about his judgments when delivered. Macphail's daughter recalled that, informally, he invited students to his home at 4 pm on Thursdays, where they were served tea and food, and given advice on the writing and passing of examinations.[97]

Macphail also stood out from his peers in his views of the optimal curriculum for medical students. In an obituary article, Charles F. Martin, a McGill medical colleague who had also been appointed in 1907 and served as dean of medicine from 1923 to 1936, stated "He was a fervent advocate of a curriculum which exposed the student as early as possible to the patient, believing that too much laboratory training in the primary years obscured the main human issues involved in the practice of medicine."[98] Paul Potter, a medical historian with doctorates in both classics and medicine, commented on this in 2003, noting that such advocacy meant that Macphail was "very much against the trend [in his own era], even revolutionary." William Osler's influence was strong when Macphail was teaching at McGill, and the overwhelming emphasis during the early stages of medical education was on science, with the first two years being spent in laboratories. It was only in 1969 that McMaster University, under the leadership of John Evans, adopted an approach similar to that which Macphail had advocated. Potter speculated that Macphail may have developed his point of view because of the era in which he entered and practised medicine. It meant that he had seen both approaches: the humanistic and the scientific.[99] As professor of the history of medicine, Macphail became well known within McGill, and in 1909 the alumni elected him to serve a three-year term on the Corporation (the forerunner of the Senate) of the University. He was "Representative Fellow in Arts," replacing John Redpath Dougall of the *Montreal Witness*, and over the following twelve years was re-elected three times.[100]

Among medical people, Macphail is chiefly remembered as founding editor of the *Canadian Medical Association Journal*. Indeed, in 1992 the journal reprinted an editorial article he had published in its first number, dated January 1911.[101] Macphail was an entirely reasonable choice, since he was recognized as having been a resounding success in his position as editor of the *Montreal Medical Journal*. The first decade of the twentieth century was the era in which medicine in Montreal attained an international reputation, and according to MacDermot (writing as a medical historian), under Macphail the monthly journal "rose to its greatest heights"[102] as an organ of the local medical community. By the latter part of the decade, Macphail and others associated with it, such as Adami, Alexander D. Blackader, and Thomas Roddick, had decided that the time was ripe for a national periodical that would attempt to represent the state of medicine in Canada as a whole, and to record the transactions and convictions of the national professional association.

On 12 September 1907 Macphail put forward a proposal for a national journal at the annual meeting of the Canadian Medical Association in Montreal, and he offered to submerge the *Montreal Medical Journal* in the new venture. The president of the association appointed him to a five-person committee to investigate the possibilities; he appears to have chaired this body. By 1910 the executive council was ready to appoint him as first editor of the *Canadian Medical Association Journal*.[103] The idea for such a periodical or a published record of the association's transactions had been floating around annual meetings of the organization for many years, and Macphail's initiative in 1907 may have been decisive in bringing the project to a successful conclusion.[104]

Macphail spent the last six weeks of 1910 establishing the new monthly. Despite opposition from interested parties in Toronto, which went to the extent of a lawsuit alleging that its name was too similar to that of another publication, Macphail's periodical appears to have been an instant success. It became known in its field for the editor's attention to matters of literary expression. In fact, Macphail – who by this time had a growing public reputation as a literary figure and for four years had been editing a highly successful quarterly, the *University Magazine* – devoted an article in his first number to "Style in Medical Writing." He began by asserting that "all important scientific observations have been recorded with a singular fitness of words" and declared that "a man who is intelligent enough to be a surgeon is also intelligent enough to learn how to write down what he wants to say in simple, accurate terms" - which is what he demanded of contributors. "Easy reading," he warned, in the sort of epigram that would characterize his writings over the years, "is hard writing."[105] He continued to edit the *Canadian Medical Association Journal* gratuitously (as he had done with the earlier medical monthly) and to keep a tight rein on its contributors until he went overseas at the outbreak of the First World War. In an obituary to him, MacDermot wrote, "His energy and personality ... set our *Journal* on its foundations."[106]

Between the years 1885 and 1907, Andrew Macphail had moved from student to professor and become a leader within his chosen profession. He had established his own family and had married into a situation that would assure financial ease.[107] In the private sphere, alongside everything else – first, combining university studies with journalism, and then combining medical work, including medical teaching and journalism, with literary production – he had played a strong role for many years in assisting his younger siblings and acting as mentor regarding their educational choices. He provided candid advice. In 1891, while entering his final weeks of lectures in medicine, he had written to William Matheson Macphail, age eighteen, to ask about his plans for the future:

> Tell me what you really want to do, what you think best for the present and in the long run for yourself, and I will try to help you to that end. You must not think there is any short cut through the fields, it is slow hard work but if you believe this and are not afraid of it you will get there in the end. Do not be satisfied with little things because they are easy and pleasant and do not be contented to make a small foundation or follow a track that won't take you anywhere and don't mind those who are having a nice time now. When you tell me what you want to do I will find you a lot more good advice and perhaps be able to tell you something that may be of advantage to you.[108]

The advice could be negative; he emphatically opposed what turned out to be an ill–founded attempt to steer a younger brother into the McDonaldite ministry.[109] When another brother got into serious difficulty of some unspecified sort in continental Europe, Macphail went to Germany personally to assist in straightening matters out.[110]

In the public sphere, Macphail had emerged as a significant figure in the medical world, first of Montreal, Canada's largest city, and then of Canada as a whole. Two years after graduation he had been appointed to the medical faculty of Bishop's. He became managing editor of the *Montreal Medical Journal* in 1903 and within a few years was advocating a national journal, a project that eventually succeeded, with himself as editor. His editing of the *Montreal Medical Journal* would have required the ability to work with people, sometimes strong personalities who were accustomed to being deferred to and getting their own way. A mixture of diplomacy, sense of purpose, and firmness would have been necessary. When the thorny issue of amalgamating Bishop's medical faculty, where he had taught since 1893, with the McGill medical faculty arose, he had shone. He demonstrated that he was willing to do things himself in order to ensure that they were done properly and also that he was willing to confront and able to overcome opposition, even to face down the apparent duplicity of colleagues and to make it part of the record. In short, he played a crucial role in seeing the process through to completion.

Macphail's appointment to McGill in 1907 provided him with his intellectual base for the following thirty years. He would become a pioneer in the teaching of the history of medicine in Canada, taking an intellectual approach that transcended the recitation of dates and names. His ideas with respect to the medical curriculum in general were so different from the conventional wisdom of the era that he can be said to have been far in advance of his time.

3

Macphail and the Cultures of Montreal

Andrew Macphail had maintained his broader intellectual activities after receiving his MD. There was a bohemian side to his life; he could not be pigeonholed as simply a typical professional man married to a wealthy woman and living within the fabled Square Mile. In December 1891 he became a member of Montreal's Shakespeare Club, and three years later he was lecturing the Caledonian Club on "The Scottish Character." The Montreal *Gazette* reported a pleasant blending of humour and seriousness in the address; Macphail did not understate the virtues of his heritage – "a love of home and country, thrift, prudence and economy, fidelity and high courage and unflinching will."[1] As early as 1895, he appears to have been doing research for two studies of Puritanism that he published ten years later.[2]

"A HOME FOR THE SPIRIT ..."

The death of Macphail's wife Georgie in 1902 marked the termination of the predominantly medical phase of his career. Although he remained active in medical teaching and medical journalism, he began to display a more serious commitment to literature, and he worked hard on cultivating his literary abilities. His interests in the years immediately following 1902 suggest a certain introversion: he compiled an anthology of verse on the theme of sorrow, which he published much later, in 1916. This focus is consistent with the romanticism evident in the titles of some poems he had composed during the years of his marriage: "Sweethearts," "Love's Retreat," "The Sigh," and "The Fountain of Love."[3] A few months before Georgie's death, he read "Sonnet of Sorrow" to a group of artists and writers.[4]

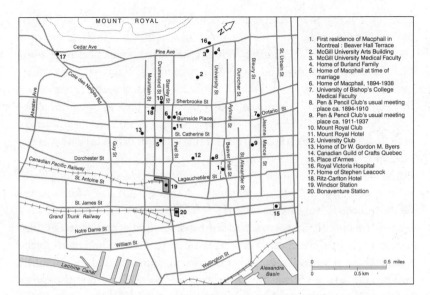

Andrew Macphail's Montreal

The group was the Pen and Pencil Club of Montreal, which had elected him to its membership in 1897 after inspecting a specimen of his work – "An article on Japan (Outing)" – submitted at the time of his nomination.[5] Macphail had published at least two articles regarding Japan, on athletics and on bicycling, in the American magazine *Outing* (one of the periodicals sponsoring his around-the-world trip in 1891), and this was probably one of them. The club, all male, which met on alternate Saturday evenings, had been founded seven years earlier with the purpose of "Social enjoyment and Promotion of the Arts and Letters." The launching of such a club may be attributed in part to what one historian of Montreal has described as a chronic lack of cultural institutions in the city.[6] In any event, each member was expected to unveil or read an original piece of work for criticism once every month or six weeks. Among the most active were artists William Brymner, Maurice Cullen, Edmond Dyonnet, and Robert Harris, poet J.E. Logan, and McGill literature professor Paul T. Lafleur. Brymner, Harris, Lafleur, and Logan had all been members since 1890, the year of the club's foundation.[7]

It was at the Pen and Pencil Club that Macphail met Stephen Leacock, who joined in 1901. So close did the men become that, in the words of

Leacock's biographers, Albert and Theresa Moritz, writing in 2002, "Until Macphail's death in 1938 he remained Leacock's chief literary mentor and confidante [sic]."[8] Another intimate, the pathologist and poet John McCrae, joined in 1905 – and it was Macphail who had moved that an invitation be extended to him. They had first met around 1900 at an autopsy, in Macphail's words, "upon the body of a child who had died under my care."[9] According to Macphail, "'The Pen and Pencil Club' ... was a peculiar club. It contained no member who should not be in it; and no one was left out who should be in. The number was about a dozen ... The place was a home for the spirit wearied by the week's work."[10] He also joined, among other groups, the St Andrew's Society, the St James Club, the Mount Royal Club, and the Royal Montreal Golf Club – the last-mentioned because of his passion for golf; a photograph of him as president of the "R.M.G. Club" survives.[11] But the Pen and Pencil remained his favourite for many years, and certainly it was the most important for his intellectual development.

The standard format at the time Macphail joined was that the members would select the "subject" for a meeting one session in advance. Those contributing were to produce something related to the chosen theme, a method that provided a stimulus and a challenge. Within a year Macphail became one of the most active members. Although it was unusual to make presentations at consecutive meetings, commencing on 22 January 1898 he did so at an astonishing eight successive gatherings, carrying on through 28 April. On six of those occasions he contributed poetry – twice they were sonnets.[12]

The meetings were convivial affairs, in part because, as Macphail noted years later when writing a memoir about McCrae, artists commented on written works, and vice versa.[13] Some even crossed over, as when artist Harris read his account of an incident he had experienced during the conflict over the Prince Edward Island "land question" in the 1860s.[14] Such a procedure almost guaranteed that the atmosphere would not become too severely competitive. There was also a degree of cross-disciplinary collaboration by members. When Captain John Try-Davies, a charter member, produced a book of stories, Harris, another charter member, illustrated the volume, and the two men dedicated the book – A Semi-Detached House and Other Stories – to members of the club "in memory of many pleasant evenings."[15]

Some perhaps unexpected topics emerge from the minutes, such as censorship and the police, a discussion provoked by the case of a Montreal policeman arresting a shopkeeper for displaying in his window statuettes like that of Venus de Medici (a modest Venus, with both hands before her

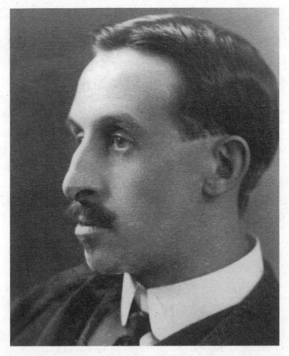

Percy E. Nobbs, 1906. Professor of design at McGill and an active member of the Pen and Pencil Club, Nobbs was a brilliant architect, a man of many diverse talents, an expert on numerous topics – and endowed with a volcanic temper.

body).[16] The minutes reveal other unpredictable aspects of the proceedings. In December 1908 Percy E. Nobbs, a well-known Montreal architect and McGill professor of design, in collaboration with a guest, "gave a fencing exhibition."[17] This was apparently a result of the fact that earlier in the year Nobbs had won an Olympic silver medal in foils. An exceptionally able and active man of many talents, interests, and passions, he deplored specialization as a curse of modernity, a perspective that would have made him a soulmate of Macphail and an embodiment of the spirit of the club. Nobbs, in addition to writing prolifically in his own professional field, later published books on salmon-fishing tactics and fencing tactics; each of them, Macphail wrote, was a serious piece of work, in effect a book for experts. The year before Nobbs joined the club, he had already published an article, "Praise of Fence," in the semi-annual *McGill University Magazine*, under his initials, P.E.N.; he illustrated it himself, for among other things

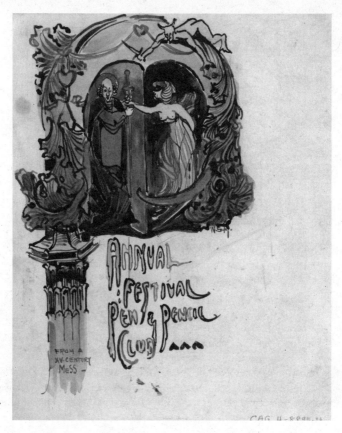

A Pen and Pencil Club menu card in 1908, front. Macphail belonged to this club of writers and artists from 1897 onwards. It met fortnightly during the colder months of the year, and as their final meeting of the season members had a "festival" for which the artists were expected to create menu cards. The initials "W.S.M." indicate that the artist in this instance was architect William Sutherland Maxwell.

he was a talented painter. During the First World War he put his fencing ability to practical use by organizing bayonet instruction in the Canadian military, and he also served as a camouflage expert.[18]

Whimsy was permitted at the Pen and Pencil Club. One of Leacock's early presentations was "Things That I Do Not Want to Read Any More,"[19] and his first had been "Opening a Bank Account"[20] - probably based on "My Financial Career," originally published in *Life* in 1895 and destined to be the lead-off sketch in his first book-length collection of humorous

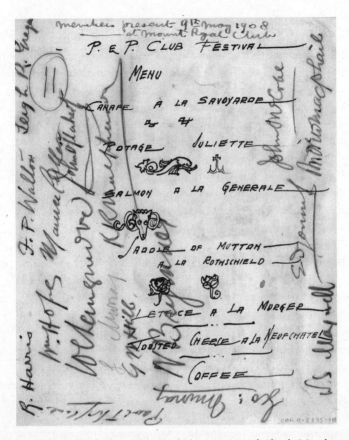

The same Pen and Pencil Club menu card, signatures on the back. Members often had those attending sign their menu cards. Among the autographs in this instance are those of Macphail, Maxwell, physician and poet John McCrae, McGill dean of law F.P. Walton, literature professor Paul Lafleur, and artists William Brymner, Maurice Cullen, Edmond Dyonnet, and Robert Harris.

pieces, *Literary Lapses* (1910).[21] Once, when the assigned subject was "Horror," Dyonnet unveiled a portrait of himself.[22] Following "a poetical study of a mermaid" by Nobbs, Macphail related having attended a mermaid in his capacity as a physician.[23] On another occasion he delivered a paper on "Superstition in P.E.I."[24]

The tone of some of the minutes suggests a lack of orderliness, possibly even a lack of sobriety, especially towards the end of a session. At the first meeting Macphail attended, the minutes record that several motions regarding the constitution were moved and lost, "and it was decided that there was no necessity for recounting [?] them in the minutes."[25] The members drank freely, with Macphail a prime instigator, moving on one occasion "that the glasses be filled" – an unusual motion even by the standards of the club. There was no resistance, though, for it was "seconded by all the members present."[26] During the Prohibition period in the rest of Canada and in the United States members made much of their freedom to drink, particularly when they had guests from Toronto the "dry." On one occasion, after entertaining the artists A.Y. Jackson and Homer Watson, "At the close of the meeting, it was noted with admiration ... that the distinguished guests from Toronto needed very little assistance in navigating the stairs to the street."[27] In 1920 the minutes recorded a discussion of the "wet" versus "dry" issue in relation to Ontario, Quebec, and the United States. With Macphail in the chair as president, "Quebec was voted to be 'the last refuge of civilization.'"[28] In the 1940s Leacock recalled, "This organization, meeting ... in the half-light of a studio, falling asleep over essays read to it, and waking up to look at pictures or drink scotch and soda, developed a life and character all its own."[29]

The Pen and Pencil was essentially a cold-weather club, for it closed down in the spring and resumed in the autumn. Each season featured a "festival," or elaborate dinner party, the final event of the year. The purpose of the society was fellowship and the provision of intelligent although not necessarily expert feedback in response to creative work, and in those terms the club was an undoubted success. It provided a sort of workshop for writers or artists to present works in progress. Leacock, for example, delivered a series of "Sunlight Sketches in Mariposa," clearly foreshadowing his *Sunshine Sketches of a Little Town*.[30]

EMERGING AUTHOR

Macphail's first book, *Essays in Puritanism* (1905), consisted of five papers he had presented to the Pen and Pencil at various meetings. The essays dealt with five individuals who represented or reacted against Puritanism: Jonathan Edwards, who "manifested the spirit of Puritanism in the pulpit"; John Winthrop, who "showed that spirit at work in the world"; Margaret Fuller, whose "career was the blind striving of the artistic sense for expression"; Walt Whitman, whose "conduct was a revolt against the false conventions which had grown up in his world"; and John Wesley, who "endeavoured to make religion useful to humanity once more."[31]

Essays in Puritanism established Macphail's position as a serious man of letters. Each piece was based on a careful investigation not only of the person's life and works but also of the period in which he (or she) lived. This was especially true of the Winthrop study, in which the "times" came close to displacing the "life." Macphail explained the rationale behind his method. The "first fact to establish in estimating a personality is the environment of the man; his class, and hence the habitual bent of his mind; his family and friends; in short, his outlook upon the world."[32] He also made liberal use of each subject's words; he desired to present the person in his (or her) own terms and own setting before passing judgment. Although the studies were certainly scholarly, they were written to appeal to a wider audience than professional scholars. Footnotes were eliminated, and the heaviness of the subject was lightened by an easy style and an ironic wit, which caused Macphail's father "often ... to give way to bursts of laughter loud & long, and that in the face of the fact that we shouldn't expect to be so affected by the subject of Puritanism."[33]

The weaknesses of the book are as readily apparent as its merits. The collection does not attempt to deal systematically with Puritanism. The characters are shown in interaction with aspects of Puritanism, but the focus of each essay remains on the individual. The result is an incomplete portrayal of what should be at the centre of the book; the closest Macphail comes to a general consideration of Puritanism is in a rambling introductory section to the essay on Edwards.[34] The opinion of the *New York Times* reviewer is worth citing at length:

On both sides [positive and negative] of his view of Puritanism he leaves an impression that he has not very thoroughly worked the matter out. One involuntarily wishes that he had done more since he has done so much, that he had made a picture rather than a group of sketches ... It is precisely because he is so clever in what he has done, and betrays here and there such insight into the obscurer phases of his subject, that one cannot help longing for more and still better ... Clearly there is considerable scope in the Puritanism these personalities are supposed to represent or to oppose, and Mr. Macphail does not entirely succeed in showing their relations to the main topic. He even gives ground for the suspicion that the main topic was a matter of title making after the sketches were composed and that the latter were not the product of a purpose to develop the topic ... [As a result, he] does not throw much new light on the

Puritanism which they [the sketches] are supposed to illustrate, [although] he does give us decidedly fresh impressions of the characters of which he treats.[35]

Almost all the reviewers praised Macphail's sense of balance in assessing the virtues and faults of the various figures. His capacity to appreciate such men as Edwards appears to have been rare among the literary men of the day, and his combination of sympathies rarer still. One critic commented that "to be just both to Jonathan Edwards and to Walt Whitman is an achievement of no small merit."[36] Most reviewers conceded that Macphail had something fresh to say on subjects that had already attracted much attention and that he said it in a fresh way. Although the poet Wilfred Campbell disagreed with much of the content and tone, he wrote that *Essays in Puritanism* "should be in the library of every intellectual Canadian."[37]

The Vine of Sibmah: A Relation of the Puritans (1906), Macphail's second book, was less successful. A novel set in the Restoration period, it was related in the first person singular by "Captain Nicholas Dexter" of Oliver Cromwell's Ironsides. The title was taken from Isaiah 16:1, 9: "O Vine of Sibmah, thy plants are gone over the sea." Marauders had ravaged Sibmah, a Dead Sea community famous for its grapes; in Macphail's novel, the "plants" are Parliamentarians like Dexter, forced to flee from the vengeful Restorers.[38] Macphail had been working on the novel for many years. One of his first presentations at the Pen and Pencil Club, in the autumn of 1897, had been a short story entitled "Cromwell."[39] By 1901 a typescript draft was complete. Dated 2 April of that year, it was entitled "Nicholas Dexter: A Puritan Soldier in the Old World and the New."[40]

The novel centres on Dexter's infatuation with Beatrix Sherwyn, a young lady he had rescued from highwaymen some ten years earlier, when she was a child. She is the ward of a prominent London merchant and alderman, who gratefully recalls Dexter's help and posts bond for him at the time of the Restoration. But the merchant is deranged and burns down his house, dying in the fire; Dexter, who was an overnight guest, leaves for the New World, believing that his love has also perished in the flames. Once in America, he discovers that she survived and is perhaps alive in another colony. Eventually, through the agency of an Amerindian war, the two lovers are reunited and married – by Dexter's most trustworthy friend, who on the last page is revealed to be Beatrix's biological father and an admiral of the late Protector's fleet.

The Vine of Sibmah abounds in the conventions of its genre, the historical romance. There are deeds of gallantry, miraculous escapes, spectacular battles at sea, tangential encounters with the great, romantic and seemingly hopeless love, and the happy ending. The narrative line is held together by a number of coincidences that can only be described as incredible: it seems as though everyone Dexter has encountered in London turns up in the wilderness in some unexpected guise. Time and again, hopes of seeing Beatrix alive are dashed, only to be revived. One reviewer commented that Dexter "figures in almost every conceivable capacity from pirate to theologian ... It is said that truth is stranger than fiction, but this book belongs to that peculiar species of fiction in comparison with which truth is commonplace."[41]

The book's reception by critics was mixed. Despite its weaknesses, it was described as one of the better historical romances of the season. Yet as Macphail noted many years later, the genre "had become belated."[42] After almost two decades of public favour, the historical romance was losing its appeal. New and more exacting standards for fiction were emerging. In the words of a London critic, *The Vine of Sibmah* "is, like most of its fellows, lacking in any attempt at psychological study. The characters are well drawn, but we may only see their clothes and their actions, and hear old phrases and old oaths upon their lips. Never once do we see into the working of their brains, or hear the beating of their hearts."[43] Stylistically, this is reflected in Macphail's overuse of dialogue and the difficulty the reader often experiences in determining who is speaking.[44]

Macphail had not been notably successful with fiction as a means of illuminating the Puritan spirit at work in New England. Perhaps the strongest impression to emerge from the book in this regard was Macphail's personal ambivalence towards Puritanism. In the United States, it was noted that although Dexter was not "the fictional Puritan" – a man of "nasal-toned piety"[45] – nonetheless, "the two most distinctive traits" attributed to the Bostonians were "Phariseeism and cruelty."[46] As more than one American reviewer observed, the Amerindians were presented as much more attractive personalities.[47] But beyond this, there is little insight into Puritanism or Macphail to be gained from reading the book.

The publication of Macphail's first two books in 1905 and 1906 brought him to a new plane of development. His first novel was his last, but *Essays in Puritanism* revealed his potential as a man of letters. In the essay or short piece he had found his genre; by 1905 he had demonstrated, in publications of Canadian, British, and American origin, his capacity as a biographical, thematic, and polemical essayist.[48] With the appearance of the two books, he established an audience and a reputation. He had attained recognition in his second career, which had now come to dominate although not eclipse his first.

MACPHAIL AND MONTREAL

Throughout Macphail's time in Montreal, it was, in terms of culture, undeniably a city divided between English-speaking and French-speaking residents.[49] In the words of historian Anthony Sutcliffe, its "dualistic character made Montreal unique in the world among cities of its size."[50] Despite the existence of "two solitudes," to use the later phrase of novelist Hugh MacLennan, Macphail appears to have been a bridge builder by inclination. At Bishop's in 1894, the year after his initial appointment, he had moved a resolution to hire additional staff in order to offer courses taught in French to provide French-speaking students with "complete facilities."[51] The initiative was ambitious and not as successful in its implementation as the sponsoring faculty members hoped. But like admitting women, opening the doors to Jewish students, and establishing a school of dentistry, it indicated that Bishop's and Macphail were open to new ideas, including one that would, in this case, contribute to reducing the isolation between the professional élites of the two linguistic communities.[52]

In the Pen and Pencil Club Macphail supported a decision in 1906 to offer membership to Henri Bourassa, the French Canadian nationalist tribune.[53] The members could have been under no illusion concerning whom they were inviting into their midst, for by this time Bourassa had established his reputation through opposing the South African War and supporting minority language rights for French speakers in the West.[54] Unfortunately, the minutes of the Pen and Pencil do not reveal Bourassa's response, and all that is clear is that he did not join or even attend as a guest. The gesture, nonetheless, is significant, and Macphail's backing of it, like his support for French-language teaching in the Bishop's medical faculty, indicates an openness to the French fact.

Among the Pen and Pencil members there were French speakers, men who were prominent in the life of the club. Dyonnet and Lafleur are the best examples, and indeed Dyonnet was probably the member who was present at the largest number of meetings over the years, for the club frequently met in his studio. But the two were untypical of the French-speaking population of Quebec. Lafleur was a Protestant, and Dyonnet was a native of France whose particular friends, according to the author of the preface to his posthumously published memoirs, tended to be English-speaking.[55] The presence and prominence of a French Canadian Protestant and a native of France – and the absence of a Bourassa – must have served to underscore for members the gap between the minority English-speaking and the majority French-speaking populations of the city.

Just as it was evident that the city was divided culturally, it was equally indisputable that the economically dominant group in Montreal was the English-speaking minority. Macphail had married into a comfortable segment of the bourgeoisie. His father-in-law, George Burland, was a highly successful and affluent businessman. The home on University Street where Macphail's wife grew up was, as noted, in the Golden Square Mile, and after Burland's death in 1907 it was acquired by the Morgans of department store fame; it has been recognized for many years as a heritage house, a significant part of the built history of Montreal.[56] Jeffrey Hale Burland, Macphail's brother-in-law, had been building a magnificent limestone mansion on Pine Avenue when he died unexpectedly in 1914. Eventually it became the home of J.W. McConnell, who was described by Donald MacKay, the author of a book on the area, as "the last of the Square Mile tycoons."[57]

Macphail was conscious of the circles he was entering, as is evident from one of his surviving letters to Georgie, written before they married, in which he refers to having made thirty-seven dollars in five days. This was, he wrote, "small enough it is true if measured by the 'millionaires' amongst whom you live but enough for two modest people who are content to love each other first and value money afterwards."[58] As a practical person, he was aware that the income of a medical doctor was not at all comparable to that of the businessmen with whom Georgie and her family were familiar. Scholarly research has established, for example, that in 1881 less than 50 percent of Montreal medical doctors owned their homes, which meant that they fell short of a standard of real affluence, although their situation was much better than the average among the general population in the city, only 15 percent of whom were homeowners.[59]

Yet according to Margaret Westley, a modern student of the former Montreal élite, a professional person such as Macphail, educated and erudite, would have had considerable prestige – "high status" – among the wealthy in Montreal, more, for example, than a retailer, even if the latter had made a great deal of money. Unlike the retailer, who in his workaday guise sought to serve and please, the professional's role was to give advice or sometimes even orders ("doctor's orders") to the wealthy and their families. Westley provides as evidence the examples of the daughters of Sir Hugh Allan and Lord Strathcona, who married professional men; and in

1912, C.F. Martin, Macphail's McGill medical colleague, married a daughter of Richard B. Angus of the Canadian Pacific Railway. Furthermore, the
exceptionally strong Scottish representation among Montreal's anglophone élite – Allan, Angus, and Strathcona were all from Scotland – carried with it an ethos that valued education and educators. Macphail's marriage to the daughter of George Burland, therefore, would not have been a
break with class norms.[60]

During the fifty-three years from 1885 to 1938 when Macphail lived in
Montreal, the city was undergoing rapid change in every sense. His immediate neigbourhood was undoubtedly part of it. MacKay has reported that
by the 1920s "people were calling the corner of Peel and St Catherine 'the
crossroads of Canada.'"[61] Men of business were transforming Montreal
and radically reshaping its very face. Scale was an important aspect of the
changes in the built environment. The size of buildings increased dramatically in the late nineteenth century and again in the 1920s, dwarfing people
and previously existing structures. This was part of an international trend
which geographers and architectural historians have referred to as "gigantism," and in its medical origin the term denoted an "excessive growth."[62] By
the mid-1920s Macphail, at 216 Peel Street, was a mere stone's throw from
the largest hotel in the British Empire, the Mount Royal, with its 1,046
rooms.[63] Only by a studied effort could he avoid seeing it on the other side
of the street, slightly to the south, as he stepped out of his home. One won-
ders how he responded to such changes in his surroundings, although,
given the political and social outlook he articulated over the years, it is
clear that he would not be inclined simply to celebrate the triumphs of
commerce. Indeed, he must have been dismayed by many aspects. Yet there
was probably an ambivalence, for he undeniably enjoyed the benefits of
metropolitan living. Although he eventually returned to Prince Edward
Island regularly in the summer, there was never any suggestion that he
would forsake Montreal for rural Prince Edward Island and live there on a
year-round basis.

One of the advantages of residing in Montreal during Macphail's time
was the fact that he could work at Canada's leading university and inter-
act with many of the most brilliant minds of the country. Among his colleagues at McGill were such people as Leacock, the political scientist and
humorist, Nobbs, the architect and polymath, and Thomas Roddick, a
transplanted Newfoundlander whom Stanley B. Frost, the historian of
McGill, has described as being in the years before the First World War
"Canada's most prominent physician and surgeon."[64] At the University

of Bishop's College medical faculty a colleague had been William Henry Drummond, the most popular poet in Canada at the turn of the century, someone whose readings and lectures were in demand across North America[65]; Drummond appears to have been a close friend, for shortly after his death in 1907, Macphail reported to James Mavor of the University of Toronto, "I miss him daily."[66] Another attraction to life in the largest city in the country was the possibility of a club such as the Pen and Pencil, which drew some of the most interesting and creative men in the dominion to it. Only a large city could offer such benefits, and in the Canada of Macphail's prime only Montreal could do so, for it was the cultural and intellectual capital of English Canada as well as French Canada.[67]

The conclusions concerning "Macphail and Montreal" that can be drawn on the strength of available evidence are limited. Macphail must have been aware of the changes occurring in Montreal, aware of who wielded economic power in the city, and aware of the dramatic cross-currents of the era. Further, he had an interest in and respect for French Canadian culture, and indeed he published the first English translation of *Maria Chapdelaine*, the classic novel of French Canadian life, with illustrations by Marc-Aurèle Suzor-Coté. In his enthusiasm for the book, he read a chapter of his translation to members of the Pen and Pencil.[68] But he and other English-speaking Canadians who shared his political perspectives, like Leacock, found it difficult to make living contact with the majority culture – witness the failed attempt to bring Bourassa into the Pen and Pencil.

Montreal was Macphail's home, although much of it was probably unfamiliar to him. What was most familiar was the Montreal of privilege and wealth – wealth that must have been astonishing to someone from the rural hinterland of the country. In the words of François Rémillard and Brian Merrett, two authors who have written about the Golden Square Mile, "Il a atteint un degré de raffinement inégalé au Canada, avec ses nombreux clubs très sélects, ses équipes sportives, les célèbres collections de tableaux de certains de ses membres, ses réceptions grandioses et ses maisons de ville et de campagne avec leur personnel stylé."[69] Around 1900, Rémillard and Merrett report, the Golden Square Mile encompassed more than 75 percent of the millionaires of Canada, and its inhabitants controlled almost 70 percent of the wealth in the country. Most of them, like Macphail, were of Scottish origin, and for the years from 1850 to 1930 it has been estimated that 70 percent of inhabitants of the Golden Square Mile had Scottish roots.[70] At the very least, this meant that in the English-speaking parts of the city of Montreal and at McGill University, Macphail's ethnicity would have been no disadvantage and would have closed few doors to him. Yet his Montreal – dynamic, educated, and enterprising – was limited, whether at his favourite club or elsewhere, no matter how much he might desire it to be otherwise. In this experience he was far from unusual. Division along linguistic lines and division along lines of wealth were realities of life in the city.

In the late 1890s and the first decade of the twentieth century, Andrew Macphail moved beyond journalism and was emerging as an increasingly serious writer. Medicine was still a major focus of his life, but increasingly he had been developing as a man of letters, taking his place with other literary and artistic notables of English-speaking Montreal. At the Pen and Pencil Club he played a central role almost from the time of his election to membership. Few contributed to the proceedings as frequently as he did, and over the years there were acknowledgements of his leadership. It was only in 1907 and afterwards that the tilt towards literary matters became absolutely decisive, and even then the habit was to refer to him as Dr Macphail.

Although for several years it was not entirely clear where the emphasis would fall once and for all (medicine or writing?), two facts were becoming inescapably clear. In the first instance, Macphail was exceptionally busy and hard-working. Secondly, through it all, whether in family matters, the medical profession, or at the Pen and Pencil Club, he was exhibiting considerable leadership ability. He was willing to take initiative (the Bishop's amalgamation, the *Canadian Medical Association Journal*), to deliver unwelcome news (advise against a clerical vocation for a brother in the face of the wishes of at least one of his parents), to deal personally with difficult situations (his brother in Germany), and to lead by example (the frequency of his contributions at the Pen and Pencil Club). Macphail was proving to be a man of great energy, bold ideas, determination, and, all in all, a force to be reckoned with.

In the years after Macphail's graduation he had demonstrated a force of character and a practical sense. At the Pen and Pencil Club he delivered poetry, prose, and, apparently, humour. In 1905 and 1906 he published his first two books, and it was clear by then that a momentum in the literary direction, as opposed to the medical, was building. The editorial aptitude he displayed with the *Montreal Medical Journal* foreshadowed his remarkable success as editor of the *University Magazine*, commencing in 1907.

4

Creating the *University Magazine*

The period from 1907 to 1914 was to be the most important in Andrew Macphail's career as a writer and an editor. Through the medium of the *University Magazine*, which he established, edited, and published out of his home at 216 Peel Street, he addressed a wide audience on contemporary public affairs, in the process articulating a comprehensive philosophy of social and political conservatism. Macphail's traditionalist ideology, asserting the importance of moral rather than material values, and rooted in attachment to the way of life he had known in his youth, found its first expression in imperialism.

This chapter will deal with Macphail's editorial and financial involvement in the *University Magazine* as the essential backdrop to treating in a systematic manner his developing world view during his most productive years.

ORGANIZATION AND OBJECTIVES

In May 1906 Principal William Peterson accepted the resignation of Charles Moyse as editor of a semi-annual publication known as the *McGill University Magazine*. The periodical had been published for five years, and in the introductory editorial Moyse had stated its purpose: "There ought to be some journal, more or less officially identified with the University, to which articles too long and too elaborate for small and frequently printed publications, can be sent ... [on] subjects of general interest in literature, art and science."[1] But as the contributors were largely McGill staff and graduates, and a significant portion of the articles were of interest solely to people with McGill connections, the potential circulation was seriously limited.[2] The subscribers numbered less than a thousand when Moyse resigned, having done most of the work and having spent several hundred dollars of his own money on the magazine.[3]

Historian and librarian Peter F. McNally has examined the *McGill University Magazine* and its contents carefully, first in an MA research paper and later in a published article. In his view, it had in its brief existence "made a significant contribution to the development of English-Canadian intellectual life, [and] Canadian magazine publishing," as well as to McGill, primarily through the diversity of its subject matter.[4] He makes this case particularly in the chapters of his MA paper entitled "Philosophy and Science" (71–84) and "Philosophy and Thought" (85–96), especially the former, which includes a lucid delineation of debates between idealists and empiricists at McGill on the nature of science. McNally suggests that in addition to reflecting a broader controversy of international dimensions, these reveal the rising importance of science at McGill and the consequent rivalry between science and arts within the university.[5] He refutes historian Samuel E.D. Shortt's dismissal of the *McGill University Magazine* as "pallid" and "a journal analogous to the alumnae [*sic*] publications at Queen's and Toronto."[6] As McNally points out in his research paper, the *McGill University Magazine*, whose individual issues were between 160 and 180 pages in length, included the features of an alumni magazine but was primarily "a magazine of general culture and opinion."[7]

If there was an area that the magazine slighted – "virtually ignored" – it was current public affairs, for McNally found only ten articles of 188 that fitted into this category.[8] Almost all of these dealt with imperialism, specifically British imperialism. "It is also noteworthy that with the exception of passing comments, none of the articles dealt with contemporary Canadian or Quebec affairs."[9] In contrast, McNally identified 31 as having "McGill University" as their subject, and 18 as featuring "McGill University – biography," together constituting 26 percent of the whole.[10] Of the biographical pieces, which focused on deceased academics and benefactors, he wrote, "With the exception of Andrew Macphail's article on Sir William Dawson, all were hagiographic in tone."[11] Later in his paper he stated that even Macphail's article could be classified as "unrelievedly flattering," its distinction from the others being that it acknowledged controversial aspects to its subject's record.[12]

Peterson, an energetic Scot with a high sense of the university's duty to extend learning and culture, was determined to have the magazine reorganized as a viable undertaking. In these circumstances he approached Macphail, who as editor of the *Montreal Medical Journal* had already demonstrated his ability to deal with brilliant and sometimes difficult personalities. Macphail had helped Moyse with some of his editorial duties and had contributed to the *McGill University Magazine* twice in the previous year. He shared the principal's belief that the journal should be made into a collective effort with a sizable editorial board. After discussing the financial aspects of the situation with the university bursar, Peterson and Macphail decided to approach prospective members of such a committee. Accordingly, on 20 June 1906, just before leaving on his annual summer-long visit to the "home-country," Peterson wrote to a number of professors and interested associates of McGill, asking them to consider the matter over the summer and to look for possible copy.[13]

By late autumn Peterson and Macphail had organized an editorial board of twelve Montrealers, including themselves. From the start, Macphail was the driving force on the committee and the man who determined the new policies and emphases. He was named editor, and many years later Stephen Leacock, an original member, recalled:

> The "board" was virtually swept aside by Andrew, as you brush
> away the chess pieces of a finished game. Historians recall to us
> the first meeting of General Bonaparte in 1799 with the Abbé
> Siéyès and the others who were to be the joint government of
> France under the new "consulate." As they came out the Abbé
> remarked to a colleague, "Nous avons un maître," – and with that
> the "joint-stuff" ended. So it was with Andrew. After a meeting
> or two, the magazine became and remained Andrew Macphail.
> Like all competent men who can do a job and who know it, he
> had no use for co-operation. We, his colleagues, were invited
> occasionally to have Scotch whiskey in Andrew's queer little
> library and then some more Scotch whiskey with cold beef in
> his beautiful big dining-room. That was all the co-operation
> he wanted.[14]

The other members were to use their contacts to find contributors; at the first meeting, for example, Peterson was asked to solicit articles from such persons as William Osler, Goldwin Smith, and A.H.U. Colquhoun. The last-mentioned was the new deputy minister of education for Ontario, a McGill alumnus, and a longtime journalist who had contributed to several issues of the former magazine; as Peterson explained, "The Board is anxious to keep our old friends and also to gain new ones."[15]

The first number of the reorganized journal appeared towards the end of January 1907 as the *University Magazine*. The following announcement appeared on the inside cover: "*The University Magazine* is a continuation of *The McGill University Magazine*, with a certain departure, and will be issued four times a year, upon the First day of February, April, October, and December. The main purpose of the Magazine is to express an educated opinion upon questions immediately concerning Canada; and to treat freely in a literary way all matters which have to do with politics, industry, philosophy, science, and art."[16] The leading articles in the first and second numbers were the journalist E.W. Thomson's meditations on "What Will the West do to Canada" and Peterson's comments on the upcoming imperial conference. Although the literary aspect of the venture was important to Macphail, he was determined that the primary emphasis should be political, a distinct departure from the *McGill University Magazine*.[17] This focus meant that the new publication avoided a problem of its predecessor which McNally has identified: it had "seemed often to have a disembodied personality, detached from any time or place."[18]

Macphail had very specific ideas about the public questions he believed required attention. For example, he was deeply disturbed by the contemporary opinion that British diplomacy had repeatedly sacrificed Canadian interests to appease the United States. As early as December 1906 he was planning a series of revisionist articles on "British Diplomacy and Canada," and over the following two and one-half years five articles on this theme appeared. In each case, Canadian protestations of ill use were dismissed, and the basic interpretation was that Canadian interests had been well protected. Macphail also objected to the equation of the imperial tie with the protective tariff; the real basis for imperial unity was sentiment, he maintained, and the introduction of financial considerations as a justification for an essentially familial tie could only debase and ultimately destroy the relationship. In short, "It is a naïve assumption that the interests of the manufacturers are identical with those of the country as a whole."[19]

Furthermore, Macphail was concerned about the course of Canada's domestic development. Since the death of his father in 1905, he had been accompanying Jeffrey and Dorothy to Orwell each summer. The renewed regular contact with his native province after an interval of twenty years gave him cause for reflection. The Island had reached a census peak of population in 1891, but had since been steadily losing people. Population declined by 5.3 percent in the 1890s and by 9.3 percent in the 1900s.[20] This would have been particularly noticeable to Macphail, for over the period 1881–1921 the absolute numbers of his own ethnic group fell by 31.7 percent,

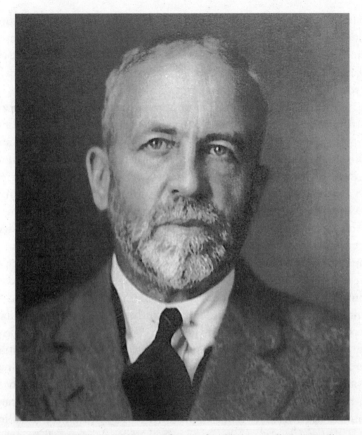

Archibald MacMechan. Longtime professor of English at Dalhousie College, MacMechan joined Macphail's editorial board for the *University Magazine* in the autumn of 1907 and remained a member until it ceased publication. He was the third most frequent contributor, behind Macphail himself and Marjorie Pickthall. He and his family were guests at Orwell several times, and he composed a Petrarchan sonnet in the host's honour, which was eventually published.

whereas the percentage of decline in the population as a whole was 18.4.[21] Accelerating regional depopulation in a period of national economic boom must have seemed paradoxical. Macphail blamed the protective tariff, the dominion's dominance over the provinces, and, ultimately, the control of the central government by the protected manufacturers. These evils were to be primary targets of the *University Magazine*. "My notion is that each Province has a definite grievance which should be removed. I think that the case of each Province should be stated."[22]

But Macphail planned to do more than simply have a set of opinions, political or otherwise, set to type. After the second number he wrote to Archibald MacMechan of Dalhousie College in Halifax that he was trying "to establish a standard of literature instead of imitation and pedantry. It is not for what I put into the Magazine I take credit, it is for what I kept out. I had a bitter passage with two important personages."[23] In the selection of contributors he was no respecter of persons or powers;[24] the quality of the submission was his sole criterion. With this receptive attitude he was soon publishing an unknown young poet, Marjorie Pickthall. When first shown her work he is reported to have exclaimed, "This means more to Canada than a new province."[25] Over the next thirteen years she was to contribute to twenty-one issues of the *University Magazine*.

Although Macphail gave his own articles and editorial services without compensation, he always paid his contributors, whether or not they wished it. In the Canada of his day this was a definite break with the past; for example, *Queen's Quarterly*, established fifteen years earlier, did not remunerate its writers. At the *University Magazine*, the average fee was twenty-five dollars, a significant amount in the early twentieth century in any part of Canada.[26] To take one measure, this was more than double the average weekly wage earned by adult males employed in manufacturing in prewar Montreal.[27] MacMechan wrote in later years that Macphail's "revolutionary policy of paying a living wage enabled the editor to rally the best brains" to the magazine and "to pick and choose ... without fear or favour." In MacMechan's opinion, the "only critical journal comparable to it in power was *The Week*; but its strength was a single extraordinarily keen and well-furnished mind [that of Goldwin Smith]. The strength of *The University Magazine* was in its corps of writers recruited all over Canada."[28]

The first number met Macphail's criterion of quality but was still largely a McGill and Montreal affair. Of eleven contributions, at least nine came from persons associated with the magazine, McGill, or the Pen and Pencil Club: two from Macphail (one over the pseudonym Angus Macfadyen) and one each from Leacock and F.P. Walton (editorial board members, McGill faculty, Pen and Pencil Club members), Charles W. Colby (editorial board member, McGill faculty), John McCrae (editorial board member, club member), Walter Vaughan (McGill bursar), E.W. Thomson (club member), and A.H.U. Colquhoun (McGill alumnus and regular contributor to the *McGill University Magazine*). As soon as the magazine appeared, Macphail and Peterson set about rectifying this situation. They accepted the invitation of interested persons in Toronto and spoke at the annual dinner of the Canadian Society of Authors on the possibility of making the *University Magazine* a "federal" venture.[29]

Armed with the first number as an example of what could be done, Macphail clearly enunciated the purpose of the journal:

> I read in the morning papers that the Manufacturers Association had stated certain views upon the tariff. I do not say that these views are wrong. I say that there is a suspicion that they are not wholly disinterested. If these views had emanated from a university, I would not say that they were right, but I should be disposed to think that they were given disinterestedly. It is our business to bring to bear upon all questions an intelligent opinion ... The Magazine must be directed not within the walls, but without ... We shall speak free. We shall tell the truth and no country, not even Canada, is the worse for having the truth told about it.

The objective was nothing less than "to produce in Canada a Magazine which will rival ... the best of the English monthlies." In this enterprise he offered partnership to Toronto and any other Canadian university.[30]

Macphail elicited a positive response from his audience, and it appears that he, Peterson, and some University of Toronto professors gathered afterwards at the house of James Mavor, a political economist. As McGill had provided the subscription list from the *McGill University Magazine* and was canvassing its graduates in order to raise the number of names to 1,500, Macphail and Peterson proposed that Toronto procure 1,000 subscribers. The Toronto academics apparently agreed and suggested to their board of governors that the university provide a guarantee fund of $1,000 for the subscriptions, which were $1 each; for example, if only $600 were obtained, the university would give $400 to the magazine. The arrangement ultimately settled upon seems to have been a simple annual guarantee of about $750, to be applied against any deficit.[31]

By the time the April 1907 number was ready for the press, Macphail was able to announce that arrangements for cooperation were being worked out with Dalhousie College as well. The origins of this link are obscure, and although in 1924 MacMechan described his college as having "stood sponsor"[32] for the *University Magazine*, this seems to have been a figurative expression. The only manifestation of the connection, aside from the authorized use of the name, appears to have been MacMechan's presence on a reorganized editorial board. There was also hope that Queen's

University at Kingston might support the journal. Dean James Cappon apparently attended the dinner in Toronto; but Queen's had its own quarterly and no connection developed, although Macphail was still hoping for it at least as late as 1911.[33]

EDITORIAL BOARD AND CONTRIBUTORS

When the third number appeared in October 1907, the editorial board had been reorganized to reflect the national character of the magazine. Macphail remained editor, but only two on the six-man editorial board were McGill men. These were William Peterson, a classicist by profession, and Frederick Parker Walton, the dean of law. At age fifty-one, Peterson had been McGill's principal for twelve years. He had studied at Edinburgh, Göttingen, and Oxford, and had already received honorary degrees from eight universities in Scotland, the United States, and Canada. Walton, an Englishman, had been educated at Oxford, Edinburgh, and Marburg. He had immigrated to Canada ten years earlier, upon being appointed to his deanship. Exemplifying the versatility of intellectuals of the era, at a meeting of the Pen and Pencil Club some years earlier Walton had delivered "Verses." In 1909 he would read a poem entitled "The Lawyer's Plaint."[34]

Of the four remaining members of the board, three were from the University of Toronto: James Mavor, William John Alexander, and Pelham Edgar. Mavor was a Scot who had attended the University of Glasgow but because of illness had withdrawn before gaining a degree; in fact, he never earned a degree. Yet his areas of interest were unusually wide-ranging, and he became a recognized authority on political economy, lecturing at both Edinburgh and Glasgow universities. He had been a socialist in his youth and a close associate of William Morris.[35] Over the years his views underwent a transformation, and he became an outspoken and vigorous opponent of public ownership and the trade union movement. Hired by the University of Toronto in 1892, he proved intensely controversial from the beginning on account of his bohemian and apparently absent-minded ways (which more than matched any stereotype of the university professor), his lack of academic credentials, and his difficulty in establishing rapport and communicating effectively with his students.[36] As a consequence, his job, in the words of historian Alan Bowker, "hung by a thread" in the early years of the century.[37]

Mavor had a personality that could be difficult sometimes, and he was prone to lasting dislikes – for example, of Leacock and the University of

Toronto historian George M. Wrong. Bowker quotes approvingly Peterson's comment to Mavor in later years, made during a dispute between them: "Your attitude ... has been marked by wrong-headedness and perversity."[38] Mavor nonetheless survived; he had local support as well as local enemies, and, moreover, he had worldwide academic and political contacts, and a considerable reputation, which helped to convey the impression that he was a person out of the ordinary in a positive sense. He has been aptly described as a "lion hunter" for his active pursuit of the acquaintance of so many leading figures in diverse fields.[39]

As a generous and indefatigable patron of the arts on the local level, Mavor made an undeniable contribution to the Toronto community. He preached art appreciation, advocated the establishment of an art gallery, and gave early encouragement to such writers as Pickthall and Ernest Thompson Seton. Moreover, about 1906 he commenced a two-volume study, *An Economic History of Russia* (1914), more than 1,200 pages in length, which Macphail's editorial abilities assisted in making more readable; it achieved immediate acclaim as a classic. Thus, in time, this complex figure with his prodigious energy would come to be recognized as being, despite the many rows in which he was involved, a bit of a treasure who helped to lead his university and his adopted city out of provincialism and into a wider world.[40]

There were three professors of English on the editorial board, each a native of Ontario who had received his Bachelor of Arts at the University of Toronto and his doctorate at Johns Hopkins. Alexander, the first to hold the chair of English at Toronto, was also, according to the literature scholar Heather Murray, "the first Canadian professor of English to be educated specifically in the subject."[41] Although educated at London and Berlin, as well as Toronto and Johns Hopkins, his reputation was largely local, where he was known as an excellent teacher who exerted great influence over the development of his students. He had worked at the University of Toronto since 1889, and while supporting the research ideal, more or less confined his writing to Ontario high school texts. Murray believes that because of his combination of university teaching and preparation of texts and curricula for the secondary schools, "how English developed in the universities in Canada, and in the public school system in Ontario, is in many respects dependent on the trajectory of Alexander's career."[42] A founder of the Canadian Society of Authors, he was well connected, brother-in-law of Byron Edmund Walker, president of the Canadian Bank of Commerce.[43]

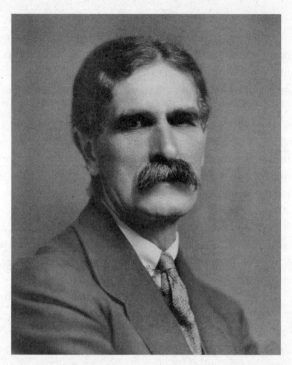

Pelham Edgar. A professor first of French and then of English at Victoria College in Toronto, he served on the editorial board of the *University Magazine* from the autumn of 1907 until 1920, by which time he was the only representative from Toronto. A close friend, he stayed with Macphail when visiting Montreal.

Pelham Edgar was the son of prominent parents, both of whose families were, in the words of historian Naomi Griffiths, "part of Upper Canada's elite."[44] His late father, Sir James David Edgar, had been a leading Liberal parliamentarian and was speaker of the House of Commons at the time of his death in 1899; he had earlier been a journalist who had published, among other works, two volumes of poetry. Pelham's mother, Matilda Ridout (Lady Edgar), was an historian who had produced a biography of Sir Isaac Brock, published in 1904 as part of the *Makers of Canada* series. A feminist, she advocated women's rights with respect to higher education, suffrage, family property, and having independent careers. In 1906 she had been elected president of the National Council of Women of Canada, an office she held until her death in 1910.[45] At thirty-six years of age in 1907,

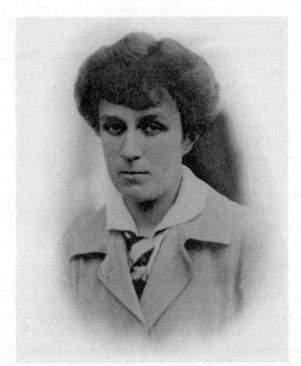

Marjorie Pickthall, author. Her work was introduced to Macphail by Edgar. Over thirteen years she contributed to twenty-one issues of the *University Magazine*. Macphail published a collection of her verse in book form (her first book) in 1913, titled *The Drift of Pinions*. Her verse drama, *The Wood Carver's Wife*, was the concluding piece in the final issue of the *University Magazine*. She considered it her finest work.

Pelham Edgar was the youngest member of the board, and in fact had been a student of Alexander; he had been teaching French at Victoria College for ten years, and would soon transfer to the English Department. An exceptional talent spotter who later "discovered" E.J. Pratt and Northrop Frye, he, along with MacMechan, was one of the ablest Canadian literary critics of his generation.[46]

MacMechan, the last member of the board, had succeeded Alexander at Dalhousie in 1889 and was also regarded as one of the most effective Canadian teachers of literature. A poet, essayist, novelist, and historian – as well as a literary critic – he was, in the words of historian Peter B. Waite, "a consummate stylist."[47] Over the years, he contributed to the *University*

Magazine more frequently than anyone except Macphail and Pickthall.[48] The author of a recent book on MacMechan has stated that his book reviews "were widely read and often ahead of their time" in their appreciation of works by such figures as Herman Melville and Virginia Woolf.[49] In 1899 his article "The Best Sea Story Ever Written" had anticipated by close to thirty years what came to be the broadly accepted understanding of the achievement represented by Melville's *Moby Dick*. He had commenced a weekly book review column in the *Montreal Standard* newspaper, "The Dean's Window," in June 1907 and continued it until his death twenty-six years later. His declared purpose was to foster a national literature that would meet international standards of quality, and his contribution would be criticism. Such a sense of mission made him a natural partner in Macphail's project.[50]

The six members of the new board were to provide Macphail with a solid nucleus of well-established and cosmopolitan writers, possessing a wide variety of experience and contacts. If Macphail (then age forty-three) is included, the median age was forty-nine and the average age forty-seven. Four were native Canadians and three were Britishers, all of whom were to die in the "home country." Three had studied in Germany, three in the United States, five in Britain, and none had had an exclusively Canadian education. Indeed, only Mavor had received all his formal education in a single country – and he was extraordinarily well travelled. Over the years between 1907 and the dissolution of the *University Magazine* in 1920, the six aside from Macphail were to make a total of fifty contributions; Macphail himself made forty-three. The three from Toronto were responsible for only fourteen of these, but they, and particularly Edgar, played an invaluable role in searching for "the young, new, unknown men"[51] that Macphail wanted. Although the new and smaller committee resulting from the association of Toronto and Dalhousie apparently never met as a group,[52] there can be no doubt that it was a substantial improvement over the board organized in late 1906.

With the appearance of the third number, the *University Magazine* and particularly the contributions of Macphail were coming to the notice of some significant imperial personages of the period. In April Peterson had suggested to Macphail that he send a copy of the *University Magazine* to the governor general. An energetic and enthusiastic man by nature, the fourth Earl Grey immediately took to the magazine, and by October he was ecstatic: in words that would have warmed Macphail's heart, he told John St Loe Strachey, editor of the London *Spectator*, "In matter, paper, type it compares not unfavourably with any of the home ... Monthlies, and in matter of Price most favourably."[53]

What excited Grey even more than the aesthetic and journalistic accomplishments of the *University Magazine* was the first instalment of the "British Diplomacy and Canada" series, with a preceding article by Macphail. With "The Patience of England," which served as an introduction to the series, Macphail defended British diplomatic manoeuvres concerning Canada: "In the main, these measures were far-reaching, just, and wise, and were inspired only by the desire to do what was best not only for the interests of Canada but for the English race as a whole."[54] Although specific Canadian interests may have been damaged on occasion, he argued, it had to be remembered that the Canadian front was only part of a much larger imperial strategy. Canadians would do well to recall that "England ... nourished and protected us as children, [and] endowed us with freedom and a kingdom when we were competent for the charge."[55]

This point of view was certain to appeal to a British viceroy, especially when his prime minister, Sir Wilfrid Laurier, had stated on 26 September, "We take the record of diplomacy of Great Britain in so far as Canada is concerned, and we find it is a repetition of sacrifices of Canadian interests ... We have come at last to the conclusion ... we would do better by attending to the business ourselves."[56] Grey believed that nothing that he or James Bryce, the British Ambassador to Washington, or any other Englishman could say would "uproot" such convictions: "This spade work must be done by Canadians."[57] Now, with the *University Magazine*'s series, the myth of the British overlord, negligent of Canadian interests, was being laid to rest by native Canadians. Grey sent copies of the October number to Strachey, Bryce, and such officials as the colonial secretary and even the private secretary to the King. To Macphail, he signified his pleasure by inviting him to Rideau Hall for two days when Rudyard Kipling would also be present.[58] Yet Macphail did not choose his articles in order to please those in power. In 1909 Grey found it "inopportune" that during negotiations for the entry of Newfoundland into Confederation, the *University Magazine* published an article ("The Two Islands") comparing the state of Newfoundland with that of Prince Edward Island, and attributing the blighted condition of the latter to Confederation and the tariff.[59]

By the end of 1907 Macphail could afford to be pleased with the initial success of his magazine. He was well on the way to accomplishing his major goals as an editor: quality, topicality, and accessibility to a wide audience outside the university. Such newspapers as the Montreal *Gazette*, the Toronto *Globe*, and the *Manitoba Free Press* frequently reviewed current numbers of the *University Magazine* and usually had warm praise for the contribution it was making to the discussion of contemporary problems. The 11 December 1907 *Gazette* remarked that an article by Warwick Fielding Chipman of the McGill law faculty on "Government by Party" was "in the best manner of the Edinburgh Review," and that the journal as a whole "takes rank with the great English monthlies."[60] In its annual assessment of Canadian intellectual endeavour, the *Review of Historical Publications Relating to Canada*, ordinarily very critical, expressed warm appreciation for the *University Magazine*, and especially for three articles by Macphail on the imperial theme: "It may be said to be representative of the educational thought of Canada … The articles dealing with Canada's political status are varied and excellent … Dr. Andrew Macphail's articles are always sane and illuminating."[61] The positive response to the first four numbers encouraged Macphail in his belief that he had been correct in reorienting the focus of the magazine. In a letter to MacMechan he wrote, "I want your frank opinion on the question – is the Magazine too political? My own opinion is that it should be more so, rather than less."[62]

There can be little doubt that Macphail was meeting a real demand in the English-speaking Canada of his day, for he often found that the strongest acclaim was gained by articles on controversial political themes. When he published his article on "Why the Conservatives Failed" in the federal general election of 1908, the Toronto *Globe* recommended that both Liberals and Conservatives read it carefully.[63] The Montreal *Daily Herald* reprinted much of the article and declared that Macphail "has succeeded during the brief term of life of the periodical in making it to rank with the best reviews of America, and of the Old Country."[64] The Toronto *Daily Star* stated that the article was so good that it should be read as a whole and could not be safely summarized.[65] When the multivolume *Canada and Its Provinces* appeared in 1914, the contributor on "The Higher National Life" concluded his section on "The Press" by stating, "In the *University Magazine* we have at last produced a quarterly periodical which may have a future of great power. [It is] at times quite equal, if not superior, to the best work on the American continent."[66]

The tendencies Macphail set in motion during the first year largely defined the path of the *University Magazine* between 1907 and 1914. He continued to seek capable new contributors and articles of immediate relevance to the Canadian situation. The base of contributors widened to the point that half of the twelve most frequent writers were non-Montrealers:

MacMechan in Halifax; Pickthall and the classicist Maurice Hutton, principal of University College, in Toronto; the classicist and theologian John Macnaughton at Queen's University in Kingston (although he returned to McGill in 1908 and moved to the University of Toronto in 1919); and the journalists Thomson and C.F. Hamilton in Ottawa. The Montreal half, aside from Macphail, Peterson, and Walton – that is, the members of the editorial board – consisted of Leacock, Chipman, and the McGill philosopher J.W.A. Hickson. With the help of colleagues, Macphail attracted non-academic figures like James S. Woodsworth and W.C. Good, and found such new talent as Daniel Cobb Harvey, G.G. Sedgewick, and C.B. Sissons.

Altogether, over the life of the *University Magazine* there were forty-six writers who contributed four or more articles or poetry selections. These may be termed "frequent contributors," and a profile of the typical one would be as follows: native British Canadian, probably born in Ontario, male, Anglican or possibly Presbyterian in religion, and almost certainly university-educated. He was as likely as not to have received his final degree abroad; if he had studied outside Canada, it was probably in Britain, but if not, it was more likely to have been in Germany than in the United States. Despite his cosmopolitan experience, he had in most cases returned to the province of his birth to pursue a career in the professions – and there was a better-than-even probability that he was a university professor. The most notable exceptions to this tendency to return to one's region were the contributors residing in Montreal, for in most cases they had come from other parts of Canada or from the old country. Although almost one-half of the frequent contributors resided in Montreal, only about one-sixth had been born in Quebec. Of sixteen who were not native Canadians, all but one had been born in the British Isles; most of these had immigrated at an age when the decision would probably be theirs rather than that of their parents, and most appear to have remained in Canada until death.[67]

CIRCULATION AND APPEAL

Macphail had succeeded in establishing a stable of reliable and able contributors. His major anxieties arose from the more mundane matters of subscriptions and revenues. From the beginning, he made it clear that he was interested in obtaining the widest possible hearing beyond the university walls. In a letter soliciting an article from Edmund Walker, as a prominent Canadian businessman, on 1 February 1907, he stated that he wished "to demonstrate that there is no gulf between the university men and other intelligent men ... Our idea is to interest all intelligent men."[68] With this in mind, he put an almost absolute ban on the use of footnotes in the journal and demanded a readable style and non-technical approach from all contributors, regardless of discipline.[69] This was another way in which he differentiated his quarterly from the *McGill University Magazine*, for, as McNally put it, certain categories of articles in that periodical "seem to have been written by academics for other academics."[70] Poetry as well as prose was welcome, and a characteristic number might include articles on travel, popular education, music, and contemporary issues in religion, as well as politics, literature, and philosophy.[71] Macphail was successful, and in an era when the Canadian academic community numbered in the hundreds, the *University Magazine* had a circulation that at one point, probably in 1912, almost reached 6,000.[72]

Circulation attained the level it did partially because of an arrangement between Macphail and G.N. Morang, a Toronto publisher. From the outset, Macphail had desired to rid himself of the business aspects of the magazine. After the expansion of mid-1907, a business manager, Charles A. Ross of Montreal, had been appointed. But this arrangement had lasted for only four numbers, and by October 1908 Macphail was on his own again.[73]

The agreement reached between Macphail and Morang towards the end of the following year was extraordinarily generous on the part of the latter: he was to collect and disburse all the money associated with the *University Magazine* gratis. In 1910 Morang, who had expressed great enthusiasm for the journal, set about raising the number of subscriptions and putting the magazine on a businesslike basis. Through an arrangement with Glasgow & Co., another Toronto publisher, he was able to raise the list to its peak of nearly 6,000, and in 1912 the price of an annual subscription was doubled from one dollar (the same as had been charged for two issues of the *McGill University Magazine* a decade earlier) to two dollars. The latter decision was a sensible and indeed necessary step, since as early as 1908 the cost of paper and press work alone exceeded 30 cents per issue. Two leading Canadian capitalists, Walker and Sir William Van Horne, used identical words – "absurdly low"[74] – when commenting in private correspondence on the old subscription fee. Walker, who had been president of the Canadian Society of Authors when it invited Macphail and Peterson to Toronto, once told Edgar, "I should like to help Dr. Macphail, but I really do not know what to do with so unbusiness-like a man."[75] Yet with the increase in price and a promotional effort directed at potential subscribers, it seemed as though the *University Magazine*'s finances, shaky until this point, were now on an even keel.

But early in 1913 Macphail discovered that Morang had in fact been keeping for himself whatever he thought was just compensation for his services – which Macphail was certain far exceeded the customary 10 or 15 percent. When pressed for a full accounting, Morang presented Macphail with a bill for about $3,000. While the dispute was going on, Morang, who held the subscription list, continued to collect the *University Magazine* money and appropriate it for his own use. Apparently legal action was eventually required in order to recover the list from him. Yet the financial outcome is unclear from the surviving evidence. During the course of the dispute, through inattention to the various details of management, the circulation fell to 3,300. Caught in the middle of this confusion, Macphail confided to his close friend E.W. Thomson, "My present disposition is to pitch the whole thing, as I am getting completely lost in small business details, which are a continual cause of worry."[76]

The financial state of the magazine had always been a problem for Macphail. Apparently, McGill gave a small amount at the beginning, but after that the only regular source of funds was the University of Toronto. This grant ended in 1910, when the Toronto board of governors, now chaired by Walker, took the association with Morang as an indication that the *University Magazine* was becoming an ordinary commercial operation. The grant had amounted to $700 or $750, but Macphail was not entirely sorry to see it terminated, for he disliked the possibility of censorship inherent in an annual subsidy. He strongly believed that Toronto should have agreed in 1907 to obtain a thousand subscribers – these could not be withdrawn at will.[77]

In addition to the subscribers and the universities, another substantial source of income, particularly in the early years, was individual Montrealers. Five hundred and fifty dollars were raised in this manner in 1908 and at least $1,150 in 1909. Some of the donors, such as Van Horne, Richard B. Angus, and E.B. Greenshields, were members of the McGill board of governors acting in their private capacities, but others were simply men of means who took an interest in literary matters. Greenshields, a businessman with varied and serious cultural interests, who had reached a stage in his life when these were starting to take precedence over his business concerns, did much of the collecting and was also one of the frequent literary contributors, publishing five poems and one article in the magazine over 1908–12. For at least the first three years this method liquidated the deficits. The *University Magazine* appears also to have made some use of personal appeals to wealthy Torontonians for funds, with Walker playing a leading role. One step Macphail would not take was to appeal to governments or incorporated bodies other than universities. In 1915, when he gave up the active editorship to go overseas, some $4,250 of his own money was tied up in the magazine. As it appears to have been supporting itself in 1914, once Morang had been removed, and as it had been turned over to him debt-free, it seems reasonable to infer that the largest portion of Macphail's loss had resulted from his once promising relationship with Morang.[78]

All in all, from the perspective of 1915, despite financial tribulations, it must be conceded that Macphail's optimism about the prospects for his magazine had been justified. Not only were there the resources to produce a high-quality, topically minded British Canadian quarterly, but as Macphail had predicted in his address to the Canadian Society of Authors, "The time is come for such a publication in Canada."[79] He had correctly assessed the Canadian reading public, and his magazine was reaching them more effectively than any previous or subsequent Canadian quarterly.[80] The triumph was his, for he had controlled the development of the *University Magazine* with a tight whip hand. Macphail very rarely accepted an article before reading it himself, and he reserved the right to refuse submissions even from his own editorial committeemen. On the other hand, his colleagues were assured that their recommendations would receive respectful attention. They were encouraged to solicit contributions and to give their opinions, but the final decision always lay with Macphail. In handling his editorial board and his authors, he showed a remarkable capacity for dealing tactfully but firmly with strong and sometimes wilful or eccentric personalities.[81]

One area in which the magazine might be open to criticism was its very British Canadian identity. Over the years few articles were published in French.[82] There is not surviving evidence of a type to permit a judgment on whether there were significant efforts to involve French Canadian authors, but given Macphail's professed admiration for French Canada over the years and his personal record at Bishop's and in the Pen and Pencil Club, it is probable that he would have welcomed any French-language contributions of quality. With his degree of control over the periodical and its contents, it would be impossible for anyone to prevent him from including French material if he had found the opportunity to do so. Writing in English, N.A. Belcourt made the case in the *University Magazine* against Ontario's efforts to restrict French-language education.[83] Macphail added a rare editorial note at the end of the article, stating that the author's "opinion ... is held by a large number of Canadians," and in effect challenging the Ontario government to state its case in the pages of his quarterly.[84] The magazine nonetheless remained British Canadian.

When the First World War erupted in 1914, Macphail, in his fiftieth year, decided to enlist. Despite an injury three years earlier that had left him almost blind in one eye,[85] he was accepted by the medical services after undergoing officers' training in Toronto. In January 1915 he made arrangements for the continuation of the *University Magazine* in his absence. A "local committee" to perform his functions was established, consisting of Peterson, Leacock, and two other longtime members of the McGill teaching staff, Charles W. Colby, an historian, and Paul T. Lafleur. The arrangement was apparently meant to endure for one year. Macphail left Montreal for Europe on 16 April 1915, and except for one brief visit did not return for almost four years.[86]

The importance of Macphail's *"University Magazine* years" is that he was successful in his objectives and was recognized as such by his contemporaries. He produced a topically minded Canadian quarterly of high quality when few thought it possible. This achievement thrust Macphail from the periphery to the very centre of the intellectual and journalistic world of prewar Canada, prompting MacMechan to remark in a letter to him in 1912, "You know everybody."[87] He could be assured that his views would obtain a wide and respectful hearing.

One factor in the success of the magazine and of Macphail himself that cannot be overlooked is his personality and hospitality. Several years after his death, Edgar provided a description:

Number 216 Peel Street came to mean Montreal to me. It was much more than a handy place to leave one's bag; it was a place where one found good talk, good cheer, and a welcome the more genuine because so unforced and natural. The house was roomy – essentially a man's house, save that from cellar to attic there was no suspicion of untidiness. The downstairs front preserved the fiction that the owner was still in active practice.[88] Arm-chair comfort was to be found in the second floor library sitting-room, and this was the expansive centre of the house - talk, picquet, whiskey, afternoon tea, what you would. A close rival in expansiveness was the dining-room. It was more formal, but here, too, hospitality thawed. One evening a half-dozen men were there after dinner. Andrew had an engagement for a couple of hours, and left us supplied with all necessities.

Towards eleven Stephen Leacock advised some supervision of the wastage, and we thought that we had done a satisfactory job when our host returned. He gave us a taciturn greeting, and proceeded, still in silence, with his restorations. I remember Leacock lighting his pipe, and solemnly saying, with the burnt match in his hand, "Here, Andrew, hadn't you better put this out?"[89]

Leacock himself believed Macphail to be "one of the most distinctive personalities I have ever known."[90]

5

National Figure

Andrew Macphail entered the world of Canadian political and social commentary with considerable force. His first articles on contemporary themes appeared in 1907, and by the end of 1909, with the publication of his collection *Essays in Politics*, he had gained a remarkable reputation in Canada and Great Britain, and some notoriety in the United States. The warmth of his reception was owing not only to the eminence of the forum he was building for himself in the *University Magazine* but also to the vigour, wit, clarity, and topicality of his writing. He articulated his interpretation of imperialism as a familial sentiment and sharply differentiated it from the contemporary emphasis on trading arrangements. While strongly endorsing the British diplomatic record with regard to British North America and affirming the essential wisdom of British institutions, Macphail presented a biting critique of early twentieth-century British society. In the process of dealing with the imperial question, he outlined what he considered to be distinctive and positive in Canada, the dangers facing the way of life to which he was attached, and his objections to the proposal that Canada follow the American path and dissolve the imperial tie. But Macphail's social views were not fully articulated at this time, for they were usually refracted through the prism of imperialism. It was only in later years that he filled in the details and added the coloration necessary to complete his portrait of the good society – the vision animating all his social and political commentary.

DEBUT: CANADA AND ENGLAND

The first two essays Macphail contributed to his rejuvenated journal were not central to his political and social thought. "John Knox in the Church of England" concerned a topic of continuing interest to him: the evangelical

Protestant tradition and in particular its Scottish manifestation.[1] "A Patent Anomaly," which appeared under the pseudonym Angus Macfadyen, focused on Canadian legislation with regard to patents and inventions.[2]

The publication of "Loyalty – To What" in the April 1907 number of the *University Magazine* represented Macphail's real debut as a political and social critic. It was the third of three articles devoted to the imperial theme, following Principal William Peterson's essay on the background and function of the imperial conference to be held in London from 15 April to 14 May, and Stephen Leacock's impassioned plea in "Greater Canada: An Appeal" for a wider, imperial conception of Canadian citizenship.

Macphail commenced his article by pointing out that on the basis of Canada's historical record there was little cause for rational concern about Canadian loyalty, which was no more to be doubted than that of Devonshire. He affirmed that Canadians were loyal to the monarch in a personal sense and were convinced of the wisdom of the British constitution and the imperial tie. But loyalty, he asserted, was like any other virtue:

> If pushed beyond the bounds of reason a virtue becomes a vice …
> Its value depends upon the ideals to which one is loyal, and the
> motives by which one is actuated.
>
> This utilitarian view of loyalty is the one which has always been
> adopted by the English people. Ever since the great events which
> happened at Runnymede, they have felt at liberty to choose whom
> they would serve. On Bosworth field, again, they had an open mind.
> They taught Charles the First the valuable lesson that a king has a
> bone in his neck …
>
> Loyalty, then, it would appear, has always been to the people of
> England a virtue or a vice, according to the circumstances of the
> case … To us in these days it appears that the loyalty of the mass of
> Russians to their "Little Father" is the cause of the unsatisfactory
> conditions which prevail in their country. In short, the lesson of
> history is that the breaking with a tradition, if it become outworn, is
> the price of progress and the safeguard against decay.[3]

These reflections were prompted by the insights arising out of at least four trips to Britain since 1891. Despite certain reservations about London and its populace, Macphail's initial impressions had been overwhelmingly favourable. He now sharpened his comments about the social extremes, condemning on the one hand "the squalor … and the brutality of the idle poor" and on the other "the inanity ... [and] the wickedness of the idle rich." The lifestyle of the latter and the growing appetite of the literate public for vulgarity were daily illustrated by the British newspapers, "giving in all their hideous details the filthiest reports of the proceedings of any divorce court in the world."[4]

Beyond these general criticisms directed at the state of British society, Macphail displayed distaste for both houses of Parliament. The Commons contained "a certain number of members whose function is to obstruct legislation, a certain number who have spent a term in prison, and ... at least one member was elected who was afterwards convicted of high treason. To ask Canadians to be unceasingly, and unreasoningly, and for ever loyal to that, is expecting too much."[5] The supremacy of such a Commons, which included fifty socialists, gave Macphail concern, especially as that body could "do evil"[6] to Canada as well as to Britain. The House of Lords he perceived as a decrepit, anachronistic institution whose political course was erratic. Sometimes the Lords appeared to act on conservative principles, sometimes out of fear of the Commons, and yet other times in the complacent belief that the power of the lower house would not be mobilized against them. A consistently progressive or reactionary upper house would be preferable, asserted Macphail. Furthermore, it "would minister to our self-respect if the House of Lords were no longer a recruiting ground for theatrical managers and the wives of American millionaires."[7]

Macphail insisted that these criticisms did not signify disloyalty to the principles of the British constitution. They were not to be interpreted as evidence that Canadians were about to join the United States or as a device for extorting trading privileges from the mother country in return for continued adherence to the empire. Like the English people in 1215, 1485, and 1649, Canadian critics were displaying "loyalty to a principle at cost of disloyalty to their Government ... The English people never committed the unspeakable treachery of disloyalty for material gain. Neither shall we."[8]

Macphail went on to deplore the way in which loyalty in Canada had become identified in the popular mind with the material interests of a particular class:

It may be because they have the facilities for making themselves heard. They have their associations, their paid secretaries, their publicity bureaus, their cable service for disseminating their views. It is they who have propagated the theory that the loyalty of Canada depends upon the benefits which they receive. They have

created a tariff as high as the country will stand. They have made it
a little higher against all the world except England, and call that a
preference, reserving to themselves the right to give equal preference
in any other quarter. Not content with free entry of their own goods
into England, they demand that the entry of goods from other
countries shall be put under an imposition.[9] If, they say, this is not
done, Canada will become disloyal, and either seek refuge with the
United States, or set up in "business" on her own account. Canada
will do nothing of the kind. If her loyalty depends upon commercial
gain, the sooner England bids her go in peace the better.[10]

Believing there was a connection between the social malaise he detected in
England and the dominance of industry over agriculture, he stated that a
"nation which is only a trading and manufacturing nation – and England
is nearly that – does not survive forever." Her ability and will to defend her
freedom were being eroded by obsession with commerce. "Traders do not
fight, they compromise … They only fight well who fight for their homes.
England has lost touch with the land, and can rejuvenate herself only by
contact with the land again."[11]

England's renewed contact with the land would come through absorp-
tion of her surplus population by Canada, Macphail maintained. He
believed such a flow of people possible because he shared the common
imperialist assumption that Canada's future was virtually limitless. Within
the lifespan of some of his own generation, he expected her population
to surpass that of England. Thus his concept of imperial loyalty was not
rooted in any sense of colonial inferiority or subservience, but in a vision of
Canada as a great and powerful nation, and in a feeling that the Canadian
role was to assist the mother country by uplifting her and returning her to
"the ancient 'truth, pity, freedom, and hardiness' of the race."[12] This was not
the imperialism of the transplanted Englishman but of the native Canadian
of British extraction who, upon visiting the mother country, had come to
the conclusion that all was not well in the land of his ancestors and that his
kin at home had strayed from "the ancient virtue of the race."[13]

"Loyalty – To What" was one of Macphail's most powerful articles, and it
indicated several themes he was to develop in later writings: Canada's prospective role in the salvation of England, revulsion at the social polarities
of industrial society, and outright rejection of material benefits as adequate
justification for the imperial tie. His second essay on Canada and imperialism appeared in October 1907, and in contrast to "Loyalty – To What" it

emphasized the mother country's positive role in Canada's development.

"The Patience of England" was the opening shot in an ongoing assault on the widely held contemporary opinion that British diplomats had not been mindful of Canadian interests when dealing with the United States. For example, the lawyer Thomas Hodgins was a prolific author who had written on British-American diplomacy as it affected Canada and had promoted this point of view, which enjoyed increased currency after the Alaska Boundary Award of 1903. The logical inference to be drawn from such an interpretation of British-American diplomacy was that it would be to Canada's benefit to enlarge her autonomy in matters of external affairs.[14] This autonomist tendency of course flew in the face of the imperialist desire to maintain the diplomatic unity of the British Empire.

Canadian imperialists responded to the challenge in a number of ways, such as founding the Empire Club of Canada to provide a forum with an emphasis different from that of the Canadian Club.[15] Macphail and the group around the *University Magazine*, for their part, decided that if the basis of the autonomist case lay in an appeal to history, they must frame a reply in similar terms. Accordingly, Macphail arranged to have James White, chief geographer of the Canadian Department of the Interior, and Duncan MacArthur of the Public Archives of Canada write a series of four articles on the Ashburton Treaty, the Alaska Boundary Award, and the Oregon and San Juan boundaries, which appeared in 1907 and 1908; two of White's three articles were published anonymously.[16] Macphail himself produced introductory and concluding essays in 1907 and 1909, and all six contributions were revisionist in the sense that they had pro-imperialist implications.

In "The Patience of England," Macphail stated that the "quality above all others which impresses the foreign mind when it reflects upon England, is her infinite patience with her own."[17] Since Canada was now a mature nation, he suggested that it was time to take stock of what England had done for her. He briefly reviewed the various crises that had developed involving Britain, the United States, and British North America, and came to the conclusion that in every instance the British course of action had been essentially correct. For example, in 1866, when the Fenians had invaded Canada from the south, Britain's response had been restrained, and rightly so, because a more dramatic gesture would only have served the interests of those south of the border who desired to use a foreign war to reunite the American north and south. "This was the moment for reticence, for patience."[18] If the mother country had appeared somewhat neglectful at the time of the Alaska Boundary Dispute, it was because she "was fighting for her life in South Africa, whilst the vultures hovered in the European sky."[19] In short, when Canadian interests had not been fully pressed it was because Britain had responsibilities elsewhere as well – and, as Macphail pointedly noted, a Canadian statesman of Sir Wilfrid Laurier's acumen had trouble enough with Orangemen and Ultramontanes, and the Manitoba Schools Question, let alone having to cope with Hindus, Moslems, Europeans, and North Americans at the same time. Taking these considerations into account, Macphail was able to give unreserved praise to British policy over the years, the crowning glory of which had been the forbearance displayed by Governor General Lord Elgin in 1849, when an angry mob, protesting the Rebellion Losses Bill, had burned the Parliament Buildings in Montreal.[20]

At the end of the series, Macphail published a recapitulation of the lessons to be drawn. It was a sizable essay, three times the length of "The Patience of England," and he began by explicitly stating the purpose of the articles: "To remove a false impression from the public mind, and … to replace it by a correct one."[21] Incorrect ideas were circulating even in high places – such as the prime minister's office – and in Macphail's view intellectuals with access to the results of scholarly research published in obscure learned journals had an obligation to participate in the popular diffusion of contradictory evidence.[22] Deploying elaborate detail, evidently based on extensive and careful reading, he defended British statesmanship particularly with regard to the Pacific Coast, the Maine boundary, and the negotiation of the Reciprocity Treaty of 1854. British diplomats had displayed cunning in exploiting European great-power conflicts, persistence in presenting claims year after year, charm in winning over recalcitrant Americans, firmness in making the best of a weak *de jure* and *de facto* case, and even disingenuousness in allowing a certain embarrassing map to "disappear" at the opportune moment.[23] Thus, at the cost of virtually no bloodshed over a period of three generations, Canada's territorial integrity had been maintained in the face of a powerful and aggressive neighbour. Macphail broadly hinted that he doubted whether Canadian diplomats could have done as well.[24]

Another contribution by White, in 1910 (when he was also secretary of the Canadian Conservation Commission), and Macphail's treatment of it illustrate the point that being a Canadian imperialist did not imply supineness in the face of British priorities. Writing anonymously again in the *University Magazine*, White condemned a proposal by American capitalists to construct a dam at the Long Sault Rapids, using a vivid metaphor: "If any part of these rapids is bonded over to a private or alien corporation, the Government will then have to deal with vested interests protected by a foreign power, which will have its hands on the throat of the St. Lawrence."[25] Without mentioning White's name, Macphail sent the proofs of his article to Laurier, strongly endorsing White's views; the scheme had so outraged him that he had told Archibald MacMechan that if no one else wrote on the subject for the *University Magazine*, he would do so himself. This was another occasion on which Earl Grey and the *University Magazine* disagreed on policy.[26] The imperial government had entered a period of attempting to strengthen links with the United States, and it tended to believe that local British North American objections to American claims or projects, whether regarding the so-called American shore in Newfoundland or the Long Sault in Canada, were potential irritants that should be removed in the interests of promoting Anglo-American harmony. Macphail and White did not want to see legitimate Canadian points of view overlooked in this attempt.

It is impossible to assess precisely the effectiveness of the *University Magazine* in fostering Canadian appreciation of the accomplishments of British diplomacy. Certainly, Grey was gratified by the new public recognition that British efforts were receiving, and his pleasure was shared by such prominent Englishmen as James Bryce, Lord Northcliffe, John St Loe Strachey of the *Spectator*, L.S. Amery of the *Times*, and the Earl of Crewe, the colonial secretary in 1909.[27] Strachey went to the point of publishing in the *Spectator* a note warmly commending Macphail's efforts. This provoked a letter from Thomas Hodgins, who demanded space for what Strachey described as "an enormously long and vehement protest against Macphail" which he "could not find space for."[28] Hodgins had also prepared articles for the *University Magazine* in response to its series, but he and Macphail were unable to agree on alterations and an appropriate schedule for publication.[29]

In Canada, the *Review of Historical Publications Relating to Canada* gave predominantly favourable notice to the series as it appeared, particularly praising the article signed by White and Macphail's concluding essay.[30] But the journal, edited by George M. Wrong and H.H. Langton of the University of Toronto, was precisely the sort of learned publication to which Macphail had complained that "correct opinions" were usually confined.[31] A more important question, given the objectives of the authors, is whether the pro-imperialist interpretation took the course predicted by Amery in "gradually percolat[ing] through the more intelligent readers into the daily papers and eventually into the minds of the public at large and oust[ing] prevailing misconceptions."[32] By 1909 Grey was writing – with his customary tendency to overstatement, if not wishful thinking – that "in future anyone who takes up this attitude [that Britain had repeatedly sacrificed Canadian interests] will proclaim himself an ignoramus or a knave."[33]

Although Macphail believed his series had put the question to rest at a scholarly level, it is unlikely that he would have advanced such extravagant claims as Grey for his achievements in public education. Canadian commentators, much more frequently than Britishers, confined their praise to the *University Magazine*'s literary and intellectual qualities, and expressed reservations about its doctrines. For example, in a press cutting Macphail kept, the Montreal *Gazette*, while carefully avoiding condemnation of the editor's desire to do justice to the British record, proclaimed itself unconvinced and pointedly brought the works of Hodgins and John S. Ewart, a lawyer and publicist strongly committed to Canadian independence, to the attention of its readers. The *University Magazine*, which in 1909 had not reached its peak in circulation, was probably sent out to some 3,000 or 4,000 subscribers, and Macphail recognized that he and his collaborators were attempting to do in two and one-half years a work of propaganda requiring a lengthy period of reiteration.[34] Within a few years Canada would be immersed in the First World War, and "old world diplomacy" would be discredited for a generation.

Macphail's third and final article in 1907 was entitled "What Can Canada Do," and he addressed himself to the problem of how Canada could best discharge her imperial responsibilities. He began by providing an overview of Canadian history for those who believed Canadians to be delinquent members of the empire:

These two centuries past, [we were] making a living as best we
might, defending our little clearings against wild beasts, our homes
against savages, and our little towns against marauders from the
United States ... It has taken five generations to raise the mortgage
from the place, and it is only now that we can send our sons to
the university without sacrificing the lives of those who remain at
home. We have had our own bitterness and sorrow. It is in these
that values are reckoned, in broken hearts, in bowed backs, and
knotted hands.
In those days England was far away and we were alone.[35]

Canada was still a comparatively new country in the first decade of the twentieth century, and the overhead for a nation of her size was enormous. With the help of James Mavor, Macphail calculated that a Canadian paid considerably higher taxes than his counterpart in Britain.[36]

After defending Canada's past record in this way, Macphail turned to the two proposals most frequently advanced for the more equitable sharing of imperial burdens: naval contributions and tariff preferences. He dismissed the suggestion that Canada should give Britain a battleship every year, for such ships would soon become the plaything of Canada's parochial politicians. "No battleship would be tolerable to us which could not safely navigate the Lachine Canal on its way to share in the festivities attendant upon the opening of the Toronto Exhibition."[37] Canada would be sufficiently occupied in providing defences for her own extended frontiers and coasts. As for an imperial preference, Macphail argued that the main benefit of the limited measure already in effect had accrued to Canadian consumers rather than to Britain as a whole – although it had aided certain British manufacturers. In any event, Britain had no need for economic favours from Canada. According to statistics he marshalled, British exports, standard of living, personal wealth, and income had been steadily rising over the past generation.[38]

Having disposed of naval contributions and trade preferences, Macphail proceeded to develop a theme he had touched on in "Loyalty – To What." He believed that there was "something further which Canada can do," thereby helping both herself and England.

> We need men, and England needs to be rid of a large part of her population. The trouble with the England of to-day is that the people – at least twelve millions of them – are half-employed, half-paid, and half-fed ... We could employ these millions profitably, but such an exodus would necessitate some alteration in the habits of the people who remain at home ... Englishmen would be obliged ... to do for themselves what is now done for them by big footmen and other indolent servants.
>
> One person out of ten in England is partially or wholly a pauper.[39]

In an uncharacteristically ruthless statement, he declared, "We will make men of them, or demonstrate that there is nothing in them of which men can be made ... If a man will not work [in Canada], neither shall he eat. January will attend to the rest."[40] Massive immigration would thus be of spiritual benefit both to those who stayed in England, whose daily habits would be purified, and those who came to Canada, who would experience a new, more wholesome way of life. Out of such a service to the mother country and her people would grow "a mutual trust and affection, which must precede any final constructive policy, either economic or constitutional."[41]

Thus, by the end of 1907 Macphail had sketched the broad outlines of his imperial perspective. With the new year he turned his attention to Canada. In January, with the Greys in attendance, he addressed the May Court Club of Ottawa on "The Dominion and the Spirit";[42] in February he published an essay of the same title in the *University Magazine*; and on 26 March he lectured to the Canadian Club of Saint John, New Brunswick, on "The Whole Duty of the Canadian Man."[43] He began by taking the broadest theme he had yet applied to contemporary affairs – the spirit that should actuate the nation in its daily work. This work might be the growing of wheat:

> It is of some importance that we should make wheat to grow. The thing which is of more importance is that we should have a right reason for undertaking that labour, and a right spirit in the doing of it. The man who makes two blades of wheat to grow where only one grew before, for the mere purpose of providing unnecessary food, is working with the spirit and motive of a servant – of a slave even … This "work for work's sake" is entirely modern; and our present civilisation is the only one which has ever been established upon that principle … With all our talk about freedom, we have only succeeded in enslaving ourselves. We have created for ourselves a huge treadmill; and, if we do not keep pace, we fall beneath its wheels. Our inventions have only added to the perplexities of life. We have created artificial necessities, and consume our lives in ministering to them.[44]

The "modern" approach to work was different from that of the ancient Greeks, who had held labour in disdain, and that of the artist, who did his work because he enjoyed it. The Canadian working in an office lived for those times when

> he is free – to do what? To escape to his little workshop or garden. The thing that keeps us in heart at our tasks during the long winter … is the hope that we may … escape to our little farms, our woods, and streams, forgetful that it is within our reach to spend the whole year in doing the things which we love to do. There is but one

free man in the world – he who creates out of the earth. If workers
work for the love of the thing, then is constituted the class of artists –
whether they work in the earth, in stone, in wood, with colours, with
sounds, or with words.[45]

For these artists-workers, there would be little distinction between work
time, in its ordinary sense, and leisure time.

Macphail proceeded to deal with the class he identified as "traders ...
whether it be composed of tradesmen exchanging their time, merchants
trading their wares, or professors trading their knowledge – for money."[46]
Modern Germany provided an example of what rule by such men could do
to a country. A generation earlier the world had looked to that nation for
leadership in ideas. "Forty years of the commercial ideal has made of the
Germans the tinkers of Europe, the bagmen of the world ... German science and learning have surrendered themselves to immediate necessity."[47]
Possessed of the spirit of Germany, Joseph Chamberlain had declared in
1896 that "Empire is Commerce."[48] Macphail warmly challenged this equation and catalogued the principles for which the great empires of the past
had been built. According to him, not one had been assembled for the
sake of money, and indeed Holland had declined in greatness as her commerce had increased in volume. Close to home, Macphail cited statistics
to show that while the British Empire had grown enormously in territory
and population between 1883 and 1897, exports had declined in both absolute and per capita terms.[49]

Despite his denial that material motives were guiding forces in British
history, Macphail was not so sanguine about the contemporary reality. He
described the voice of the trading class as "the dominant one in Canada
and in all parts of the Empire to which we belong."[50] He even declared
the history of modern civilization to be the story of how the ethic of the
trader had "led to the corruption of public life and to personal misery, to
the political lobby and the social slum."[51] Thus, the trader's business was of
concern to more than the economist and the trader himself; it had debased
the quality of political, social, and personal life.

In the face of this cheapening and homogenizing threat, Macphail
declared, "We in Canada have the opportunity of making a new experiment. We have not entirely abandoned ourselves to the dominion of work
and the desire for money."[52] Canadians were essentially a rural people,
although for the past generation they had been turning away from the
countryside. He conceded rural life to be mere existence as long as it was

lived in poverty. But things had changed on the farm, and comfortless existence was no longer the order of the day. Indeed, the question was now
whether the farmer would succumb to the temptation of planting his additional grain of wheat for any reason other than enjoyment. At stake was
whether "we would save our soul alive, [whether] we are to have any meaning in history."[53]

Rural people were distinguished by the healthy interest they took in the
affairs of their neighbours. In a sense, a rural community was an enlarged
family, and in Macphail's view national life was "merely the sum of family
life."[54] Hence it was an easy step for him to portray his proposal that "we
should make of Canada a refuge for all within the Empire who are in distress, for the unemployed, for the discouraged"[55] as the logical extension
of his desire for the development of a distinctive Canadian identity. His
immigration policy would "purify and enrich the race."[56] At the same time,
native Canadians should strive to "keep our spirit right and our heart from
rotting with luxury or with poverty."[57] The alternative to regeneration was
a world dominated by those "twin sisters ... the factory and the slum," he
asserted. "If these continue to be our ideal of achievement, then, having
achieved nothing but slum and factory, no one will ask who or what we
have been – 'More than he asks what waves / Of the midmost ocean have
swell'd, / Foam'd for a moment, and gone.'"[58]

"The Dominion and the Spirit" was one of the richest and most suggestive of Macphail's early essays. Not only was he applying his critical powers
to the Canadian reality, but he was sketching in broad outline the basic
social and moral assumptions underlying his troubled diagnosis of the
state of the empire. Yet in 1908 he was hopeful as well as worried, and thus
there was reason to speak publicly of "The Whole Duty of the Canadian
Man." Macphail believed that at Canada's stage in its development the
most urgent responsibility of citizens was to assist in governing. He denied
that there were special mysteries involved in public life, comprehensible
only to those who had taken politics as a vocation. To refrain from openly
taking positions on public issues for fear of offending those in power was
to play the sycophant or slave: "The obligation of expressing our opinions
publicly is at the basis of all free government ... The Government has done
its duty when it acts upon the opinion which it hears. If one section of the
community is dumb and another is vociferous the government must not
be blamed if it assumes that only those have opinions who are willing to
express them."[59]

Making his argument more specific, Macphail stated that almost three-quarters of Canadians lived on or near farms. These people, he said, would benefit from lower prices. Yet a minority resident in cities determined the tariff policy of Canada, with dire consequences for the cost of living of all Canadians. Armed with calculations made by Mavor, Macphail claimed that Canada was the world's most expensive country in which to live, and Montreal the most expensive city. Over the previous ten years commodity prices had increased 67 percent and the cost of living some 40 percent. Wages had risen almost as rapidly as prices, but "those who have no commodities to sell and do not earn wages, are beginning to find their situation intolerable."[60] Macphail was referring to the plight of the professional middle class, to which he and his medical and academic colleagues belonged. The interests of these people, like those of the farmers, lay in lower tariffs. "But we never say so."[61] Macphail analysed the current situation as government by and for an interested minority, and as taxation without representation: "The Manufacturers Association appears to think that the taxing power lies with them and I do not think we are all represented in their Councils."[62] At times, he said, he felt that "imperialism," a derivative of the Roman word *imperium*, meaning "a centralized sovereignty and an acquiescent tax-paying dependency"[63] – was an unfortunate word for what he advocated; yet taking a realistic look around him, he was not so sure that it was inappropriate.[64]

In his address Macphail repeated much he had already written in the *University Magazine* about such matters as British diplomacy, naval contributions, the nature of the imperial bond, and the relationship of factory and slum.[65] All these concerned the civic duty of the Canadian. At a higher level was his duty to God, a subject Macphail would leave for the present to clergy. His most interesting and revealing comments concerned the family, a level of obligation he described as being second only to the religious. "In all civilized societies," he declared, "the family is the unit."[66]

> Originally each family was more or less self-contained and mutually supporting. The man procured food from the forest or from the soil, and was aided in these occupations by his boys who became competent at a very early age. The woman dressed the skins, and made them into garments, and prepared the food for eating …
>
> At an early age the girl too, was initiated into these mysteries. She was self-supporting from her childhood; and, indeed, added to

the wealth and comfort of the family. The child, instead of being
a burden, was an asset …

Into this community of families comes the manufacturer
with his machinery and his love of money and his formulas
about efficiency, saving of labour, industrial progress and
commercial development. Every turn of his wheels disintegrates
the family by destroying the multifarious occupations of every
member of it … The country has grown rich but the family is
destroyed …

The care of the offspring has been handed over to male and
female hirelings – physicians and nurses – and thus a wide
outlet for the physical and mental activity of the woman has
been effectually stopped. Deprived of the care of her children
the woman has suffered a diminution of her affection and it
has been replaced by a noisy sentimentalism which is equally
disastrous for mother and child.[67]

The lesson to be drawn was clear: "We have failed, and must fail worse
according as we turn away from the ideal of the rural life." It was only in
the countryside that the family flourished, and Macphail was certain that
the well-governed and usefully occupied family was the basis for all good
government, whether at the level of school district, parish, or nation. The
better the family was governed, the less government would be required
at other levels. In ancient Greece, the only sense of public duty had been
to the city, and at that time local patriotism had been sufficient. "But
with us our means of communication have become so rapid that neither
family or [sic] city can live to itself, and we require a larger polity."[68] It was
with this new, more complex society, bursting with anarchic energy, that
Canadian "man," often from such a background as sketched by Macphail,
had to come to terms.

Macphail in his Saint John address took his critique of modern civilization a step beyond pointing to a rather vague "trading spirit" as the cause
of the malaise. Now the embodiment of the enemy became the manufacturer, who was perverting the British ideal of self-government and destroying the very basis of civilization, the family. With this wide-ranging lecture, Macphail had begun for the first time to reveal the positive vision
forming the basis for his social criticism.

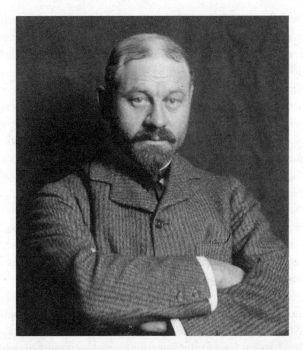

Andrew Macphail. This photograph is part of a set taken of Pen and Pencil Club members; the date is unknown. Macphail appears to be in his middle or late forties. If so, he was editor of both the *University Magazine* and either the *Montreal Medical Journal* or the *Canadian Medical Association Journal* at the time.

THE "AMERICAN WOMAN"

With the composition of "The 'American Woman'" later in the spring of 1908, Macphail enlarged upon the central themes in his Saint John address. He had made direct contact with Strachey through the agency of Grey, who appears to have been a close friend of the editor and when in Canada rented his London house to him. Macphail seems to have requested the intercession of Strachey with the editors of the *National Review* or the *Nineteenth Century*. But in reply, Strachey asked Macphail to reduce the article in length, divide it into two sections, and submit it to the *Spectator*, signed, under "Correspondence." This, he took pains to emphasize, was the journal's form of signed article and not the equivalent of a letter to the editor. Given the controversial nature of the essay, he expected a great deal of criticism but was willing to risk it "as I think on the whole your view is right," he told Macphail. "I may say that we almost never publish articles in two divisions and I only suggest this now because I am so very much struck by the ability of the article."[69]

Macphail accepted the suggestion, since the *Spectator* under Strachey's guidance had become London's leading weekly and was "perhaps the only weekly taken seriously throughout Great Britain, and in the United States."[70] No doubt he was also influenced by the fact that he had been reading the *Spectator* for many years – thirty years, he told Grey, which, if accurate, indicates that he had had been reading it as a student at Prince of Wales College.[71] He began the first section by explaining that by the "American Woman" he meant a social type not confined to the United States and not including most American women. The defining characteristic was that the woman lived in "luxurious idleness"[72] as a result of the ongoing destruction of the family and the pre-emption of its everyday functions by industrialism. He claimed that in his choice of a title he was only reflecting a contemporary literary convention that identified most wayward heroines in novels as American women or offspring of American women. Yet the sensitive American reader could be forgiven for suspecting that something more lurked behind his use of the term, for in focusing on such indicators as rising divorce rates and falling birth rates, Macphail employed a wealth of American examples.[73]

The articles consisted of a dissection of the social mores, taste, and personal conduct of the woman removed from her "natural" role within the family. Beginning with the proposition that "an organ, an animal, or a species cannot exist independently of its function," he observed that all the "primitive functions" of modern woman except one, childbearing, had been "usurped."[74] Deprived of her proper role and condemned to idleness and restlessness, the woman was led to seek a new identity outside the home. To Macphail, the world beyond the family was the natural domain of man, and for a woman to adapt to it would mean taking on the characteristics of a man, with a consequent loss of authenticity. The result would be a diminution of those qualities – gentleness, deference, and quietness – which constituted the only effective basis for her influence: feminine charm. This charm was not the result of "excessive talkativeness, nor that distortion of the countenance in public places which is called laughter. Not intellectual attainment nor the artistic temperament ensures its possession." Rather, it was found in the woman who "suffers long and is kind, who envieth not, who vaunteth not herself and is not puffed up, who doth

not behave herself unseemly, who seeketh not her own, is not easily provoked, who thinketh no evil, beareth all things, and believeth all things."[75]

Thus Macphail's lengthy essay on modern woman revealed how deeply
he considered the effects of industrialization to have penetrated daily life.
The personality of the woman was being distorted beyond recognition,
for the domestic tasks in which her basic nature would find fulfilment
were being taken outside the family. The woman was the primary victim
of the attendant unhappiness, and Macphail acknowledged that the forces
behind this transformation were not of her making. Indeed, they were
directed by men. In a later, expanded version of the article, he wrote that
the "Greek attitude ... is in the main correct: whatever the woman is or
does, is the fault of the man."[76]

"The 'American Woman'" was an extension of the analysis Macphail had
offered in his Saint John address.[77] When the articles appeared, they were
accompanied by an editorial note dissociating the *Spectator* from some of
his statements. While describing Macphail's first article as "so vivid, so suggestive, and so incisive in style, and ... in so many particulars so timely and
so wholesome," Strachey took public exception to Macphail's suggestion
that the traditional duties of women constituted their only proper role –
"a view as erroneous as it is conventional."[78] On the following Saturday, in
a reply to a letter protesting Macphail's first article, he felt compelled to
reiterate his belief that Macphail was guilty of "occasional exaggerations
and injustice," and that his views on the low birth rate of American women
were "now and then much too strongly expressed." Nonetheless, Strachey
agreed that the propagation of the species was "the main function of the
woman in the world."[79]

The publication of the articles was delayed until October, partially
because of the controversy they caused at the journal's office and partially
because of Strachey's desire to leave them until after his holidays so that
he would be present to deal with readers' responses. In late November he
wrote to Macphail, "You will be interested to hear that we have been del-
uged with violent letters of protest from old readers of the 'Spectator' in
regard to your Letters. Plenty of them tell us they have read the 'Spectator'
for thirty years but will never read another copy." In the same letter, he confided to Macphail that he had come to have second thoughts about the
identification of the type as the "American Woman."[80]

The appearance of "The 'American Woman'" articles in the *Spectator*
brought Macphail substantial international attention. From the United
States alone he received more than a hundred columns of commentary,

"most of it absurd."[81] It was one of the more controversial essays to appear in the influential but rather staid *Spectator* of the early 1900s, and it undoubtedly made a considerable impression on Strachey. He wrote to Grey, "I am glad I published the articles and I believe they did good in America as well as here ... Macphail strikes me as a man of great ability and with a real mastery of style ... I cannot help thinking that he is destined to make a real mark as a publicist." Yet Strachey feared that Macphail occasionally let "his love for a telling sentence lead him a little too far."[82] He asked the governor general for information about his new contributor; the indefatigable Grey met the request and promptly sent Strachey's letter, marked "confidential," to Macphail.[83]

It is apparent from Macphail's correspondence with Grey and Strachey that he greatly valued the favourable opinion of the editor of the *Spectator*. Despite his critical comments on the state of British society, he sought to meet British standards and attain British recognition. The mother country was still the centre of his intellectual universe, and in this he was not alone. Certainly, his prominent appearance in the *Spectator* enhanced his reputation among Canadians. R. Tait McKenzie – who had been his roommate in his student days at McGill and was now a physician building a distinguished career as a sculptor and as a pioneer in physical education at the University of Pennsylvania – wrote, "This will be your formal entry upon the world's stage as an essayist, and I congratulate you."[84]

Indeed, "The 'American Woman'" did mark a turning point in terms of the exposure Macphail's views received. By early 1909, Strachey was soliciting an article on Canadian trade policy. He had probably seen two articles by Macphail in the *University Magazine* of the previous year focusing on the Canadian tariff: "Protection and Politics," in the April number, and "Why the Conservatives Failed," in December. If so, there can be no doubt that Strachey would have found them congenial, for he described himself as a free trader "by religion."[85]

PROTECTIONISM AND AMERICAN INSTITUTIONS

"Protection and Politics" emerged in the wake of the financial crisis of 1907 and dealt with the origins and consequences of protective tariffs in the modern world. Adducing data from German, French, American, and Canadian history, Macphail contended "that Protection is a political device, that at times it may be a valuable weapon of defence, rarely a commercial necessity, and not often an advantage to the community as a whole."[86]

Protection had been adopted in the United States in order to exert political pressure; in Germany, to consolidate the political support of agrarian interests; in France, to reinforce national distinctiveness; and in Canada, to resist political pressure from the outside. In his version of the Canadian case, Macphail liked to leap directly from the abrogation of Reciprocity in 1866 by the United States (partially for annexationist reasons) to the adoption of the National Policy tariff of 1879.[87] Although, he argued, a protective policy could serve a legitimate national purpose, its source lay in historical circumstances, not in the recognition of a principle of eternal validity.

The origins of protection might be political, but its consequences were also economic and moral. Protection had always involved the collusion of an interested class, since it "restrains competition and so saves the trader alive."[88] Prices were no longer established by market forces; trusts were organized, and "price stability" (on the seller's terms) became the order of the day. As a result, the panic of 1893 had not been accompanied by an immediate decline in prices, and following the panic of 1907 the prices of many consumer goods had in fact risen dramatically. Hence the professional middle class with its fixed incomes, already staggering under the blows of inflation in times of prosperity, was finding that downward trends in the business cycle no longer afforded relief. But the professional men were "the most dangerous to the settled order of things ... [for they had] the habit of exercising their minds, of forming opinions, and arriving at conclusions."[89]

Although Macphail maintained a certain detachment in tone when dealing with the origins and economic results of protection, he was scathing in his denunciation of the political and moral consequences. Protection had always been implemented with the expectant aid of an interested class. Eventually, to ensure the continuation of their favours, this class would build a "machine" to provide political security for their benefactors. In the United States, where the average rate of duties was 19 percent, the Republicans had been in power for forty of the past forty-eight years; in Canada, with a rate of 16 percent, there had been three governmental changes in forty-one years of national existence; in England, where the rate was 5 percent, there had been nine such changes over the same period. Beyond political stagnation lay other dangers. Macphail was certain that every nation required an aristocracy of some sort. Protection created an aristocracy of wealth, composed of "merchant princes," "copper kings," and "iron magnates," whose public behaviour gave "a glamour to the criminal courts."[90] The deportment of this aristocracy and the standards of entry into it led Macphail to declare that moral issues were involved. Employing his strongest language to date, he denounced

> the ineffable blessings of Protection – legislators bought as one
> .would buy a drove of swine, men who have grown rich under
> Protection divorcing the wives of their poorer days and publicly
> consorting with harlots, their sons committing murder in public
> places with impunity. Corruption of public life, and the degradation
> of society to a condition of savagery, is – so runs the feeling –
> too high a price for the people to pay for the enrichment of an
> interested class.[91]

This moral content, he wrote, could well be the catalyst that would awaken the long-suffering Canadian public from its political slumber.[92].

A dominion general election was held on 26 October 1908, and Laurier won his fourth consecutive mandate. In December, with the widely acclaimed[93] essay, "Why the Conservatives Failed," Macphail attempted to explain the seeming confirmation of the status quo by Canadians. After subjecting Robert Borden's campaign to a detailed criticism, which included many shrewd and amusing observations on electoral politics, Macphail arrived at the heart of the matter:

> The Conservatives failed because their campaign was too picayune.
> The issues which they presented were too small. In reality there are
> only two questions which could vitally interest the country: whether
> it shall be handed over entirely to manufacturers for exploitation,
> and what arrangements shall be made by which Canada shall take
> her proper place in the Empire … There are now in Canada two
> pseudo-Conservative parties, both standing for the same privileges
> and for the interests of the same class. It is little wonder, then, that the
> voters neglected to exchange the one for the other.[94]

Borden had had nothing of substance to say on the imperial question, while Laurier was able at least to point to the British preference. Although Macphail rejected any suggestion that imperialism was primarily a trading relationship, he nonetheless took note of the fact that Laurier had not demanded favours from the British in return. He had acted in the spirit of family affection, which was the true basis of the bond; the preference itself, given unilaterally, was a material manifestation of that sentiment.

Macphail repeated his earlier opinion that the real beneficiaries of the preference were Canadian consumers. Therefore reform-minded electors could support the Liberals, "signifying, in a poor blind way, their allegiance to the principle of a freer trade."[95] Borden had declared in favour of protection for all Canadian industries, which had alarmed rather than reassured voters. "The country apparently is willing to endure the burden which it carries; it is in no temper to allow that burden to be increased."[96] Yet the Conservative leader's "oracular utterances" had suggested to the electors that his policy would do just that.[97]

Macphail concluded his essay with a highly critical review of the Conservative record over the previous two decades. In their fervour to send men to South Africa, they had stampeded the Liberals into precipitate action, which was contrary to the spirit of self-government. By opposing the Grand Trunk Pacific Railway, they had raised the suspicion that they really were in the pocket of the Canadian Pacific Railway. With their divisions over the Manitoba Schools Question and their failure to support the minority in the Autonomy crisis of 1905, they had deserted the tradition of Macdonald, whose "guiding principle … was the maintenance of good will between races and between the holders of creeds … To deprive any section of the community of its privileges is the exact reverse of the Conservative tradition."[98] To be successful in Canada, asserted Macphail, a party must "recognize frankly and absolutely that the rights of the French are exactly the same as the rights of the English … There must be no air of condescension or superiority, because politically all are equal."[99] His essay concluded with the statement that the Conservatives would continue to fail until they returned to conservative principles.

Early in 1909 Macphail made a brief but pointed contribution to the *American Review of Reviews* entitled "How Canada Looks at American Tariff-Making." He provided a short history of Canadian-American trading relations, informed his audience that Canadians were well aware of the growing American sentiment in favour of freer trade, and stated that many Canadians would welcome a mutual lowering of tariff barriers. But there was one reservation: "They will make no proposals, and they will have nothing to do with any proposals, which would put England at a disadvantage."[100]

Macphail provided Strachey, an ardent free trader and imperialist, with a précis of his *American Review of Reviews* article. Such sentiments, and those expressed in the two essays in the *University Magazine*, pleased Strachey, for he believed that "it is purely a delusion to think that Canada, because she

does very good business with the United States, will want to allow herself
to be absorbed by the Union. People are not governed by those reasons."[101]
He requested that Macphail compose for the *Spectator* an 800-word "Letter"
outlining his point of view.

In "A Canadian View of Reciprocity and Imperialism," Macphail reiterated his opinion that when Canadians came to adjust their commercial
relations, they would refuse to sacrifice British interests. Thus there was
no prospect of their entering into exclusive reciprocal agreements with
the United States. The British preference was inviolable partly for senti-
mental and patriotic reasons but also because of what Macphail termed
"the lesson of 1866." Economic dependence on the United States at that
time had meant considerable disruption when the Americans abrogated
the agreement. Yet Macphail believed that Canadian self-interest would
sooner or later lead to the decision to admit American goods at lower
rates. Such a move would in no way undermine Canada's relationship with
the empire. "The worst enemy of Canada is the man who declares that,
if we are permitted to trade with the United States or with Germany, we
shall become Americans or Germans."[102] It is little wonder that Strachey
declared the article to be "excellent."[103]

In his *Spectator* "Letter," Macphail had broadly hinted at reasons other
than considerations of *realpolitik* for Canadians to be wary of too close an
association with the United States. He virtually stated that the American
government was an instrument of the manufacturing class. Although
more and more Americans seemed to desire freer trade, "the rigidity of
their institutions protects the Government against public sentiment."[104]
The previous month, with the publication of "New Lamps for Old" in the
University Magazine, Macphail had focused his attention directly on the
American polity, its problems, and their origins.

The immediate stimulus for Macphail's reflections on the American
experience was the movement in Canada for autonomy from Britain. The
nautical metaphor "cutting the painter" (severing the rope attaching the
bow of a boat to a ship, thus separating the two vessels) was often used,
and Macphail proposed to examine what that had entailed for the United
States. By separating themselves from Britain and the guiding light of tradition, Americans had been forced to devise a paper constitution. The results
were there for all to see. Some institutions, such as the Electoral College,
were long since moribund. The practical working of the others was a standing caution to all who would attempt to mould political institutions to a
plan rather than let them develop in response to events.

With a President installed for four years, an executive chosen
arbitrarily, a senate elected, no one knows how though all suspect
how, and safely ensconced for a term of years, with a popular
assemblage reduced to the level of a debating society which is
powerless to do anything but talk, the people are helpless until their
moment of despotism comes around again. That is why there is no
public opinion in the United States and no political discussion in
their newspapers ... Argument does no good unless the conclusion
can be enforced.[105]

In contrast, traditional British institutions ensured that a government
"can be turned out at any moment."[106] American municipal government
was a public disgrace, but the proposed solution was worse: "to take [it]
out of the hands of the few citizens who do control it and to give it over
to 'Commissioners', men who in the Greek cities were called tyrants."[107]
Macphail concluded that there was "less government of the people by the
people in the United States than in any community of white men with
whose history [he was] acquainted."[108]

Although these evils, directly traceable to defects in American constitution making, were bad enough, there were still more. Institutions that were
imposed consciously and arbitrarily had their effect on social conduct.
When basic laws were so obviously man-made and not the outgrowth of
the wisdom of the ages, lawlessness was rampant. Macphail cited American
judges on the corruption of criminal and civil procedures, and provided
examples of lynch law being practised openly, even by public figures and in
some cases in retribution for exercising freedom of the press.[109]

The result was that "their best citizens"[110] were acknowledging the failure
of the experiment in life, liberty, and happiness. The lesson for Canadians
was clear:

A community which lays the axe to its communal roots may
continue to exist and even to increase in bulk. But it cannot possess
any real vitality until the wound is healed or until it send down new
roots into civilisation again ... Cut off from the stream of European
civilisation and from the institutions which the genius of our race
has created, and left to our own devices, we should certainly commit
acts of equal folly ... A people in much the same situation as ours,
though more numerous, wiser, and richer, have not, after a century
and a half of experiment, evolved a political condition which is

satisfactory to a sane man ... A nation must grow from the roots, and in this process of growth a thousand years are as one day. A nation crawls on its belly, slow as a glacier.[111]

Macphail did not pretend that the situation of Canadians in 1909 was fully satisfactory. They were, in his opinion, "living under the government of an interested class,"[112] but in contrast to Americans they had flexible British institutions at their disposal. Should the public become aroused – as they had not in 1908 – they had the means to make their indignation effective.

"New Lamps for Old" was a vigorous polemic defending the British connection and purporting to demonstrate the superiority of the ancestral institutions over their American counterparts. As such, it was accorded a warm reception by prominent Englishmen. Amery, Grey, Strachey, and Rudyard Kipling all expressed their agreement. Strachey considered the article "brilliant"[113] and commended Macphail for "the pluck and courage with which you speak out to your countrymen on all subjects."[114] Principal Peterson's only regret was that "it will appear just at a time when I was going to suggest an effort to increase our circulation in the United States!"[115]

ESSAYS IN POLITICS

In the late summer of 1909 Macphail published a collection of his papers entitled *Essays in Politics*. Nine of the ten contributions had previously appeared in the *University Magazine*. The other, receiving its first exposure, was a lengthy piece on "The Psychology of Canada." The purpose of the essay was to examine certain proposals for strengthening the imperial bond and "to make some observations upon the psychology of Canada, to show forth the working of the Canadian mind upon the great question of Imperialism."[116]

Macphail began by pointing out that caution in the pursuit of even the most laudable objectives was the essence and supreme lesson of the British political tradition. He then turned to the question of defence. "We cannot share in the glory of the Empire unless we share in its danger and, to put it bluntly, in the expense of it."[117] Although he still insisted that the capital expenditures involved in establishing Canada on a firm basis were sufficient excuse for her not having contributed in the past, he now believed that the country had entered a new stage of development. As a result, Canadians were at last able and willing to contribute to their own defence. But this would raise a host of political problems: not only would there

be internal Canadian issues to be resolved, but any new defence arrangements, particularly if they involved "contributions," would bring into question the constitution of the empire. Many thorny matters would have to be
dealt with, and Macphail confessed that he had no easy answers – he could
only point out the stumbling blocks.[118]

Macphail spoke with more finality on the proposal that the mother
country give Canada a "preference" in entering her markets. This would
simply be protection under another name, which was unacceptable. In
this essay, Macphail discoursed for the first time on the regional effects of
the National Policy. According to his calculations, the Maritime provinces
had lost some 218,000 people over the previous twenty years, and most of
them had gone to the United States. "These provinces," he wrote, "contain
a population of nearly a million persons, and they are the most intelligent
in Canada. They form a decaying community. They are intelligent enough
to be aware that a community must at times make sacrifices, but it is rarely
the duty of a community to perish supinely."[119] The "ultimate cause" of the
plight of the Maritimers was that they were being denied access to their
"natural markets."[120] But the danger of annexation was a thing of the past
and hence there was no longer a justification for an economic policy with
such dire social consequences.[121]

Macphail discerned a tendency towards freer trade in both the United
States and Canada. A lowering of American customs barriers within eighteen months "may be accepted as a fact."[122] In Canada the manufacturers
had been riding high for a generation or more. They "have claimed that
they were the people of Canada. The utmost of their claim now is that they
are the 'East' and that they have created the 'West.'"[123] But westerners as well
as Maritimers were coming to perceive their interests as opposed to those
of the manufacturers. The protectionists were also facing opposition on a
class level: organizations of Canadian farmers and workers had recently
declared in favour of freer trade. Thus if Britain adopted protection, she
would not only be exposing herself to public corruption and a higher cost
of living; she would be joining "a lost cause."[124]

Aside from these practical arguments against Britain's adoption of an
imperial preference as a means of cementing the empire, Macphail saw a
more basic issue. Contrary to Joseph Chamberlain's assertion, empire was
not simply commerce. Macphail did not object to material interest being
one of the pillars of imperialism; but imperialism was composed also "of
loyalty to a noble tradition, of affection for kinsmen who yet occupy the
old homes, of a wider patriotism, of a desire to be full partakers in the

glory of a remembrance of old achievements."[125] He argued that imperialism based on trade was at the mercy of the highest bidder, and that such
imperialism "appeals only to traders. We in Canada are not traders. We
are farmers; at least 62 percent of us live on or near the soil."[126] If imperialism continued to be identified in the public mind with protection, it
would share the eventual and inevitable fate of protection. Hence it was
important to understand that "Imperialism is in reality a way of looking
at things, a frame of mind, an affair of the spirit, a singleness of purpose
in making of the material at our command something new and good, by
a process of decentralisation and co-operation. It is born of affection, and
until it free itself from the vindication of business cunning and brute force
over moral ideas, it will not make a near appeal."[127] This was Macphail's
most eloquent articulation thus far of what imperialism meant to him.
Whatever the motives of imperial decision makers, such imperialist intellectuals as Macphail and Strachey did not attempt a materialist rationale
for imperialism and certainly did not identify its essence with "the determination to conquer, dominate and exploit."[128]

Beyond the themes outlined for the first time or enlarged upon in "The
Psychology of Canada," the importance of the appearance of *Essays in Politics*
lay in what its reception revealed about Macphail's growing reputation.
The *Review of Historical Publications Relating to Canada* gave the book the
place of honour in its volume devoted to 1909, and endorsed Macphail's
general arguments on British diplomacy, protection, and the nature of the
imperial tie. It praised his sense of humour, his "shrewd and searching"[129]
powers of analysis, and referred to him as "this master critic."[130] Nonetheless,
it detected and documented "some exaggeration and inconsistency"[131] and
found structural weaknesses like those of *Essays in Puritanism*: "The book,
which is a collection of essays written at different times and seasons, suffers from the consequent lack of unity and definite purpose. It is a little too
much of a patch-work quilt."[132] Yet the notice closed with the declaration:
"There is nothing which we should more strongly urge upon a citizen of
Canada than a careful perusal of these candid and thoughtful essays."[133]

Essays in Politics was particularly well received in Britain. The
Fortnightly, Contemporary, Saturday, and *National* reviews, in addition to
Strachey's *Spectator*, all took favourable notice of Macphail's collection.
The *Contemporary Review*, for example, stated that his "incisive prose
style reveals a mind of extreme ability stored with the best literature and
trained by direct observation."[134] British reviewers seemed as much struck
by Macphail's mastery of language as by his arguments. One wrote, "Half

poet and half rhetorician, he is always an artist in words – and verbal artistry is so rarely produced by a 'new country' that it would be wrong to undervalue it."[135] American reviewers tended to focus on the comments relating to their country and, understandably, did not share the enthusiasm of their British counterparts. The *Baltimore News* criticized Macphail for generalizing on the basis of isolated incidents and stated, "By a similar process of reasoning, Canada's own degeneracy could be proved from materials furnished by this very book."[136] Although resenting the superior tone adopted towards American life and institutions, the reviewer praised Macphail's criticism of the protective system and pronounced the book generally thought-provoking.

Both directly and through friends, Macphail learned of the approval of his book by such eminent Englishmen as A.J. Balfour, Lord Cromer, Kipling, and Strachey. Probably because of this information and the appreciative reviews, he decided to make a flying visit to Britain in late 1909. While there, he was the guest of Kipling and spoke at a dinner at the Athenaeum that was arranged by William Osler, who was then at Oxford University. During the brief visit he was able to observe some of the campaigning for the January 1910 general election and to test his impressions of the British political scene. One disappointment was that he did not meet Strachey, who was in Switzerland at the time, although he did have lunch with the literary editor of the *Spectator*, Charles L. Graves.[137]

The *Review of Historical Publications Relating to Canada* had predicted that Macphail's volume, because of its critical orientation, would receive more acclaim in Britain than in Canada. Kipling had praised the book "forasmuch as it dares to indicate that the new countries also have duties,"[138] and he had warned Macphail that the Canadian response would probably be "sensitive."[139] The periodical and Kipling appear to have been correct. Indeed, one favourable Canadian reviewer commented on the disparity between the British response to *Essays in Politics* and "the comparatively small honor yet accorded in Canada."[140] But there is no doubt that the book was noticed and taken seriously at home. Late in October Macphail received a letter from Laurier: "I am now gone [*sic*] over your volume through & through."[141] E.W. Thomson reported that the prime minister had been deeply impressed by its "power and brilliancy and success."[142]

In Andrew Macphail's first three years as a Canadian political and social commentator of national repute, he had centred most of his writings on the imperial theme. His attachment to the empire, as one British reviewer of *Essays in Politics* remarked, was romantic to the point of being quasi-religious.[143] Yet at another level Macphail was radically critical of the contemporary imperial reality, both "at home" and in Canada. This dissent was rooted in a critique of industrialism and its effects on Canada, which he was only beginning to articulate in his comments on modern woman and the family. The primary vehicle for his views was his own creation, the *University Magazine*, and he contributed to ten of its first eleven numbers. On the one hand, its scholarly and literary standards enforced a respect among the Canadian intelligentsia for the opinions expressed in it, and, on the other, its topical subject matter and comparatively wide diffusion and influence ensured that even the prime minister believed that it was in his interest to take note of its point of view. Owing to his journal, his sharply defined convictions, his arresting manner of expression, and his prestige in Britain, Macphail was rapidly assuming a pre-eminent role within Canada as a publicist with university credentials.

6

Against the Moderns

The years 1910 and 1911 were Andrew Macphail's most productive in terms of the volume of his writings. He published almost fifty articles and articulated in detail his attitudes on modern woman, education, trends in theology, and that fount of modernity, the United States of America.

Macphail set forth his views on woman, education, and theology most comprehensively in *Essays in Fallacy*, published in June 1910. He had put much careful consideration into the book, and in later years described the essays as having "made for more correct ... thought. That alone is sufficient reason for liking them."[1] The perspective was strongly traditionalist, in harmony with his own past and in anticipation of many of his reflections in later years.

The book opened with two essays on woman – the only topic of the three with which Macphail had already dealt extensively in print. The first and longer was an expanded version of his 1908 *Spectator* article, "The 'American Woman." In an introductory "Note" he explained that "the limit of space imposed by periodical publication compels a condensed form of statement, and does not permit of that ... wealth of illustration by which a free asperity of expression may be obtained, and full conviction enforced."[2] He used his opportunity to compare the spread of the "American woman" phenomenon to the flourishing of various types of rats, to introduce material from ancient Rome and Greece and modern Turkey and China, to enlarge upon his criticism of the "American woman" as mother, to increase his statistical examples, particularly American ones, and to present the early Christian view of woman. This additional evidence did not alter his thesis: the "present situation of women is a result ... of all those forces, industrial, economic, and social, which go to form what we call our civilization."[3]

It is difficult to accept the second essay, "The Psychology of the Suffragette,"[4] as a fully serious piece of writing. Ostensibly the purpose was to discover "why such women as so desire should be permitted to vote, to hold office, and to engage in public life." He stated, "To warrant such an important departure from the established order of society, nothing less than a fundamental reason will suffice; that is, one which has been valid ever since the advent of life upon the earth, or, at any rate, of beings which have the appearance of movement."[5] He proceeded in a partially allegorical, partially tongue-in-cheek, and partially solemn manner to list what he considered to be the fundamental characteristics distinguishing woman from man: dependency, lesser sensitivity, lesser intelligence, greater selfishness, unreflectiveness, lack of sympathy, and lack of a moral sense. Devoted to externals in her attempt to win recognition, woman developed neither a true sense of beauty nor what Macphail referred to as "character" – which in his mind had been the cardinal achievements of ancient Greece. Indeed, he stated that the rise of the "feminine ideal" tended to coincide with the decline of civilizations and the degeneration of arts and letters.[6]

Macphail did little in his essay to extend the analysis he had presented earlier, although he briefly reiterated his belief in man's responsibility for woman's plight. The paper was more striking for its vituperative than its intellectual qualities, and may be taken as a polemical postscript to his earlier writings on modern woman. Yet it also revealed what appear to have been genuine fears on Macphail's part – that women, if admitted to the political process, "would become unconscious dupes of the wily intriguer, or willing victims of the honest reformer who is himself deceived."[7] In his view, woman had over time "developed a kind of ethic of her own, which was entirely adequate for the circumstances in which she was placed, but breaks down hopelessly in a wider sphere of activity."[8] Thus his biting sarcasm in dealing with women who stepped beyond their proper realm should be understood in light of a remark later made by his friend, the like-minded James Mavor, who stated that the contemporary feminist movement should be treated either with "complete reticence" or with "overwhelming ridicule."[9] In "The Psychology of the Suffragette," he was throwing down the gauntlet – a challenge that would eventually be taken up.

In 1914 Macphail published in the *University Magazine* an article entitled "On Certain Aspects of Feminism." In it, he claimed to have no quarrel with women who succeeded in the conventional professions and trades:

"These have succeeded by sheer capacity and by long years of industrious preparation. Such women are everywhere received as comrades ... They are freeing themselves from conventions which grew up in a different environment."[10] But on the other hand there were the feminists, women whom he believed to be symptomatic of two of the worst evils of the modern age: the "American woman" phenomenon, and the passion to reform society.

> This desire on the part of the few women, who are otherwise
> unoccupied, to share in the work of government arises from sheer
> conscientiousness. They honestly wish to atone for their failure,
> through no fault of their own, to perform that function which
> is exclusively theirs ... These women with their fine natures,
> approaching the masculine type are deficient in the instinct for
> husband-getting. They are obliged to turn to other avocations,
> and they find them already preempted by men. Coarse women
> always marry.[11]

While conceding that feminists were of higher intelligence and attainments than most women, he stated that this complication contained the seeds of its own solution: the average woman would "in due time deal with the aberrants who have risen above the line ... as faithfully as [she] has dealt with the aberrants who have sunk below the line on account of diminished intelligence and too grossly animal passion." He put his trust in the "cruelty of the female."[12]

Having described "emancipated women," their origins, and probable fate at the hands of "normal women,"[13] Macphail proceeded to assail their reforming zeal and the causes they espoused. He particularly objected to their campaign against prostitution, which he characterized as "the harrying of the harlot."[14] Not stopping at reiteration of his point that legislation of morality tended to corrupt the legal process and undermine respect for the law in general, he indulged himself in no-holds-barred sarcasm at the expense of the reformers: "They have a just and instinctive dread of the competition which is offered by the members of that ancient and dishonourable profession, those women who toil not nor spin, especially at a time when the desuetude into which these occupations have fallen leaves so many other women also in a condition of idleness."[15]

There can be little doubt after reading "On Certain Aspects of Feminism" that Macphail's words were at least partially calculated to anger and draw a response from feminists. For example: "The most obscene novels are

written by women and by the least highly specialized males."[16] Thus it is
unlikely that he was greatly surprised when the Montreal Local Council of
Women wrote to the editorial board of the *University Magazine* protesting
that he should "abase his art in an article such as this, to a moral and intellectual plane so far beneath him ... We find much that is an offence to
good taste as well as to good morals."[17] One member of the board, Mavor,
sent the protesters a sharp response, fully endorsing Macphail's expressed
views on feminism: "The movement in its various and divergent branches
has assumed a form which appears to me to involve ... a profound danger
to the progress of humanity."[18]

It is certain that Macphail was personally acquainted with at least
one of the two signatories, Octavia Grace Ritchie-England. She had been
a member, with him, of the McGill graduating class in arts for 1888 and
was the spouse of F.R. England. The latter had been a teaching colleague
of Macphail throughout his twelve years at Bishop's and had served with
Macphail and William Henry Drummond on the committee that had
negotiated the amalgamation with the McGill medical faculty. As early
as 1888 Grace Ritchie had demonstrated – in the words of Stanley B. Frost,
official historian of McGill – "considerable strength of character" in defy-
ing the principal, Sir William Dawson, over the content of her address as
valedictorian of the first McGill class of female graduates, the issue between
them being her plea that female students be admitted into the Faculty of
Medicine. Despite the principal's having censored the reference out of the
written version, she included it when she delivered the address, causing
a bit of a tumult. She went on to become the first woman to receive a
medical degree in the Province of Quebec, graduating from Bishop's in
1891. Three years later she was appointed an assistant demonstrator of anatomy at Bishop's, and in 1897 she married England, a widower.[19] Macphail's
rather chilly response to the letter signed by her and by Anna Scrimger
Lyman in the spring of 1914 was a terse, formally worded note, sent by
return mail, expressing his thanks for the interest in his journal, the helpful comments, etc.[20]

To Macphail, in 1914 the world was already suffering from "too much
reformation."[21] Enfranchised women, unschooled in the ways of the
world and moved by emotion rather than the wisdom born of knowledge
accumulated through experience, would be all too likely to support every
proposal that could be masqueraded as a reform. The fact that they were
now demanding the suffrage, rather than pleading for it in a respectful
fashion, was simply one more reason for refusing it. "It is the untempered

enthusiasm of women which alarms them [men] ... Their militancy in the one cause is proof that it would be employed in others."[22] Thus, concern for the survival of the conventions of civilization, rather than prejudice, underlay male opposition to female suffrage and emancipation. The alteration of woman's place in the world was one of those nineteeth-century experiments that should never have been set in motion.[23]

In an important article published in the 1990s, historian Veronica Strong-Boag identified Macphail as a key antifeminist in the era of first-wave feminism in Canada, bracketing him with Goldwin Smith and Stephen Leacock.[24] She observed that "Canadian antifeminism is a fighting creed"[25] – a generalization that certainly applies to Macphail's writings. Admitting that antifeminism is a complex phenomenon, she pointed to the need for analysis of Canadian antifeminism. As described by Strong-Boag, it is an antimodern ideology, with a strong tendency to appeal to nature for justifying sex roles, and to interpret challenges to these roles as revolutionary – for the antifeminist writers, catastrophic – in their implications for society. One of the consequences would be "problematic men," no longer sure of their own identity.[26] Macphail was undoubtedly, in late twentieth-century terms, sexist in the sense that he believed there was a man's place and there was a woman's place in society; that they played complementary roles; and that this was the way gender relations should be ordered, regardless of the fact that it involved limiting the activities and options of women.

On the other hand, Macphail did admit of exceptions. In his 1914 article he had expressly stated that those women who had succeeded in the professions and trades had done so through sheer merit and hard work and that they were "everywhere received as comrades" as they liberated themselves from archaic conventions. There is independent evidence to support his personal record in this respect. In the unpublished memoirs of Roma Stewart Blackburn, the first woman called to the Prince Edward Island bar,[27] she singled out Macphail for the assistance and encouragement he had given her in her efforts to become established in the business world when she moved to Montreal in the interwar era: "He undoubtedly did more than anyone in the way of urging, advising and helping. He offered recommendation, hospitality, and help in finding suitable residence. He couldn't have done more and to him I owe immeasurable gratitude."[28] These words, written in the early 1980s, came from a woman who in the same manuscript documented the blatant discrimination she had experienced in law school at Dalhousie University[29] and who subsequently became an activist in the women's rights movement of Quebec.

In Macphail's own memoirs, he repeatedly acknowledged the saving humanistic influences of women, his grandmother and his mother, in his early life. It may also be relevant that he had arrived as a student at Prince of Wales College and McGill University in each case one year after females had first been admitted. Thus, from an early part of his life he was accustomed to the presence of women of strong character and women who were able to compete as equals, even if he did think of them as exceptions.

Yet as may be expected, Macphail's record is not unblemished. His daughter, who revered him, reported to the present author that she had wished to follow a career in medicine, but he had not permitted it. Nor would he allow her to become a nurse.[30] No one who knew Dorothy Macphail Lindsay could doubt that she had the capacity – the intelligence, judgment, and force of character – to pursue a professional career successfully. Evidently Macphail, who had two sisters with university degrees, one of them a physician, was not comfortable with the idea of his own daughter, whose abilities he must have recognized, having an independent career. She remarked that her father may have feared that she would become a "bluestocking."[31]

Dorothy Lindsay recalled an occasion in the prewar years when, having become interested in politics, over dinner she had attempted to question him about contemporary public affairs; this was "not well-received." He was very silent at meals, with his whisky on the table to accompany the food, and she guessed, more than half a century later, that he was thinking of his next article. In any event, he did not welcome the intrusion.[32] Such discussions and decisions over her future would have occurred in the period when Macphail was writing his most forceful antifeminist material, and no doubt the last thing he desired was to have his daughter embarrass him by becoming an active feminist. This prospect was not impossibly remote. Mavor's daughter Dora had served as an usher in Massey Hall when Sylvia Pankhurst visited Toronto in 1911, and by the next year she was seriously contemplating a career as an actor, despite her father's obvious misgivings; in fact, Mavor was "desperate" in his desire to divert her from this path.[33] Mavor's own evolution in attitude illustrates the sort of factors which may have come into play in the reasoning of such men: in earlier years he had favoured women's rights, but a turning-point had come in 1903 when he met some feminists during a visit to Chicago and he "observed with distress, though without surprise, that their own households suffered sadly from the public demands upon their abilities and their time."[34]

Macphail's antifeminist writings have, of course, survived, and they have had much more currency than the evidence from Blackburn's memoirs and interviews with Macphail's daughter. In the 1990s in Prince Edward Island, as Macphail became increasingly accepted as an icon of such values as the traditional rural way of life and sustainable agricultural practices, he emerged as a symbol of the Island itself. Consequently, other aspects of his record received more scrutiny, and on occasion he came in for criticism in discussions around the time of International Women's Day.[35]

There is no doubt that Macphail took the women's movement of his era seriously. Like Mavor, he interpreted it as representing a challenge of the most fundamental sort. In fact, he had signalled this in his "American Woman" pieces in the *Spectator* by using the words "nature" and "natural" more frequently than in any previous writing; and he utilized the "organic" metaphor for only the second time. When a writer begins to describe social institutions in transhistorical terms, he unveils his most basic beliefs. The imagery matches exactly the sense of "a world at risk,"[36] which Strong-Boag has identified as being at the core of visceral antifeminism, and this alarm is doubtless at the root of the extreme language Macphail used regarding feminism and suffragettes. His caustic reference in the 1914 article to "the least highly specialized males," cited earlier in this chapter, is also of a piece with the "problematic" male identity which Strong-Boag presents as one of the dual spectres haunting the antifeminist writers.

Yet being a good editor, Macphail at the same time made space in the *University Magazine* for the contrary point of view. Immediately preceding his attack on feminism was an article by the Toronto suffragist Sonia Leathes entitled "Votes for Women."[37] His piece made no reference to Leathes's and thus was not presented – at least, not explicitly – as a refutation. On other occasions as well, arguments in favour of women's rights, including female suffrage, appeared in the *University Magazine*, prompting Deirdre Byrne, a recent student, to describe it in her research paper as "an inclusive 'conservative' periodical." Byrne cites articles by, respectively, John Macnaughton (explicitly favouring female suffrage), F.P. Walton (forcefully advocating married women's property rights in Quebec), and, perhaps most interesting, cardiologist and medical historian Maude E. Abbott, whose contribution Byrne characterizes as "a tribute piece to the long tradition of women in medicine,"[38] an article which the *University Magazine* published eleven years before McGill admitted women to its medical faculty. Like Ritchie-England, Abbott had been denied admission to McGill's Faculty of Medicine, and she had obtained her MD degree from Bishop's, three years after Ritchie-England, in 1894. When the first females graduated in medicine at McGill in 1922, Abbott treated them to a celebration at the Ritz-Carlton Hotel.[39] "That Macphail would be so willing

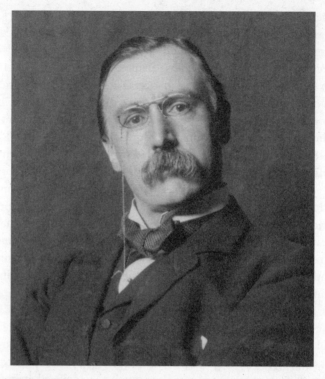

Frederick Parker Walton. Dean of law at McGill, he was an active member of the editorial board of the *University Magazine* from its beginning in 1907, and also a frequent contributor, until he left Canada in 1914. Unlike Macphail, he supported female suffrage; he was also a strong supporter of married women's property rights in Quebec.

to publish views opposing his own is astonishing, given the deep-rooted sexism inherent in some of his statements."[40] The conclusion of Byrne's paper was that "at a time of great upheaval ... *The University Magazine* was open to the expression of a diversity of views ... [based upon] principles of consideration and inclusion."[41] In fact, Macphail was using his quarterly as a true forum for discussion of contentious issues and not simply as a personal pulpit, even on the question of women's role in society – clearly a subject that aroused deep feelings in him.

Macphail's interactions with the independently minded women of his era could have their lighter aspects. In 1911 he received the following request from Frances Fenwick Williams, a female Montreal writer:

My new novel – "Theodora" – is almost completed. As it is of a
serious cast I have introduced you in the guise of a comic character
to brighten things up a little. In the capacity of Prof. Grubbs, author
of a play on "Women" you and your remarks afford much innocent
mirth to the hero, the heroine, and their friends. Needless to say,
whenever you open your mouth and make a remark on my sex you
are promptly "squashed" by somebody. Do you mind?

The libel law in Canada – in Quebec, anyway, – is stringent. I
should like to be assured that you will not make any base attempt
to collar the proceeds of my work. When you see how amusing you
really are I am sure you will not blame me for immortalizing you
in print.[42]

Although the letter, dated 6 September, which Macphail kept in his files,
is marked "Ans. Sept 11th," it is not clear whether he gave such assurance.
In 1915 Williams published a book with the title *Theodora* in England and
apparently, in the same year, the same book with a different title, *A Soul on
Fire*, in Canada and the United States.[43] A copy survives in the McLennan
Library of McGill University.

Set in contemporary Montreal, *A Soul on Fire* features, among other
things, references to suffragettes, to Henrik Ibsen, and to debates among
women in clubs over such issues as child labour. There is an obvious sympathy with the suffrage movement. The book includes as a minor figure a
Prof. Lant, who had published "Woman Explained" and whose position is
portrayed as retrogressive in the extreme. For the most part, his views are
dealt with through the device of other people talking about them or mentioning them in letters. One character writes:

You know his theories about women – that they are only fit to bear
children, spin, and do the menial work of the world? Oh, yes – I beg
his pardon! – and obey their husbands! He is rapidly converting me
to Suffrage; the Pankhursts ought to pay him a rattling good salary to
advocate their cause. Well! we got into conversation and he had the
nerve to tell me that the Greek women were the happiest the world
has ever seen because they were shut up like small-pox patients (my
simile, *not* his!) and seldom saw anyone but their husbands.[44]

Later, the same woman remarks that "he is a nice man to talk to – not
a bit like his books."[45] With one exception, Prof. Lant does not express his

opinions directly in the novel, and on that one occasion he is promptly responded to.[46] He disappears from the plot before the halfway mark in the 316-page book, and he is certainly not a major figure in the novel, which focuses much more on the occult than on social issues.[47] But his views bear great similarity to those Macphail expressed.

The letter Williams wrote to Macphail and the role he played in inspiring her character Prof. Lant may be taken as an indication of the notoriety he had acquired among contemporaries as an antifeminist. Strong-Boag has made the point that Macphail and the other leading early antifeminist writers she cited, Leacock and Smith, were dominant figures in the small English Canadian intellectual élite of the era and that there were no women of comparable stature. Consequently, their views would have been well known and probably widely discussed – in some instances perhaps with sharpness of temper – among those concerned with the issues surrounding the women's movement.[48] Satire, such as that offered by Williams, has been characterized by the sociologist T.B. Bottomore as "a form of criticism practised by the impotent who know that they are impotent."[49]

EDUCATION

Macphail's third essay in *Essays in Fallacy*, "The Fallacy in Education,"[50] deserves particularly careful attention. Prior to publishing the book, in his writings Macphail had made surprisingly few comments on education for a university professor who came from a family with a long history of formal learning. But there was at least one early public indication that Macphail was a traditionalist in curricular matters. On the occasion of the presentation of the first Anderson Medal at Prince of Wales College in 1896, a Charlottetown newspaper reported, "The only training, he [Macphail] said which is fitted for boys and girls is the one based on classics and mathematics."[51] In "The Dominion and the Spirit," he had briefly discoursed on the utilitarian approach to education that found so much favour among capitalists: "The charge which they bring against us is that the education which we give to our children makes of them merely educated men, and not men of business. It is the 'business man' who understands education. The boy must be illiterate, empirical, disdainful of all knowledge which is not the result of personal experience. The New Education is the thing, and Germany is the place where it is made."[52] Yet in "The Psychology of the Suffragette" he had digressed long enough to indicate that he did not believe that the distinction between "them" and "us" was absolute: "Higher education, as it is called with a certain degree of assumption, ... consists in an increased capacity for the recollection of unrelated statements."[53] These two themes – the demands of the outside world on educational institutions and the pedagogical failure resulting from the acquiescence of educators – were central to his critique of modern education.

It is perhaps indicative of Macphail's seriousness of purpose in this essay that he immediately came to the point: "The fallacy in education ... [is] that the information which a child acquires must have in itself some utility apart from the educational value which lies in its acquirement."[54] By way of contrast, he considered that the proper aim of education was making "a man different, and better than he was before ... [that is,] the upbuilding of character."[55] In 1911 Macphail was to give a slightly more expansive definition of education: "the training of taste and character, the symmetrical development of body, mind and imagination."[56] But the emphasis remained the same – on the development of the person, not on utility. The means to this end was the discipline of the pedagogic process.[57]

For educational content, Macphail favoured the classical curriculum – a view clearly at variance with the modern attitude "that the study of the classics is useless, and that study alone is valuable which has something to do with science."[58] Yet he insisted that the conventional dichotomy between "classical" and "scientific" education missed the point. The issue was "between any education whatever and no education at all."[59] He believed that "all education is one. Science merely aims at establishing the orderly continuity and development of created things, and classics the continuity of the intellect and the emotions; it becomes thereby a part of science itself." What was really in question was the purpose of the process: the intent of the modern curriculum was not "that the boy shall be educated ... [but] that he shall be efficient in the calling which he is to follow."[60]

Macphail identified the traditional approach with England and stated that "Englishmen were the best educated men in the world. They acquired a tincture of learning, a sense of fairness and of duty, a contempt of low conduct. They feared God, honoured the king, and loved their country. They had character."[61] Over time it had been discovered that "in spite of this character or by reason of it, they did not get on in the world as well as those who had a different education or none at all," such as the Germans and Americans, who were "beating" the English in some fields.[62] The schools of the United States had been saturated with utilitarianism, leaving many well-schooled Americans illiterate, a fact that Macphail demonstrated with an impressive array of examples. He conceded that Americans recently had been doing well in business, but attributed this to their natural resources and large internal market, not their schooling.[63]

Educational systems had their effect on nations and their capacities. He characterized the United States as a cultural desert: "In America to-day – and Professor Leacock has reminded us very forcibly that Canada is in America, – where there is neither art, nor literature, nor education, fifteen thousand professors are lecturing before a hundred thousand students in the higher institutions of learning."[64] Quantitative schooling gave no assistance to communities in governing, for with their illusions of omniscience they tended to ignore the lessons of experience. But the young Englishman, even if he knew nothing else, "had suspected from his classical studies, slight though they were, that there were people in the world before his time, and that their civilization was different from his own."[65] Consequently, he acquired a certain humility in the face of the past and a humanistic tolerance of other peoples and creeds, which was of inestimable value to an imperial nation.

> That man alone is educated who is competent to enter into the heritage of all the ages, by living over and integrating in himself the intellectual life of the race at the various levels of its achievement. By watching eagerly and disinterestedly the whole pageant of humanity unfold itself, he will get a grasp of the plan and purpose of it, and by knowing it learn to love it. Life has no meaning unless one can see the whole of it; and the present can be freshened only by a new sense of its vital connexion with the past … If a man would enter into the kingdom, he must go to school as a little child in the childhood of the race, and use the classics as his book.[66]

The business of scholars was not to train their charges for specific professions but "to act as mediators between the living and the dead"[67] – that would be social utility enough.

The classical curriculum had a related social significance: as well as drawing the potential out of the individual, it drew him out of the vulgar mass, in effect providing a ladder into an élite.[68] Historian A.R.M. Lower, in his book *Canadians in the Making*, relates a relevant anecdote based on a comment by Macphail's brother Alexander: "One wintry day in Kingston … [Alexander] was seated before his comfortable fire with a couple of younger men. A workman was visible through the window, shovelling the snow as it fell. 'Sandy' turned to the young men, indicated the contrast presented by the two sides of the window and said one word: 'Latin!'"[69]

Unlike "practical" subjects, classics could not be learned by halves or short cuts. Nor, in Macphail's words, could they be learned by "the boy who has no mind." And the latter would be under no illusion that he knew what he did not know.[70] Macphail stated approvingly that the "main result of the English method was that boys with minds which were capable of improvement were educated and became leaders of men. The boys without such minds were relegated to their own place without loss of time to their teachers or waste of their own. The aim of the American method" he insisted, "is to bring the whole mass up to the same level, with the result that there are few leaders and many ill-educated."[71] In short, education if it was to be true education was for the few and not the many, just as it had been in Orwell district school and Prince of Wales College.

Macphail believed that the "school is a late product of civilization and a sign of the complexity of life."[72] Originally the child's character had been formed within the family. The school had arisen as an adjunct to the home, with the schoolmaster placing strong emphasis on obedience, truthfulness, precision, and industry. Over time, interesting and potentially useful knowledge came to be included in the curriculum, and it grew in proportion until the acquisition of information had become the focus of the "educational" process. To make matters worse, the schoolmaster as an exemplar of the sterner virtues was steadily being replaced by the schoolmistress. In an essay published elsewhere in 1910, Macphail had noted that all but 2 of 163 teacher trainees in residence at McGill's Macdonald College were women. "For imparting information, women, or letters, or phonographs will do,"[73] he stated, but the immature and probably celibate young woman was scarcely adapted to the task of building character in rough young boys. If faced with disobedience and unruliness, she was likelier to burst into tears than enforce her will with the strap. Impressionable boys might come to see this as the appropriate method of getting their way. Such examples would certainly not be the means of instilling manliness. Macphail went on to express his doubts about the value of education for women and his concern about coeducational classes. Suffice it to say that his arguments were in line with his general views on women; for example, he feared that in mixed classes boys would acquire bad mental habits from contact with girls. In another essay in which he touched on the debilitating effects of female teachers, he suggested military drill as "a useful corrective."[74]

Not only did "the fallacy of utilitarianism" fail to inculcate proper values in the young; it contained "the paradox that he who seeks shall not find."[75] Education that attempted to do all things would end by doing nothing well. A craft could only be learned by practice, not by reading printed symbols on a sheet of paper. In taking boys suited for the crafts out of their natural environment during their formative years and placing them in schools that strove "to develop a mind which is not there to develop,"[76] the state was destroying craftsmanship. Since the craft had to become a part of the man, a craftsman could never begin too young. If talented enough, he might also become an artist. "The history of aesthetics teaches us that a fine craftsmanship underlies art, and that artists are bred only from a race of craftsmen." As a result of the decline of crafts in the modern age, art was now "sterile."[77]

The educational system had become job centred rather than person centred. The extreme case was "technical education," which seemed "designed to make of a boy a more subservient tool, a less reluctant part of the machine which we have created for ourselves."[78] With tongue in cheek, Macphail gave his approbation to a system of schooling recently established by the railwaymen of the United States: young boys were being recruited to be trained in the making and working of machines. The result was that at an earlier age than before, men were becoming integrated cogs in the industrial system. This only reinforced Macphail's contention that "if our direct aim is not to make the individual more sensitive, more beautiful even, but consciously to attempt to make him more efficient, better qualified for his job, we shall end by treating him as if he were a jack-plane or a chisel."[79]

At the other end of the educational spectrum, the universities were also surrendering to utilitarianism. "The ancient belief [had been] … that a University exists for the preservation and advancement of learning and for the formation of character."[80] American universities had long since given up any pretence of such a justification. In the United States the university was "put to the question: 'Do you pay?'"[81] Its response was to do everything possible to convince the public of its direct usefulness. The result, which Macphail documented at some length, was a failure to produce educated men. In another essay published in 1910 he lamented, "The whole tide and force of events in a new country is set against the scholar, and in favor of the plumber; against the university and in favor of the trades-school. It has become, in reality, a question between Plato and phosphates, between life and the manipulation of materials."[82]

Matters were different in England, but even there the enemy was at the gates. A "Joint Committee of Oxford University and Working-class Representatives on the Relation of the University to the Higher Education of Work-people" had in 1908 issued an ominous report. Its general orientation was to make the learning of the university more accessible to workers as members of the working class, rather than as potential escapers from the common herd. In Macphail's words, "It state[d] the case for direct utility"[83] and "arrived at the conclusion that in a University education alone lies the sovereign remedy for all social ills."[84] Writing to St Loe Strachey in 1909, he had declared that he regarded the assumptions behind the report as "folly worthy of wrath and curse, and of every scoff and jest at one's command."[85] His own lengthy remarks on the report and other innovations, such as adult education and university extension programs, would meet this prescription.[86]

Macphail concluded his essay by relating the confusion about the functions of the university to the general social flux he detected in the modern world, the condition that had given rise to the "American woman." The workman was best advised to remain at his bench, for a "man who is a rail-splitter or a tanner by nature and environment will not split rails or tan hides well if to-morrow he expects to be called upon to preside over the councils of a nation." Macphail was certain that "we can attain to a civilization once more, [only] by each one doing his own work and doing it well, by going about it quietly all the days of his life."[87] This general purpose would be best served by a system that was classical in content and spirit; only those who wanted and could profit from an education would get it.

> It is as near as town-dwellers may come to that which many a boy has received to perfection in a country home with its multifarious occupation, brought up by intelligent, well-to-do, and godly parents with the assistance of a good schoolmaster armed with a short stick or a dichotomous piece of leather .... [This] system would lend itself admirably to the creation of that love of country which is called patriotism by inculcating the obligation of defending it; it would harden the habits into morality and develop the feelings of submission and dependence into good manners and religion .... That was the practice in the Greek schools. The pupils were trained to fear the gods, to honour their heroes, to speak the truth, to defend their native land.[88]

"The Fallacy in Education" was one of Macphail's most important statements of his convictions. In his sharp distinction between those who could think and therefore were fitted for leadership, and those who could not and therefore should cultivate their gardens, he revealed much more explicitly than ever before an élitist tendency that was to develop over the years into a strong distrust of democracy. By focusing on such consequences as the alleged atrophy of craftsmanship and artistry, and the potential in the modern process for dehumanization, his critique illustrated the breadth of his approach. His brief concluding remarks, asserting connections between his educational ideal, a rural setting, and civilization itself, suggested the direction of his thought towards an eventual condemnation of modern society. Macphail was taking up threads from such pieces as "The Dominion and the Spirit," "The Whole Duty of the Canadian Man," and "The 'American Woman,'" and beginning to weave them into a coherent world view. Education in its proper sense and serving its proper purposes was a vital part of the integrated whole. The stern schoolmaster brought out the best in a boy; the classical content divorced from any apparent utility discouraged all but the best minds; the system's selective process would provide a means for the best to attain positions of leadership.

MODERN THEOLOGY, NEW CHURCH

In Macphail's essay on education he had hinted at his concern for what he appeared to interpret as a decline in religious sentiment: "Education divorced from religion ends in lawlessness, defiance of authority, and ill-manners in every relation of life. It is the negation of all discipline." Yet he had at once qualified this by stating, "Of course I am not speaking with praise of those schools in which a system of traditional theology and organized ecclesiasticism is mistaken for religion."[89] Nonetheless, he had gone on to endorse at least one aspect of such professedly religious schools: the teachers were usually men. In previous essays he had also indicated that he was acutely skeptical of all systems of theology, and that his own religious tendency was syncretistic rather than sectarian.[90]

With "The Fallacy in Theology,"[91] the 166-page concluding part of *Essays in Fallacy*, Macphail articulated in detail his position on spiritual matters. He began by noting Cardinal Newman's definition of theology as "the science of God." Professing to be a scientist, the modern theologian had been expected to prove what he said about God, just as the geologist had to prove what he asserted about the crust of the earth. In Macphail's words, this "attempt to make God a subject of speculation ended in failure. Nothing was proven ... The theologians took into their hands the carnal weapon of science; they perished by it."[92] The fallacy in theology was the resort to scientific methods in dealing with a spiritual matter; science would succeed in promoting religion no better than politics or force had. Theological conjecture in the modern age tended to end in futility or worse, for it promoted atheism in scientifically minded persons who observed the theologians' failure.[93]

After giving a negative appraisal of modern theology, Macphail went on to define religion as "an affair of the whole man." Its essence was "the conscious adjustment of conduct to the divine will."[94] The revelation of this will to an individual and its apprehension by him required emotional and spiritual acquiescence; "Pascal ... sums it all up in the inimitable words, 'it is the heart which is the judge.'"[95] The connecting link between the religious man's conduct and his emotional oneness with God lay in his beliefs. The defining characteristic was that he was concerned with his relationship to God and not only with this world. Any attempt to explain this assumption – at once a product of feeling and belief – that man was part of a whole lying outside the realm of his knowledge constituted a theology. This was the proper field for theological investigation, and Macphail took the view that any religion required at least an implicit theology. Yet he maintained that the essential component in religion itself was belief – not knowledge, proof, or reason. Theologians, although playing an important supportive role in religious affairs, must not appropriate all to themselves. In this way, by avoiding overlap with science, religion could again appeal to men of intellect.[96]

Macphail next dealt at length with the development of Pauline theology. He interpreted its doctrines of justification, sacrifice, the logos, and the bodily resurrection in an historicist manner as arising within a framework dictated by the Jewish theologians with whom Paul had to debate and the philosophically minded Greeks to whom he had to appeal. By providing the necessary means for the survival of the new persuasion, and even promoting moral conduct on the part of the early brethren, the system had served early Christianity well. Although much of Paul's theology had been assembled opportunistically, it had also advanced the cause of religion, the essence of which he had accurately, in Macphail's view, described as residing in the individual life rather than in particular rituals or ceremonies. Yet by the second century Paul's doctrines had hardened into a formal creed to which all "Christians" had to assent. The demands of the institutional church then began to stifle the religious sentiment at the basis of Christianity; the ultimate result was that "the theological interpretation of the blood of Christ was substituted for the person of Jesus."[97]

In the concluding sections of his essay, Macphail proposed "to apply to present conditions the considerations which have been put forward."[98]

The legitimate aims of theology, he wrote, were "to find out the meaning of life ... to help people in their efforts to believe what they have always believed ... [and] to establish the identity of the new with the old, and the unity of the present with the past, to bring present knowledge into harmony with old surmise, and bind the ages each to each in piety."[99] He lamented that "the theologians of our generation have failed us. They have allowed the people to scatter in the highway ... or, like obdurate mariners, they held their course too long and cast away the ship."[100] A theology that was appropriate for one age was unlikely to meet the needs of another; Paul's arguments were more relevant to the church historian than to the contemporary theologian. While dismissing the "new theology" with its pseudo-scientific pretensions, Macphail nonetheless declared that theologians urgently needed to come to grips with the questions of creation and evolution if modern man was to have an adequate sense of his place in the world. "The theology which we have is unreal, and ... an outworn theology will not do for a living church."[101]

Lacking a credible theology, the Protestant churches of the day were failing in their ministry. The clergy perceived this lacuna and had lost their sense of purpose. "Being uncertain of their vocation, they have jumped to the conclusion that their business is the propagation of ideas."[102] But religion was an affair of the emotions, not of the intellect, and the true function of the minister was "to create a condition of mind from which religious emotions will arise."[103] Thus modern theology had not only proved futile in its own terms but, by its failure and allurements, had distracted the clergy from their appointed task. What was the proper course for the individual in such a situation? "Probably the best that can be done is for each of us to endeavour to be as religious as he can, with a faith that out of this communized feeling will arise in due season a new theology and a new church."[104]

Although "The Fallacy in Theology" displayed an impressive erudition on Macphail's part, what he left untouched in such a lengthy and wide-ranging paper may be as important and revealing as what he wrote. He paid no attention whatever to the concerns of the rising social gospel movement and indeed in later writings was at pains to reject it. Religion was a matter between the individual and God, with the church and theologians as mediators; the condition of society did not enter the picture except as the occasional stimulus to religious feelings. He explicitly endorsed the Roman Catholic concept of a house of worship as "a place of calm for the senses, a retreat from the world of thought," and stated, "By the contemplation of heavenly things the transitory and perishable will seem of less importance than they now appear to be; and men will turn from them with hatred and full purpose to endeavour after a new obedience."[105] Later in 1910 he added that in such a religiously charged atmosphere, "social problems will be solved by neglecting them."[106]

In an article Macphail published in the *University Magazine* in 1913 entitled "Unto the Church," he expressed his unease with the priorities of contemporary Protestant churches in no uncertain terms. He looked with particular disquiet on the movement to form a united Protestant church – the "New Church." It was not the idea of church union in the abstract to which he objected; rather, he believed that the unionists held an erroneous view of the church's proper role in the world. Macphail harboured no doubt on the matter: the "church is a house of prayer – that, and nothing more, now, or at any other time."[107]

The men of the "New Church" movement had an entirely different concept: their institution would be activist and reformist. Macphail thought they should have learned from recent clerical attempts to legislate morality, which had not succeeded in "inculcating the virtues of purity and temperance."[108] By categorizing vices as crimes and passing unenforceable laws, "all law is brought into contempt and the guardians of the public safety are corrupted."[109] Yet in early 1913 an international body of Presbyterians met in Montreal and took as its own what Macphail described as "a political programme which has never yet been equalled in comprehensiveness." By adopting such "propaganda," he wrote, the church would become "merely a political party, attempting to change the environment of men instead of their characters."[110] He was especially scathing in his references to those who desired to engage in "social service" and "uplift the poor." These people were "idle and ignorant busybodies,"[111] usually

> celibate females who regard prolificacy as a proof of profligacy, and inculcate secretly the false aspects of the Malthusian doctrine. They corrupt the life of the poor at its source, and bring dissension where harmony previously prevailed. Knowing nothing of motherhood, they instil the belief that the bearing of children is the last infamy that can be imposed upon a woman. … Passionless themselves, they are insensible to that pleasure which lies in the indulgence of passion, even of those who are commonly described as low.[112]

Their only accomplishment would be to make the poor discontented with their lot, thus creating misery where there had been none before. Poverty was really a question of character, not of environment; nor, it seemed, was it a matter of inadequate wages. Yet scholars writing since the 1970s have documented the grinding poverty, from which there seemed little means of escape, that existed just a few city blocks from Macphail's home in Montreal during his time. They have, in fact, traced it to the level of wages – an economic reality that seems not to have registered with him.[113] "The true method ... is to righten the individual and demonstrate that all things of real importance follow in due course from that."[114]

Macphail was particularly adamant about the proper concerns of the church because, in his view, once it had opened its doors to worldly considerations, there was no limit to the role they would play. His most damning evidence in this respect came from his own city: "Nearly all of the holy places for Protestants in Montreal have been desecrated by the churches themselves. Within the past few years seventeen churches have been sold, and five others are in the market. All denominations have been equally culpable."[115] The former churches were now stores, cinemas, hotels, morgues, and the like. The churches had not met the challenge and probably had not even perceived it. Macphail noted that the Roman Catholics, who had maintained the traditional concept of a church as an otherworldly place, had sold none of their churches.[116]

In *Essays in Fallacy* and such subsequent articles as "On Certain Aspects of Feminism" and "Unto the Church," Macphail's treatment of woman, education, and religion displayed a common concern for the family, school, and church as inculcators of social virtues and values. A strong conservative bias was revealed in each essay. The woman should remain in the family circle and occupy herself with her daily tasks as housekeeper and mother, yielding deference to her spouse in all matters. The school, if correctly conducted, would complement the home, instilling in young men a healthy sense of discipline and humility. The church that was performing its proper duties and confining itself to them would further the habits of obedience and submission to forces beyond the self. Family, school, and church would unite in producing persons of high character and corresponding standards of conduct. But Macphail's book was a catalogue of the destructive impact of contemporary social forces and tendencies on these institutions as embodiments of his ideals. Modern society was becoming increasingly alien to his values.

Essays in Fallacy was well received in 1910, which would seem to indicate that its rejection of much that was modern struck a responsive chord.

Most reviewers tended to agree with H.W. Boynton, the American critic and biographer, that Macphail's style "marks him as a follower of the best traditions in literature."[117] The predictable exceptions were women's publications and some of the ecclesiastical press. The former tended to respond in kind to Macphail's sarcasm and vituperation. At least one exponent of the "new theology" virtually accused him of being an atheist: "The Fallacy in Theology" was allegedly "a denial of the facts ... of the Christian religion ... Mr. Macphail is ... arguing for that shadowy and impalpable dogma of the modern world, that nothing is really true."[118]

Several reviewers stated that they believed "The Fallacy in Education" to be the outstanding achievement of the book. Rudyard Kipling had predicted that the essay would be "very detestable to all right minded men" but added that "it's dead cruel true."[119] The writer for the New York *Nation*, despite a generally critical notice, conceded, "No one has punctured more forcibly the fallacy of utilitarianism as a university ideal."[120] The most perceptive review appeared in the *Manchester Guardian*, which described the book as "critical and negative, with a strong conservative disbelief in progress." The review praised Macphail, saying, "He sometimes achieves a real freshness of outlook ... [The] pithiness and lack of bombast or verbiage are rare and welcome features." Yet it added that Macphail's "immature knack of running away after every hare that he chances to start makes his essays much longer than they need be, and is the chief obstacle to their enjoyment."[121] Most reviewers treated the book as the idiosyncratic product of a man with strongly traditionalist convictions and the ability to express them powerfully.[122]

Since substantial portions of the book appeared in the *University Magazine*, the *Spectator*, the *Cambridge Review*, the New York *Sun*,[123] the Montreal *World Wide*, and the 1909–10 volume of *Empire Club Speeches*, this series of antimodernist tracts attained a comparatively wide circulation. Furthermore, Macphail was at the same time expressing closely related ideas in *Saturday Night*. Thus his conservative social views were increasingly coming to occupy an equal position with his imperialism as a basis for his reputation and influence.

Macphail was doubly honoured about the time of the publication of *Essays in Fallacy*. On 10 May 1910 the Royal Society of Canada announced that he had been elected to their section 2, and indeed he was the only nominee to receive enough votes before the annual meeting to ensure election. Less than a month later, Goldwin Smith died at the end of a long career as doyen of Canadian criticism. When asked to give a eulogy, Macphail described him as "an example of fidelity to one's own convictions, and of courage in expressing them."[124] The Toronto *Globe* and other newspapers immediately began to speculate on Smith's most likely successor, and they appear to have fixed on Macphail. When giving notice of a forthcoming series of his articles, *Saturday Night* declared, "Dr. Andrew Macphail, we have no hesitation in stating, is a prototype of Dr. Goldwin Smith ... No other can fill the gap."[125] One journalist wrote that Macphail had shown that he was not afraid to deal with national subjects in a broad, comprehensive manner. "His style is almost as perfect as that of the Sage of the Grange, and his opinions have given rise to almost as much controversy in the columns of the daily press."[126]

Andrew Macphail had established himself as an articulate critic of modern trends on a broad front in the years after 1909, when he published *Essays in Politics*. His second collection, *Essays in Fallacy*, made clear his forceful opposition to the moderns in matters of gender relations, education, and the role of religion in society. As when he wrote on the imperial relationship, his essays attained recognition outside Canada, especially in Britain. Macphail did not avoid controversy and even appeared to provoke it deliberately. His words were particularly provocative with regard to the feminism of his era; yet in the *University Magazine* he provided space for advocacy of the cause by a number of persons, and in his dealings with independent women his record appears to have been less reactionary than some of his writings would suggest. Nonetheless, there can be no doubt that he stood on the conservative side of the contemporary debates on feminism, education, and religion. He did not support gender equality, utilitarian education, or the social gospel – in fact, he opposed all three with vigour.

7

Concerning the United States

AMERICAN CIVILIZATION AND THE *UNIVERSITY MAGAZINE*

Recognition was coming to Andrew Macphail as he was emerging from a spirited and well-publicized polemic on the subject of the United States. Although most of his earlier comments on American matters had taken the form of digressions from or illustrations of other themes, the cumulative effect was that he had left little to the imagination of his readers. An examination of some of the articles on American themes by other contributors that he selected for the *University Magazine* reveals views similar to his own. In October 1907 Archibald Maclise had published an essay on "The American Newspaper" in which he declared, "The best literature in the United States to-day is found in the advertisements."[1] These in turn were condemned as being misleading at best and fraudulent at worst. Stephen Leacock contributed two unflattering assessments of American culture and education in the first three years of the journal. He conceded that at least in the field of humour the Americans had excelled; yet given the general sterility of their intellectual life, he did not forecast a bright future even in this case. His criticisms of American education were similar to those of Macphail; he believed it to be suffused with the spirit of commerce, and he expressed a strong preference for the British system.[2]

Since the *University Magazine* contained no articles countervailing this tendency, American writers came to believe that the journal was, in Macphail's words, "animated by malice and misled by prejudice"[3] vis-à-vis the United States. In February 1910 Macphail replied to the charge with an essay entitled "Canadian Writers and American Politics." He began by explaining that these writings were part of a general emergence from parochialism and stated that it was understandable that Canadians' gaze should

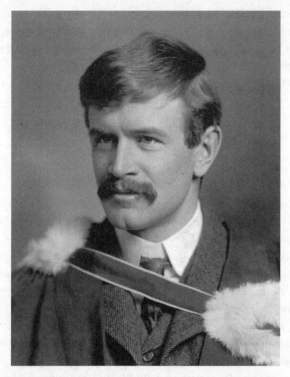

Stephen Leacock. Most famous as a humorist, Leacock was professor of political science at McGill University and a frequent writer on contemporary issues for the *University Magazine*. This photograph was taken in 1902, the year after Leacock joined the Pen and Pencil Club. Shortly after Macphail's death, he published an unmatched evocation of Macphail's personality. .

fall upon their neighbours. He admitted that there was much to admire in the United States. "But the American voice of admiration, wonder, and praise appears to the stranger so entirely adequate for all the needs of the case that he does not feel the necessity for adding his small voice to the general chorus ... Because Canadian writers do not adopt this creed they are convicted of prejudice."[4]

Macphail emphatically denied that Canadian writers or the Canadian people at large harboured malice for the American people. They inhabited largely the same environment and faced many of the same problems, and thus had every reason to inquire how their neighbours had fared.

It is our right. The book of history is open to the world for all to read, and if we find words of warning on the page we shall not rightly be convicted of prejudice if we transcribe them for our own use ...

Infection spreads ... It is not the sign of prejudice but of a desire for self-preservation to fly the yellow flag over a plague spot. It becomes then a duty for Canadian writers to warn the people as impressively, and even as violently as they can.[5]

The most obvious symptoms of disorder in the United States were the corrupt practices of the courts and various levels of government. In a letter to Archibald MacMechan, also in February 1910, he wrote that the "heaviest charge I have against them [the Americans] is that they have made the idea of democracy hateful to the world. They had an opportunity and deliberately chose the evil."[6] Again Macphail related these problems to the severance from Britain, to the reliance on theory rather than experience, and to the democratic assumption "that men who know nothing about anything else may know all about government."[7] But there was another fundamental cause: according to his calculations, more than half the people in the United States "do not belong to the race whose native tongue is English."[8] This was particularly true in the large cities, where between 65 and 80 percent were of non-American parentage. Furthermore, the trend was accelerating: between 1899 and 1908 the United States had received some 7.4 million immigrants, of whom only 10.8 percent spoke English. In an earlier essay Macphail had stated that new countries such as the United States were "a fertile ground for the development of the worst features of the various races which come to exploit it."[9]

The consequences of racial mixture were only beginning to be felt. Macphail cited American military authorities on the non-martial qualities of a heterogeneous population. At the same time, Americans had shown a distinct tendency to criminality and contempt for the rights of others, an attitude that had carried over into their conduct of international affairs. In another country, such primitive behaviour and attitudes on the part of the masses might have been restrained by the growth of an élite of enlightened leaders. But the democratic ethos prevented such a development, and the result was "a population capable of provoking war but not of waging it."[10]

As an indication of the decline of American civilization, Macphail cited the deterioration in standards of English speech.

Everywhere [in the United States] there is evidence of the evasion
of those difficulties which aliens find with the consonants of our
language. The shibboleth of the English is the letters th and j, and
the sound of them is now rarely heard in the land. From Galveston
to Chicago th is pronounced t, as in the common expression "what t'
hell," Jimmy becomes "Chimmy," Journal, "Choinal," world, "woild,"
they "dey" – each race avoiding the crux in its own peculiar way.
American writers now write English as if it were a foreign tongue. It
is not the language of daily speech and when they write it they find it
unfamiliar, hard, and inflexible.

We must free our minds from the delusion that the amiable,
sweet-tempered, amusing, kindly, educated men whom one meets
in the universities, clubs, churches, offices, and homes of the cities of
the United States are characteristic of the nation as a whole. They are
merely the saving remnant who hate corruption and covetousness,
who regard divorce as always a calamity and usually a disgrace. To
these our hearts warm and our hands are stretched out.[11]

The lesson for Canadians was plain: if they followed the American example
of indiscriminately encouraging immigration as they seemed to be doing,
Canada would become a replica of the United States. Already Canadians
were faithfully emulating other American patterns of behaviour:

Our notion of "developing the country" is to eviscerate it, mining
the phosphates and nitrates from the soil under a pretext of farming,
ravaging the shores for fish, and felling the forests with ax and fire.
When this work is accomplished - What then? Nothing but the
record of a lost race in a dead sea, known as America. A nation which
does nothing for civilization is a parasite. Better for us that we should
remain a parasite upon England than a parasite upon a parasite …
Possibly we shall do neither.[12]

Although Macphail's judgments were uncompromisingly stern, he
insisted that they arose not from malice but from a legitimate concern for
Canada's own destiny and a neighbourly solicitude for the United States.
His sources were American, for "the best Americans"[13] were beginning
to express similar fears. In any event, it would be good for Americans to
know what others thought of them. He concluded by suggesting that the
people of the United States appoint a commission composed of such men

as Leacock, Rudyard Kipling, and George Bernard Shaw in order to obtain a consensus of world opinion.[14] Kipling clearly shared Macphail's point of view and cheered him on: "The article on the U.S. is good, discerning and truthful; and I think we need more of that."[15]

Some American writers thought the content of Macphail's article vitiated the force of his denial of anti-American prejudice. The Boston *Herald*, for example, conceded that he had made some valid points but complained that he was "an extreme critic" and had exaggerated the extent of American venality, lawlessness, and illiteracy.[16] Nonetheless, Macphail returned to the attack in the April 1910 issue of the *University Magazine*. G. Lowes Dickinson, a fellow of King's College, Cambridge, and one of his nominees for a commission, had recently published some reflections on the United States, which Macphail used as the basis for an article. During a visit to North America in 1909 Dickinson had lectured in Montreal, where he met Macphail, Leacock, and Principal Peterson. It is apparent from a letter he wrote to Macphail two days later that he had found the company congenial: "It is not often one can 'converse' on this continent, & the occasions are precious."[17] When Macphail visited London later in the year, Dickinson was one of the notables with whom he lunched.[18]

"As Others See Us" was essentially a digest of Dickinson's "Letters on America,"[19] interspersed with comments by Macphail, who began by suggesting that for the purposes at hand Canada could be considered part of America. To Dickinson, the cardinal fact of American history was that America was a continent of competitive, scrambling pioneers. Never had any society so wholeheartedly abandoned itself to the principle of *vae victis!* The result was that it was now "the paradise of plutocracy," he said: "American politics are controlled by wealth, more completely, perhaps, than those of any other country."[20] In his opinion, England was more democratic than America, and unless the American people could devise countervailing forces, a new industrial feudalism would arise. He lamented the absence of manners and the tempering influence of religion, and declared, "All America is Niagara. Force without direction, noise without significance, speed without accomplishment."[21] Reflective callings did not command respect, for "in America, broadly speaking, there is no culture … there is no life for its own sake."[22] In concluding, Dickinson noted that his comments had been uniformly negative, and his explanation for this probably applied equally to Macphail's attitude: "All the things I dislike in modern civilization are peculiarly prominent in this country; and I have been more interested in civilization than in America."[23]

The *University Magazine* maintained a steady offensive on the subject of the United States. In 1910 James White and Arthur V. White published articles in the April and October numbers opposing, respectively, the plan of American interests to build a dam at the Long Sault Rapids and the proposed export of electrical power to the United States. Each author based his argument on the way in which American monopolists had ravaged their own country, as well as the general principle that the vital natural resources of Canada should not be put under the control of aliens. Macphail himself felt so strongly about the issue that in February he had told MacMechan that if he could not get anyone to write exposing "this monstrous plot to seize the resources of Canada,"[24] he would do so himself. As mentioned earlier, when he did obtain an article from James White, he sent the proofs to the prime minister.

Following these two articles, in December Dean Walton dealt with a matter of continuing fascination to Canadian critics of the United States: the comparative divorce rates of the two countries. The article was based on a paper delivered in August to the International Law Association meeting in London where, according to one report, it had "provoked the longest discussion of the conference."[25] Armed with a multitude of statistics, Walton estimated that the American rate was more than 320 times that of Canada and argued that "divorce, as an institution, has its headquarters in the United States."[26] The fundamental reason, in his estimate, was that "the modern spirit" had penetrated that country more fully than any other, and, like Macphail, he believed that the breakup of the family was a step backwards from civilization to savagery. Walton also associated the prevalence of divorce in the Republic with the growth of the feminist movement.[27]

In February 1911 Macphail published his last major article on the United States for several years. "Certain Varieties of the Apples of Sodom" was a revised version of an address of the same title delivered on 5 January to the St James Literary Society of Montreal. Its content was largely a reiteration of his previous criticisms of the American way of life, with minor elaborations and an increased sharpness of expression. For example, the American approach to developing a country was "not easy to distinguish from a sustained act of piracy,"[28] and the immigrants from southern and eastern Europe had "brought their filthy European vices with them in the steerage."[29] Macphail was careful to point out in the former case that his comment applied to "all new countries" and thus included Canada.

A new element in his critique concerned African Americans: "We have heard it said that all men are born equal. There can be no social equality when intermarriage is out of the question, and without the possibility of social equality political equality is impossible. The law was unable to protect the negro and is now unable to protect the white."[30] The contradiction between the liberal ideology of Americans and the actual treatment of the African American minority by the Euro-American majority provided an inviting target for conservative critics of the Republic. In a letter to Earl Grey later in 1911, Macphail recalled reading that "when Patrick Henry delivered his famous 'give me liberty or give me death' speech, he crossed his wrists in imitation of a shackled negro whom he *saw* before him in the outskirts of the crowd."[31] Macphail's earlier references to African Americans had left some doubt about his sympathies: in the previous year he had declared them "unfit to exercise the functions of free men."[32] He had nonetheless expressed revulsion for slavery, lynch law, public torture of African Americans, and race riots.[33]

"Certain Varieties of the Apples of Sodom" was most notable for the disillusion with democracy it displayed. Indeed Macphail, like Dickinson, professed to be more concerned with the universal questions posed by the condition of the United States than with the particulars of the American case. The Republic's political system required a continual effort of the populace to remain informed and alert, he wrote. This had not been sustained, and into the vacuum had stepped the tyranny of the political boss and the party. From the assertion that all were equal was drawn the inference that all were equally suited for public office. With the entrance into popular assemblies of "the poor and ignorant ... [among whom] the corruptor finds his readiest clients,"[34] deliberations deteriorated in tone until "men of independent views and independent means"[35] found the atmosphere unbearable and left public life. Gresham's Law (in summary form, the principle that "bad money drives out good"),[36] operated in politics as well as in finance. Macphail believed that all the legislatures of the day were failing to attract the men they should. Canada and the mother country faced the same perils, for the United States was but the extreme case. The only corrective he could prescribe was that "the intellectual men descend from the pedestals which they have erected for themselves, and the rich men return from wallowing in their own pleasures."[37] By pointing out the degeneration of the Republic, he hoped to do his part "to goad its 'best men' into action"[38] and to open Canadian eyes to the dangers inherent in following the American path.

It is apparent from Macphail's articles on contemporary affairs in 1910 and 1911 that he detected at home many of the vices he decried abroad. The

intense partisanship and abusive language displayed in the 1909–10 session
of the Canadian parliament led Macphail to remind members of Burke's
comment that "a man may be a patriot and a gentleman at the same time."
One speech by the minister of finance had suffered sixty-eight interrup-
tions. Members who engaged in such conduct were "the worst enem[ies] of
the people."[39] As early as 1908 Macphail had considered publishing a digest
of scurrilous remarks made in the House of Commons as a deterrent to
the culprits. He found another symptom of the decay of Canadian democracy in statutes passed by the Ontario and Alberta governments expropri-
ating certain private interests and denying them access to judicial appeal.
"The declaration of any legislature that the courts shall be closed has a
sinister sound."[40]

IMPERIALISM, RECIPROCITY, AND THE DOMINION
ELECTION OF 1911

The most frequent vehicles for Macphail's commentary on current
Canadian issues in these years were two weeklies, *Saturday Night*, published in Toronto, and the *Canadian Century*, published in Montreal.[41]
With these writings, and also with some articles in the daily press,[42] he was
making an attempt to reach directly a wider audience than the readership
of the *University Magazine*. They were relatively short tracts and amounted
to concise attempts to bring general considerations to bear on immediate
issues or specific events. In them, he primarily pursued three general subjects: the parallels between Canadian and American courses of development; a popularization of what he had earlier written on the imperial
theme; and, perhaps most importantly in his own mind and for his own
development, trading relations with the United States. Aside from the vul-
garization of political life, Macphail stated that Canada was following the
American example in the wasteful use of resources and in recruiting aliens
for this enterprise of destruction. He believed that Canada was about a century behind her neighbour but would do the same work in shorter time
because she could draw on American expertise. He welcomed the establishment in 1909 of a Canadian Conservation Commission but lamented
its lack of funding and a strong mandate. "An unpaid commission, which
is not executive nor administrative, whose functions are chiefly to collect
information, offer advice and frame rules of conservation, will doubtless,
in time produce an effect, that is, … when there is nothing to conserve;
but in the meantime the waste goes on." He caustically added, "We have

progressed this far: we are beginning to insist that our resources must be destroyed within the country. That is the intent of the law prohibiting the export of pulp wood."[43]

In several short articles on imperialism in 1910 Macphail said little that was new. He reiterated that Canada's loyalty was a matter of the spirit, not "loyalty for the sake of the loaves and the fishes."[44] He ardently defended the record of British diplomacy relating to Canada, advocated the encouragement of immigration by the English poor, and dismissed as naïve in a premillennial age the idea of an independent and secure Canada separate from the empire. The most effective way of assuring Canada's safety was not to recline in the shadow of the Monroe Doctrine but for Canadians to start pulling their weight within the empire by contributing to its defence. This course of action would be the prelude to remodelling imperial institutions in order to reflect the new reality of the coming of age of Canada and whatever other dominions followed her lead. It would also be consistent with Canada's heritage, and again the United States was held up as a horrifying example of the perils facing a people who repudiated their past.[45]

With the publication in 1911 of "Imperialism: The Problem," Macphail stated with striking clarity his perception of the dimensions of the imperial question:

Eventually we came to understand that a nation no more than a man can live to itself, and that entire pre-occupation with personal affairs ends in meanness and corruption, and that selfishness is the destruction of self. The path by which nationality is attained lies quite otherwise. It is only by doing its work in the world that a nation is justified; and it governs itself best when it makes the larger duty its first concern ... A condition of [national] helotage is not favorable to the development of the individual character ... The individuals which compose that [helot] nation inevitably develop the qualities of the servile; and servility is worse than barbarism ... As we are at present, we are subject to all the perils of the Empire, and denied many of its advantages; and even if those advantages are moral more than material, they are none the less important.[46]

An article entitled "Imperialism: The Solution" followed a week later and was essentially a repetition of Macphail's previously expressed opinion that the time had come for imperial reorganization, and that the place to begin was with a regularized provision for mutual defence: "Once the

separate States unite to tax themselves for [this] purpose ... all the problems now facing the Empire begin automatically to solve themselves." The
new element in his argument was his insistence, arrived at by a process of
elimination, that Canada alone was in a position to take the initiative. The
results would be well worth the effort, since "our status in the world being
defined, the full consciousness of a deserved citizenship would make itself
felt in every public act. Responsibility would sober us and ennoble our
character, and in the larger light of obligation we should address ourselves
anew to domestic problems, and solve them better, because they were felt
to be a part of an Empire and world obligation."[47]

The political development that excited Macphail most in these years
was the Laurier government's adoption of a policy of limited reciprocity
with the United States. Earlier he had unequivocally condemned the operation of protection in twentieth-century Canada, blaming it for raising
the cost of living, corrupting public life, depopulating the Maritimes, and
tainting imperialism. After the 1908 general election he had written that
only two issues could arouse the Canadian people. Now, three years later,
the Liberals, who had deserted their principles in 1893, were raising one
of them – whether the protected manufacturers could continue to have
public encouragement in going about their business.[48]

From the first, Macphail welcomed the Fielding-Taft reciprocity agreement of January 1911 as a measure designed for the common good rather
than an interested few. He believed the terms to be favourable to Canada and
even saw a benefit in the method of concurrent legislation: instead of both
parties being bound by a treaty whose provisions might over time become
disadvantageous, each retained its fiscal independence. Hence, the arrangement would exist only as long as it was of benefit to both countries. Sir
Wilfrid Laurier had declared, "Whatever we may be able to accomplish with
the United States, nothing we do shall in any way impair or affect the British
preference"[49] – which Macphail thought would be sufficient rebuttal to any
accusations of disloyalty. His optimism was unbounded, and he wrote, "This
is the beginning of the end ... It does not matter much whether these sched-
ules pass into law or not. If these do not, more thorough-going ones will."[50]

In Macphail's enthusiasm for reciprocity, he muted his criticisms of the
United States and published a number of articles emphasizing the new
spirit of amity in Canada's relations with her neighbour. All sources of friction had been eliminated through a series of six treaties, agreements, or
conventions between 1908 and 1910. In these circumstances, the times were

ripe for an extension of autonomy in external affairs with respect to the Republic, for there was little risk of serious negative consequences flowing from Canadian inexperience.[51] He also perceived in progressivism a revival of American public conscience, which might in future make the United States an example rather than a warning to Canada.[52]

When a general election was held on 21 September 1911, the Liberal Party entered the contest with a majority of forty-three. Macphail thought the Liberals had every prospect of success: they had a prestigious leader, an impressive record, and in the public mind they were associated with prosperity. Yet they lost by a margin of forty-six. Macphail did not believe the defeat could be accounted for by the accumulation of minor causes that were certain to beset any government long in office. Rather, in an article in the *University Magazine* entitled "Why the Liberals Failed," he argued that the result had turned upon the single question of reciprocity. The issue had not been decided on its merits for, like Macphail himself, the protected interests had interpreted the limited measure as the thin end of a wedge. Given this threat to their privileges, "Everything else was subsidiary and merely a question of method ... The naked truth is that the government was defeated by the charge that all who dared to support it were, *in posse* or *in esse*, disloyal. And this simple ruse succeeded."[53]

Macphail did not doubt the bona fides of the mass of people who professed to have voted Conservative for patriotic reasons. He found "something noble in this attitude ... In all sincerity many good and loyal souls were seized by a genuine alarm that their nationality was in danger."[54] He went on to say:

Any one who fails to appreciate the entire genuineness of this feeling of alarm must miss the whole significance of the result ... [The election] disclosed to us the anomalous nature of our citizenship; and all our political troubles arise from that ...

These terrified Canadians distrusted not the Americans but themselves, and they disclosed to the world that they had no faith in their own citizenship ... Any nation which yields to anything less than overwhelming physical force deserves the fate which comes upon it ... We have suffered many things at the hands of the exclusionists these sixty years past; but this is the worst, – to cast upon us the stain of a merely mercenary loyalty. The cause of these vagaries again lies in the nature of our citizenship.[55]

Thus the election had revealed the dangers inherent in the existing undefined relationship to the British Empire. Because Canadians did not have a firm sense of their position in the world, they had allowed themselves to be stampeded by unscrupulous politicians. The result of the election left Macphail so profoundly disillusioned by what he considered to be the prostitution of imperialism that he momentarily questioned that sentiment itself: "If Empire has come to mean the renunciation of freedom, even in the matter of trade, and if loyalty to the King is inseparable from loyalty to protection, then the Imperial problem is not so simple as it appeared to be before September twenty-first."[56]

The years 1910 and 1911 had been among the busiest of Andrew Macphail's life, and it is probable that they were the years in which his views on contemporary issues attained their widest diffusion. As well as writing some fifty articles and editing the *University Magazine*, he had been engaged in the conversion of the *Montreal Medical Journal* into the *Canadian Medical Association Journal*. In December 1910 Grey had brought to his attention a school journal issued by the New Zealand government for use by children in the common schools. Macphail responded to the hint by proposing a Canadian publication that would appear ten times a year and be distributed to every schoolchild in Canada. It would include articles in both French and English and be controlled by an editorial board appointed by the provinces; the board would choose an editor, and Macphail intimated that he would be available for this task as well. The purpose would be to interest Canadian children in their country, and he stated, "To let it [the project] fall directly into the hands of the provinces would, I think, be fatal. We should then have nine journals, possibly contradictory, instead of one expressing correct opinions in clear tones."[57] Macphail went to the extent of obtaining estimates of the costs from G.N. Morang, but the project appears to have progressed no further. Despite its abortive nature, this undertaking gave further evidence of Macphail's concern in these years to disseminate "correct opinions" as widely as possible. He was particularly excited in this case by the prospect of access to the French schools of Quebec.[58]

Macphail's vigorous optimism in establishing two national journals and seriously considering a third within a five-year period was of a piece with the Canadian climate of opinion at that time. His own quarterly published articles promoting the idea of a national library for Canada, the development of local repertory theatre, and improvements in copying, storing, and making accessible historical documents related to Canada.[59] The country was coming of age, the future seemed boundless, and the mood of "Canada's century" found its expression in a proliferation of agencies for cultural betterment and promotion of national – as opposed to parochial – feeling. Grey was an embodiment of this energetic spirit, and in 1907 he had inaugurated dominionwide festivals of music and drama, providing a trophy for each. Macphail heartily approved, declaring, "The effect of these competitions will be to maintain a high standard of speech and manners, as there is a tendency on the part of all communities to acquire peculiar and vulgar dialects. The church, the schools and the stage are the three agencies on which they must rely to maintain a high standard of diction and to preserve the purity of speech." Grey's initiatives would also aid in "the establishment of a common sentiment on matters of common interest."[60]

In addition, Macphail spent active summers in Prince Edward Island. He conducted experiments in the culture of potatoes and tobacco, and participated in community projects. Consequently, for both the 1908 and 1911 elections he was seriously considered as an independent candidate for the dual-member federal riding of Queens.[61] Macphail's active involvements in such spheres as medicine and Island agriculture are significant both in their own right and as indicators of his breadth of practical interest. But his primary importance in 1910 and 1911 remained as an intellectual critic of contemporary events and tendencies – a second Goldwin Smith, in the minds of some. He made no apology for the negative tone of his comments; in an address to the University Club of Montreal, he had argued that it was the business of university men to "tell the truth" about all current topics: "We are a class set apart. We have elevated ourselves into the exploiting, the parasite class ... But we can justify our existence by telling the truth even about ourselves ... It will not do any longer to stand by and declare that we are holy men who would be defiled by coming in contact with the world, preferring to sit in a well and gazing at the stars."[62] He saw around him a world in a state of flux: women leaving their proper station in the family, clergymen turning the church away from its legitimate calling, educators losing sight of the very meaning of education, the American experiment in undisciplined liberty disintegrating; and Canadians, who lacked a clear sense of who they were, following false gods and being deluded by false prophets. In such a situation, the duty of the professor outside the classroom was to continue doing what he did in his daily work – to seek the truth and to replace confusion with a comprehensive understanding. If this activity led him to be critical of contemporary reality, so much the worse for contemporary reality.

Articles critical of the United States appeared from time to time in the pages of the *University Magazine*. If Macphail had been asked why it was the focus of so much criticism in his own writings and that of the contributors to his quarterly, his answer would probably have been that it was because it was the epicentre of modern trends within the English-speaking world, and that the criticism was not the result of animosity against the United States per se. Macphail was familiar with the Republic, for he had travelled to many parts of it at different times in his life, and thus his views were not rooted in ignorance through lack of contact. Nor were they linked to a sense of grievance derived from the Loyalist tradition, nor to economic protectionism. Thus, not tied to what Macphail referred to as "hereditary hatred"[63] of the United States or to economic self-interest, his critique was one of social mores, political practices, and the plutocratic domination of American life in general. It added up to a definite distaste for Americans' way of life as he understood it.

EYES INJURED

All of Macphail's activities were sharply curtailed by an accident that occurred on 18 June 1911, the night he had planned to leave for Orwell. A soda bottle exploded in his face when he was opening it and the glass entered both eyes. His daughter, who was present when the accident occurred, went for help, which arrived from 346 Mountain Street, three streets west of Peel, within about twenty minutes in the form of Dr W. Gordon M. Byers, a lecturer in ophthalmology at McGill. Macphail spent some weeks in hospital, where the same specialist, Byers, "performed a brilliant operation on my eyes." One eye remained bandaged for months, and in a note (probably written in the mid-1920s) to a letter received from Kipling, he stated that because of this accident, "I lost the sight of an eye."[64] According to Macphail's daughter, if he had not been wearing a pince-nez, it is probable that he would have been totally blinded. As it was, he was up and about by mid-July, and went to Prince Edward Island near the end of the month.[65]

Although Macphail in his correspondence sometimes tended to make light of the significance of this accident, there can be no doubt that it had a serious negative impact on every aspect of his life. To his great frustration, he could not learn to drive an automobile; he was prevented from pursuing his favourite game of golf; and he could not spend nearly as much time as before on intellectual work. His left eye was more severely damaged than his right, and with it he could distinguish only light and darkness. He contracted glaucoma in the left eye, and periodically suffered a great deal of pain. At such times, he was forbidden to read or write. During these periods, which could last for weeks or months, he composed articles mentally and awaited an abeyance of pain to write them out. Nonetheless, he resisted pressure from physicians to have the eye removed, in case something should happen to the better eye. He learned the exact position of everything in his Peel Street house in order to be able to guide himself in the dark, for on at least one occasion he was warned of possible blindness. In the words of his daughter, who often read aloud to him in the periods when he could not use his eyes, "He suffered the tortures of the damned" as a result of this injury, which continued to trouble him for the remaining twenty-seven years of his life. To others, the only sign that his eyes were troubling him was a black patch over his left eye.[66]

8

The Conservative and the Maritimer

Andrew Macphail continued to develop his traditionalist critique of modern North American society in the years from 1912 to 1914. In addition to his response to such immediate issues as the naval question, two broad tendencies can be discerned in his writings. He increasingly condemned the entire urban and industrial way of life, and he drew out the conservative and anti-reform, anti-activist implications of his positions on such subjects as the church and feminism. But he went beyond these largely negative statements and presented his reflections on an alternative way of life and its embodiment: the farmer, more specifically the Prince Edward Island farmer. These affirmations of faith bring us to the heart of Macphail's social thought, the assumptions at the root of his variant of Canadian imperialism.

POST-1911 DISILLUSION: TARIFF, NAVY, POLITICS

Macphail's positions on major political issues between the reciprocity election of 1911 and the First World War are largely predictable from his earlier writings. He continued to advocate freer trade with the United States and to press for Canada's taking a permanent and responsible share in imperial defence, which he came increasingly to perceive as crucial for the future content of the British connection.

In the month following the 1911 election Macphail was approached by both John Redpath Dougall and E.W. Thomson with a view to rallying the low-tariff forces. Dougall, the editor of the *Montreal Witness*, a newspaper which Macphail had long regarded highly, declared that a comprehensive educational campaign was required. He proposed the formation of a tariff reduction league centred in Montreal and possibly led by Macphail. This organization would function as a pressure group after the manner of the

Single Taxers and other single-issue organizations. Thomson, an Ottawa journalist and writer of both realistic and humorous fiction, was perhaps Macphail's closest confidant outside his immediate family; years earlier, he had been among the very few Macphail had told of the impending death of his wife. He suggested a weekly newspaper edited by Macphail and himself, "with plenty of courage and wit – which you, and to some degree, I, could supply, as none others could."[1] The idea of such a newspaper would seem to be consistent with Macphail's other projects for dissemination of "correct opinions" on a national scale: the *University Magazine*, the *Canadian Medical Association Journal*, and the school journal proposal. But the plans aborted. Macphail's eyes were troubling him, and as Dougall noted, "Money does not flow towards free trade advocacy, but away from it."[2]

A general air of gloom seemed to envelop the low-tariff camp. Thomson, who was close to Sir Wilfrid Laurier, reported that there was "no fight left in the damned Grits – Laurier gallantly puts up an air of making one – but he is for pimping to the tariff-grafters as of old – and Fielding's paper, Halifax Chronicle, indicates him in the same frame of mind."[3] Macphail shared Thomson's doubts concerning the steadfastness of the Liberal Party and even considered discontinuing the *University Magazine*.[4] But he did not let his quarterly die, and in early 1912 he re-entered the battle with a number of articles centring on the trade question.

Appearing in the *University Magazine* and *Saturday Night*, Macphail's pieces focused on the proposal that a tariff commission be appointed. He began by asserting that almost half the Canadian electorate was still convinced that the tariff should be reduced, thus causing continuing uncertainty among Canadian capitalists. "Therefore we can understand how important it is to them [the capitalists] that the tariff should be taken out of politics and entrusted to a commission of their own creation." Yet "nothing ... touches the people so nearly as the tariff." Canadians, as a result, had every reason to scrutinize carefully the method of appointment and the powers of the commissioners. Even if these details met the approval of a vigilant public, Macphail's own fear was "that a commission which honestly advised the payment of higher duties would become as great as Diana to the Ephesian silver-smiths, and that its decrees would be imperative as if they had been let down from heaven." On the other hand, if it were to "demonstrate that ... duties should be lowered, then its conclusions would be considered merely academic." Thus he believed that the recommendations of the commission would be "hortatory or mandatory according to the circumstances of the case."[5] Indeed, the latter would be the more probable, for a "commission which is appointed to administer a system quickly becomes identified with the system ... They [the commissioners] are apt to impute their own excellences to the system which they administer." Consequently, he suggested that the taxing power remain with Parliament in form as well as substance – after all, if reciprocity had been the decisive issue of the last election, each member had been elected a tariff commissioner.[6]

In other essays Macphail continued to advocate lower duties between Canada and the United States, and sought to disentangle the tariff question from the general problem of the threats and challenges of contiguity to the Republic. He argued that Canada had less to fear from trade than from the increasingly civilized tone of American life – indicated in part by the election of Woodrow Wilson as president in 1912. Canadians with an appreciation for the finer aspects of life might in the future leave for the United States, just as some of Macphail's generation had moved to Britain. Hence this "force of attraction" and what it revealed about the backwardness of Canadian social life should be of more concern than trading relationships. And his views on whose interests were served by the debasement of public discourse were wellknown.[7]

As an advocate of a low tariff, Macphail was clearly at odds with most imperialists and conservatives, including members of his editorial board. Principal Peterson and Dean Walton had been disturbed by "Why the Liberals Failed," and had succeeded in having Macphail hold the number until Stephen Leacock could prepare a more orthodox article.[8] When Macphail came to articulate his position on the naval question, he again faced criticism within the imperialist camp, and became involved in an extensive debate through the mails with Archibald MacMechan. Macphail's essay, "The Navy and Politics," appeared in the *University Magazine* of February 1913, and Peterson again had strong reservations, which he published as "A Supplement." His comments amounted to a defence in conventional terms of the policy Robert Borden espoused.[9]

Although as recently as 1907 Macphail had endorsed Thomson's position that Canada should confine itself to coastal defence, since 1909 he had believed the naval situation to be "most portentous,"[10] and he had argued that a more comprehensive defence policy was needed. The contents of the *University Magazine* from 1909 to 1913 reflected this concern. Aside from Macphail's piece and Peterson's "Supplement," there were six articles on the navy, with three (two of them by Leacock) occupying the place of honour.[11] But Macphail had an additional, non-military rationale for his advocacy: he believed that such a policy could and should be the first step in reworking the imperial relationship. Indeed, this may have been the more important consideration, for in December 1913 he told MacMechan that he suspected the recent war scares had been manufactured for profit: the "sinister figure of the financier was always in the background. They sold their bonds in the enthusiasm which they created."[12]

Whatever Macphail thought of the crises of the period, he believed the opportunity for imperial reorganization was tantalizingly real. In 1909 Borden and Laurier had agreed on the necessity for a Canadian navy separate from the British fleet, and both had opposed a policy of contributions. But in the next year Borden changed his position: he advocated a unified fleet, declared that no permanent policy should be adopted without a mandate from the electorate, and stated that contributions would be justified should an emergency arise. Laurier had remained in favour of a Canadian navy, saw no obligation to consult the voters, and introduced the Naval Service Act, which created the Department of Naval Service. Macphail supported this policy, which he believed to be the beginning of Canada's assumption of a mature role in imperial defence. Although he may have differed with the government over details, he accepted it as a sincere recognition of the principle that Canada had permanent responsibilities. It was an initiative from which much else might come, and in his opinion it could even mean the dawning of a new era for imperial relations.[13]

Canadian politics would not let this be. Borden, the Quebec *Nationalistes*, and an unfortunate accident combined to discredit the government's plan. "The Canadian navy went on the rocks. The Imperial movement also came to a standstill on September 21 [1911]."[14] Borden's appeal to a sham imperialism on the naval as well as the trade question nauseated Macphail: "This parade of holy sentiments for party purposes is like using sacramental dishes for the feeding of swine."[15] Once in power, Borden waited over a year before announcing his substitute for Laurier's policy: an emergency donation to the mother country of $35 million for the purchase of ships, which would then be Britain's responsibility.

As leader of the opposition, Laurier denied there was an emergency and held to his previous position: "a permanent policy of participation by ships owned, manned, and maintained by Canada."[16] Macphail shared Laurier's doubt about the reality of the alleged emergency, heartily approved of his consistency, and dismissed as an evasion of responsibility Borden's policy – or non-policy, for the Conservatives argued that it was an emergency measure, not a permanent commitment or recognition of principle. The Conservative proposal was a symptom of the general malaise of Canadian society, since it appeared "like a 'business proposition,'" argued Macphail, "and to business men payment in money is the easy and obvious way … We are relieved of the bother of building ships, and sailing them, and fight- ing them."[17] He wrote to MacMechan, "My own view has always been that we should get at the underlying principle of the thing"[18] – and it was pre- cisely this that he saw Borden refusing to do. Once again Macphail had found himself in adamant opposition to orthodox Canadian conservatism and imperialism on a major issue of the day. He had considered not pub- lishing "The Navy and Politics," and in a letter to the University of Toronto historian George M. Wrong he lamented, "I seem to be the only Tory left in the world."[19]

The performance of the Conservatives on the naval question was doubly iniquitous: not only did their proposal evade the basic issue, but their manner of dealing with the Liberals served to embitter Canadian politics and carried the danger of distorting Canadian political develop- ment. When the bill to provide contributions to the British Admiralty was debated in the House of Commons, the Liberals resorted to obstruction- ism and the government responded with closure. But the Liberals held the high card: their majority in the Senate rejected the bill. Borden, being more concerned with retaining his own majority in the Commons than with obtaining a mandate to deal with the "emergency," did not seek a dis- solution. Consequently, when war came in 1914, there was no Canadian navy, no contributed ships, and no permanent naval policy.[20]

Macphail did not blame the Liberals: "In the past two years [1911–13] they have suffered much provocation. The basest passions were deliber- ately aroused against them and the holiest sentiments were invoked for their defeat." But he feared that the Conservatives' demagogic use of the loyalty cry would drive the Liberals into a false position: "The danger to the Liberals now is that the question of method shall develop into a ques- tion whether or not Canada is to remain a part of the empire at all … The naval question is not the final question." The fundamental issue, Macphail contended, was that of self-government: who was going to decide on the use of whatever Canadian naval forces would be called into existence. "Self-government can be obtained in only one of two ways, by organic union with the Empire, or by independence. These are the only alterna- tives. All other proposals are mere subterfuges for evading the issue." The Liberals had to choose between the two possible courses, and Macphail was concerned that "they may find themselves forced into an untenable position without knowing it, and without being prepared or willing to defend the place into which they were thrust by their own logic."[21] He warned that

> Liberal politicians and journalists who speak from the lips outward, repeating their formulae, – autonomy, self-government, happy as we are, vortex of militarism, dove of peace, entanglements, internal development, – would do well to take thought and consider where the logic implicit in these words will lead them. For these words do possess a logic of their own, no matter how lightly they are spoken. In time they will harden into a creed which will fasten itself on to the Liberal party ...
>
> Independence as the destiny of Canada is an arguable alternative but the Liberals should be quite clear in their own minds that it is towards independence they are heading when they proclaim self-government as their creed and organic unity as their anathema.[22]

As in his statement of his views on education in *Essays in Fallacy*, Macphail's tone was deadly serious. Indeed, MacMechan wrote to him concerning this article: "I liked you better than usual in these arts, because your Puck of banter deserted you."[23]

Macphail's disillusion with the Conservatives was part of a larger disillusion with Canadian politics. In early 1913 he told Wrong, "The liberals ... have no minds and they have no courage. The party is shot through with protection .... The conservatives ... are not conservatives at all, they are what I call Septembrists. You can have no politics in a country which is dominated by a financial issue."[24] This attitude was reinforced by experiences closer to home. With his help on the hustings, his younger brother Alexander, although a professor of engineering at Queen's University, had in the autumn of 1911 contested and won a provincial by-election in the Prince Edward Island district that included Orwell. While nominally an independent, Alexander was known to be favourably disposed to the local opposition, and his election and that of a Conservative for the dual-member riding cost the Liberal government its majority. There was undeniably an element of poetic justice in the role the Macphail brothers played in defeating the Liberal government, for it was a successor to the provincial government that had taken power in 1891 and reduced the salary of their father, a known Tory (then superintendent of the Asylum for the Insane), by 25 percent.[25]

This was Andrew Macphail's first direct experience in "practical politics," and he was initially enthusiastic about the result, particularly as it was instrumental in bringing to office as premier an old classmate from Prince of Wales College, John A. Mathieson. It had been Mathieson, one and one-half years his senior, who had taken the shy boy from Orwell with him to the college's Shakespeare Club. He had taught in the neighbouring village of Kensington during Macphail's period in Malpeque, and their friendship endured until the younger man's death. But Mathieson began his tenure by choosing his cabinet to represent religions and counties, and within a month the Macphails were considering opposing the government and attempting to persuade some Liberals to "go independent." The premier, perhaps suspecting the political loyalty of his old friends, and not intending to be shackled or turned out of office by "independents," called a general election for January 1912. In the wake of twenty years of Liberal rule, the Conservatives won by an overwhelming majority, and although Alexander was returned by acclamation, the result deprived him of his political leverage. Politicians, to Andrew Macphail, were distinguished by "their poverty of thought, their incoherence of mind, and lack of system."[26]

BUSINESS VALUES, DEMOCRACY, AND THE MILITARY ETHOS

What was at the root of this "divorce of patriotism from politics"? Macphail's answer became increasingly clear and insistent: the intermingling of business and politics was to blame, since they were "in direct antithesis. The ethic of the one is love of money; the ethic of the other is love of men. Business deals with questions in narrow detail: politics considers them abstractly in relation to the well-being of the community." Macphail went on to argue that the "essence of democracy is the proportional representation of all interests in the community. The weakness of all democratic legislatures lies in the predominance of the business element."[27] It was this that accounted for jobbery in public life and the manipulation of imperial sentiment for party purposes. The consequences were morally catastrophic and socially divisive: "Self-reliance was destroyed. Sectional jealousies were created. The country was arrayed against the town."[28]

More broadly, to Macphail, the business spirit was a poison sapping the vitality of the Canadian organism: "It cannot understand that there are whole categories of subjects beyond its control. With its passion for organization it destroys what it touches. Everything fine, – religion, friendship, love, education, literature, art, newspapers even, – wither and die at the first touch of its breath."[29] When Gustavus Myers's *History of Canadian Wealth* appeared in 1914, Macphail "read it with secret shame"[30] but circulated it among his friends.[31] In his indictment of business ethics, he also cited another contemporary American muckraker, Lincoln Steffens, writing in the *Metropolitan Magazine* concerning the corrupting influence of business on politics in the United States.[32]

Macphail discerned a cure for this malaise, albeit an extreme one: "War," he wrote in early 1914, "is the price which a nation pays for salvation from its internal exploiter … Politics in Canada is unreal because it is dissociated from … the obligation of self-defence … because, in short, it is without the mainspring of patriotism."[33] He did not believe that war would be a terminal experience for his Canada; rather, it would be a cleansing process. In writing of this drastic redress, Macphail assumed the mantle of prophecy: "It is righteousness alone – not building railways with borrowed money, calling upon aliens to be fruitful and multiply, and possess the land – which exalts a nation."[34] Yet such warnings were apparently not welcome: "They say: 'Why should the man tell truth just now, when graceful lying meets such ready shrift?'"[35]

What, precisely, was the truth that required telling in early-twentieth-century Canada? More specifically, what was truth to Macphail, a middle-aged Scottish Canadian, born into a Calvinist family and socialized in the rural hinterland? He increasingly saw the contending forces as city and country, producer and parasite, farmer and non-farmer. The contemporary crisis had originated in the Industrial Revolution, with its invention of the steam engine and other labour-saving devices, "those monsters which we have created for our own oppression."[36] Society had fostered the delusion that machines could be made to do all the work, and men had been attracted to cities to tend them. In 1912 Macphail reported that over the previous decade the rate of increase of Canada's urban population had been almost fourfold that of the rural population. But it had all turned into a grotesque nightmare. The son of the farmer or village artisan had lost the freedom to go about his work as he pleased:

> [The] Lancashire cotton spinners who broke up the first beginnings
> of the jenny in Hargraves' house were profoundly right. By a sure
> instinct these prescient people had a sagacious knowledge that
> their children's children would be destroyed; and the event has
> fallen out as they described. The descendants of these free men are
> now imured [*sic*] in factories by a process of imprisonment which

is only voluntary by name. If it had the appearance of being under compulsion they would surely go mad. They have become helpless in any task but the tending of machines, too helpless to revolt, because if they revolted they would surely starve.[37]

The urban environment was overcrowded, vulnerable to disruptions and contagions, and notoriously ungovernable. Municipal administrations throughout North America had shown a remarkable propensity for corruption. The result had been the rise of the Galveston plan of commission government which, according to Macphail, was simply a confession that cities were incapable of self-government. Such a debacle could not go on forever: "Humanity always proceeds in a straight line until it arrives at an impasse, and it will reach the end of the machine age just as surely as it reached the end of the age of stone and the age of bronze."[38] He detected "signs that the end is near at hand. Industrial unrest is merely an expression of blind dissatisfaction." These rumblings were pregnant with hope for Macphail, since they proved that "the cry of nature has never been stilled."[39]

As yet, this impulse – at once an expression of discontent with the complexity and artificiality of the city and a longing for an existence closer to nature – was spontaneous and uninformed by the new realities of rural life. "A generation has grown up in Canada which knows not the land and remembers only the middle period of poverty and misery which followed the exhaustion of the virgin soil, forgetting, however, the earlier days when the earth yielded her treasures upon the slightest solicitation when the farm was a world in itself, inherited from father to son, which supplied within itself all human needs, and diverse occupations yielded a multifarious interest."[40] Macphail argued that this generation had not yet realized that regeneration of the soil through mixed farming, artificial fertilizers, scientific rotation of crops, and conservation of moisture had brought back "the older order," in which "the intelligent farmer" could become, "if not rich, at least independent."[41] Of one thing he was certain: the "safety of the city depends upon a continuation of the factory system a little longer, until all knowledge of the crafts shall have perished from amongst men."[42]

Macphail's total rejection of urbanization and industrialization in these years was accompanied by an increasing disenchantment with other symptoms of progress and movements for change, whether in politics, the family, or spiritual life. Democracy, feminism, and the "New Church" were all interpreted as aspects of the disintegration of an earlier, more orderly, and secure way of approaching life, when persons and institutions had played out their allotted roles in a world they accepted as given. Democracy, Macphail wrote in 1912, "is not so cock-sure of itself as it was in the first flush of its youth ... Whilst the business was to pull down what our fathers found to be good and useful, democracy succeeded admirably. Now that all is levelled, hope has given way to perplexity, and glee to stupid amazement."[43] Establishing reformed institutions in the people's affections had not proved as easy as instilling doubts.

Through an address delivered in 1913 to the first meeting of the Canadian Political Science Association, Macphail dealt directly with the popular prestige of contemporary political institutions. The villain was not the common-garden politician whom Macphail had already criticized so extensively for muddling the great issues of the day. At least the political practitioners knew that "the thing which has grown is better than the thing which is made ... and that an anomaly which works well is better than a logical system which is contrived in advance of events."[44] Rather, he attacked "the doctrinaires and professional reformers," "the amateurs," "the theorists," and "the logician."[45] By their carping and their attempts to reduce the art of government to neat formulae, "they destroy public faith in the institutions of the country, and so are the worst enemies of the people."[46] The theorist should, in effect, put up or shut up: "If he thinks the people are not properly represented, it would appear to be his duty to strive to represent them, and not solace himself with railing at those who have been selected."[47]

In reaction against what Macphail interpreted as the destructive levelling spirit of the period, he turned to advocating the sterner virtues, particularly those of the soldier, who "is coming into his own even in Canada." He thought men wanted their sons subjected to military discipline, which "makes for obedience, self-reliance, and courage, qualities which are as essential in civil as in military life." He declared, "The school-mistress with her book and spectacles has had her day in the training of boys; and sensible parents are longing for the drill-sergeant carrying in his hand a good cleaning-rod or a leather belt with a steel buckle at the end. That is the sovereign remedy for the hooliganism of the town and the loutishness of the country."[48] He urged that Canada adopt universal military service, since the "value of a military training lies in its effect upon the individual ... A nation which is good in war is good in peace; and a nation which is no good in war is good for nothing."[49] He contrasted the values of the military lifestyle to "the perverted virtue of the trader and the misapplied industry of the world." If this was "militarism," then he advised advocates of military training not to shrink from using the word. The results would be well worth the effort, since "a man cannot have the spirit of a civilian at one moment and of a soldier at another."[50] He even rhapsodized that "the military idea … inspires all organization. Obedience is beloved. A woman is 'ordered' by her physician. A nurse goes on 'duty.' A boy adores a 'uniform.' A captain of militia is a wonder to himself."[51]

These were heady words for a man not given to enthusiasms. But the danger was great: "Those who would lure us away from our established institutions are really inviting democracy to stretch out its neck so that some tyrant may the more effectually place his foot upon it."[52] Macphail had no doubt that parliamentary government was the best political system, at least for British peoples, and he opposed all contemporary signs of change, such as the rise of third and fourth parties. The two-party system, and Parliament itself, were more than a matter of chance:

> This barrier which divides men into two main parties is not a thing of human invention. It represents a division in the stream of human thought … Upon the one side are those who believe in destiny. They observe that there is a chain of cause in nature, that there is a compulsion in the way things grow, and that they proceed by the path that is ordained. These are the Conservatives. On the other hand are those who are worshippers of chance, who rebel against this Calvinistic interpretation of nature, and seek by every path to escape from the fate which is laid upon them. These are the Liberals. The one is content with order: the other is desirous of change … All political confusion arises from this, that Conservatives are not content to remain conservative, and Liberals liberal.[53]

If such was the case, politics in Canada were indeed confused, for in December 1913 Macphail and the *University Magazine* were reproached for partisanship by both Liberals and Conservatives.[54]

In these years Macphail was exhorting conservatively minded Canadians to maintain their traditional ways in religious, social, and political life. He saw little cause for optimism and in 1914 remarked to MacMechan, "Certainly we in Canada have made a mess of things and no man can see the issue."[55] Gone was any trace of national egotism in reference to the United States: "For a generation we have been the thank-Gods of America. We were not like those republicans and sinners." But times had changed. Writing in 1914, he declared, "Within the past five years events have demonstrated that their [Americans'] public conscience was not dead but sleeping; and any one who thinks to the contrary may ask of their numerous makers and administrators of law, who are now in gaol."[56] If anything, the Americans were now providing examples for Canadians to emulate. The high tide of progressivism seemed evidence of at least partial repentance. In Canada, the "Great Barbecue" continued unabated.[57]

PRINCE EDWARD ISLAND AND THE MARITIMES: PRESENT AND PAST

The northern version of the gilded age was not an era of prosperity and expansion for the Maritimes. While central Canada and the West grew enormously in population and economic output, the Maritime provinces stagnated. For example, in the first decade of the twentieth century the population of Canada increased by more than one-third; in Nova Scotia and New Brunswick the increases were 7.1 and 6.3 percent, respectively, and in Prince Edward Island there was a decrease of almost one-tenth.[58] More and more, Macphail came to reflect on the changing regional balance within the dominion and on the disparity in conditions between central Canada and his native region.

No doubt a partial explanation for the greater prominence of the Maritimes in Macphail's writings can be found in his involvement in the multivolume *Canada and Its Provinces* series. As one of eleven associate editors, with such scholars as Walton, Wrong, Thomas Chapais, and W.L. Grant, his role was to edit papers for the two volumes on the Maritimes and to write the section on the history of Prince Edward Island.[59] Yet Macphail's concern for questions relating to the Maritimes and especially his beloved Island went beyond that of the detached academic researcher. In 1910 he had written:

> When a middle-aged man goes amongst his very own people, he realizes afresh that he is not a native of Canada but of his own province. Dust we are; but it is the dust of the place where our fathers lie buried of which we are formed. It is hard for a man who has been born in Prince Edward Island, we shall say, to look upon the plains of Saskatchewan and the mountains of British Columbia as being equally precious with his own red soil and green fields. He has heard of the St. Lawrence; but to him the Orwell and the Hillsbourough [sic], rivers of the Island, are better than all the waters of Canada.[60]

These sentences had been primarily calculated to deflate the pretensions of Canadian "nationalists" and "autonomists," and to affirm the existence of a distinctively Maritime frame of mind.

> A nation is not a process of thought, but the result of inexorable circumstances which are not amenable to human control. A nation which will endure creates itself, as slow as a glacier and as ungovernably as the course of the world. ... To come to the point, England - by which he [the Prince Edward Islander] may mean Scotland - is nearer to him in miles than Calgary, Edmonton, or Vancouver, and in affection than is Drummond-Arthabaskaville.[61]
>
> Canada exists for him merely because it is a part of England. If it were not for that, the very name of it would be utterly meaningless, much more so than the "States" where many of his people sought refuge from the early hardships which the confederation of the colonies imposed upon them.[62]

In succeeding years Macphail would add new dimensions to his writings on the Maritimes and articulate a positive social vision that he closely associated with his province.

As well as his essay on Island history, Macphail furnished volume 13 of *Canada and Its Provinces* with a ten-page introduction on the Maritimes. Drawing on the work of MacMechan and W.O. Raymond, the contributors for the mainland, he presented Maritime history as a unity, describing how in early times the fate of the area had been uniformly dependent on and marginal to outside forces, and how later the struggle for responsible government had taken a similar course in each of the colonies. The result was that "after a century of bickering the three provinces had achieved a system of government which was entirely satisfactory to them." Macphail clearly found this period to his taste, for he wrote that while the local inhabitants exercised the freedom of self-rule, the important role of Government House in the small communities "did something to alleviate the rawness of colonial life. The people were furnished with certain standards. A society created itself in which some amenity and graciousness was preserved."[63] Here, in short, were three miniature replicas of the old country.

The colonies were also blessed with prosperity in these years. They were progressing rapidly and drawing closer together. "Between them there was a community of sentiment and a community of interest which had developed a local patriotism."[64] Macphail went on to insist that on the basis of this common feeling, Maritimers had determined in the 1860s to reunite old Acadia. The Canadians had then intruded their plans into the Charlottetown Conference but had been met with local hostility. Canada was distant and was burdened with a history of rebellion, riot, racial tensions, and annexationism. "It was the cry of ancient loyalty against a transfer of allegiance."[65]

Yet the Maritimers had entered Confederation. Why? Macphail's marshalling of evidence suggested conspiracy or, at least, venality on the part of local leaders. The post-Confederation years were presented as a period of protest and decline. Uncharacteristically, Macphail did not commit himself on whether the economic deterioration had resulted from Confederation. But he commented cryptically, "Just because people reason that an event happens in consequence because it happens in sequence, politicians need to be scrupulously careful to refrain from cajolery and force." He concluded the essay by declaring his belief that the exodus of people from the region was coming to an end, and by asserting, "No part of Canada is occupied by so carefully blended a race ... true to their allegiance and to their institutions."[66]

Although giving due prominence in his larger article to the Island's neo-feudal system of land tenure, whose dominance was unique in English-speaking British North America, Macphail's account of the British period in general, the development of colonial society, and the advent of Confederation was very much in keeping with the themes of his introductory essay. Prior to 1873 the Island had been "flourishing. The people ... had complete control of their own affairs and a militia quite adequate for their defence. The import duties ... were sufficient for all public needs, and they could be altered or abolished to suit any contingency that might arise. There was no public debt."[67] The serpent in this Eden, as in contemporary Canada, was the intermingling of politics and finance. Bankers with a heavy stake in the solvency of the Prince Edward Island Railway had manipulated the people into the larger and more secure financial realm of Canada. "In this illumination the politics of the confederation appear only as a sinister farce."[68] The tendency to discern recent parallels was also evident in his treatment of the Island loyalists, whom he denounced in terms almost identical to those he applied to the Ontario loyalists who had gratified their "hereditary hatred"[69] in 1911: "For many years they existed as a community bound together by a common hatred, and the 'loyalist vote' was regularly trafficked in by the politicians."[70]

Only one and one-half pages in seventy-one were devoted to the four decades after the province's entry into Confederation. Rather than dwelling on "the decay" at length, Macphail contented himself with pointing out that three-quarters of the exodus went to the United States, and noting that the Island's population was falling despite its having the largest average family size in Canada.[71] By way of contrast, he wrote some twenty-five pages on the French regime, partially because he believed this early period had been neglected by previous historians. His account showed insight, and he was unsympathetic to the expulsion of 1758: "Whatever causes existed in Nova Scotia for the deportation of the Acadians, in Isle St. John there were none associated with the conduct of the inhabitants."[72] Once again, the fate of Acadians had been determined by outside events. The British officials who made the decision were either ignorant or guilty of "the grossest misrepresentation."[73] This section was not superseded in Canadian historiography until the publication in 1926 of a monograph by Daniel Cobb Harvey, a protégé of MacMechan who had contributed two articles to the *University Magazine* – and who had written to his mentor from Oxford University in early 1913, "From a mere boy I have been keen on *The University Magazine*; and it has been my ambition to 'get into it.'"[74]

Macphail's article gave evidence of assiduous research into published and unpublished primary sources, and of his acute critical faculties in dealing with the material. Yet there were serious flaws: a tendency to didacticism and a trait he shared with almost all historians of Prince Edward Island before or since – an extreme reluctance to acknowledge the importance of religious divisions in Island political and social life. Indeed, he managed to avoid the subject entirely. This being said, it remains nonetheless true that "The History of Prince Edward Island," more than any of his previous work, revealed an aptitude for serious historical research and writing. Historian J.M. Bumsted, writing in 1983, described the article as "one of the best-written pieces of provincial history ever produced."[75]

TOWN AND COUNTRY

Two issues that Macphail believed to be closely connected to the regional question were relations between Ottawa and the provinces, and between town and country. In writing of Prince Edward Island he had stated, "This province is not alone in the belief that it is suffering from the bonds of confederation. From British Columbia also comes the cry for 'better terms'; from Manitoba the demand that its boundaries be enlarged."[76] As early as 1907 he had declared that each province had its own grievance. The reason for this accumulation of discontents was the ascendancy of the dominion over the provinces. He conceded that in the wake of the American Civil

War the Fathers of Confederation had desired a strong central government, "but it was never intended that ... [this] was to be employed for the
destruction of provincial political life." Through the power of the purse,
the dominion had made the provincial assemblies into "mere adjuncts,"
and through the power of appointment it chose senators, judges, and lieutenant governors.[77]

The irony was that this domination did not promote a community of
feeling within Canada. A nation was not created by deliberate acts of will;
it had to grow into a unified and harmonious whole. The only remedy for
this constitutional impasse was a policy of radical decentralization. If the
powers to tax and to spend were left largely to the provinces, the dominion
would "cease to be regarded as an alien power to which tribute must be
paid, and to be attacked so that a part of that tribute may be disgorged."[78]
This loose federalism, with its emphasis on provincial autonomy, would
allow a free and natural growth of pan-Canadian sentiment. Concerning
the powers of appointment, Macphail stated, "No human being to-day has
more power than the premier of Canada ... Such authority is too great
for any one man to wield. The possibility of naming the man who is,
nominally at least, to wield this power is too great a temptation to those
extra-constitutional entities which prevail in all democracies."[79]

The unnamed powers of course resided in the cities, whose features
Macphail had already described. But it was not simply the existence of areas
of high concentrations of people to which he objected. He linked urbanization with depopulation of the countryside and impoverishment of rural
social life: "The society in the country has nearly perished. Schools are failing with a falling population. Churches are obliged to unite through sheer
weakness."[80] He was also convinced that the changing balance between
town and country entailed a rising cost of living – which in 1913 he estimated as having amounted to 51 percent over twelve years.[81]

Yet the dichotomy of urban and rural life involved much more than
numerical and financial considerations. "There is always a latent dissension
between town and country,"[82] Macphail maintained, and it was the ten-
sion between the values associated with each that prompted him to write
The Land: A Play of Character, in One Act with Five Scenes.[83] The emphasis
throughout this drama is on dialogue rather than action, and the conversations are saturated with didacticism concerning the mores of the business
world, the effects of wealth on its possessors, the qualities of the farmer,
the urban environment, modern education, the family, and, above all, the
proper place of woman. In fact, a website devoted to Canadian adaptations

of William Shakespeare's works has identified *The Land* as: "a loose adaptation of *The Taming of the Shrew*." The writer, Gordon Lester (described as "Project Manager" for the Canadian Adaptations of Shakespeare Project), accuses Macphail of "a disturbing and cynical misogyny" and finds the play to be "a reminder of how Shakespeare was, and can still be, used to promote misogynistic and similarly hateful ideologies."[84]

Most of the leading characters in *The Land* are unhappy, materially oriented city dwellers who privately yearn to renew contact with the soil. The end comes with a decision to exchange the tedium, idleness, and joylessness of the city for the peace and freedom of work on the land. This choice is presented as the sovereign remedy for domestic disharmony arising from the phenomena associated with the "American woman." Even Macphail's description of the personae and the contemporary Montreal setting is heavily weighted. The play opens in "the room of a rich man who has himself no taste but has sense enough to employ men who have, when taste is required. The room was designed by one expert, built by men who gave value in their work."[85] Although called a library, "it retains few of the characteristics of a library, and resembles rather an office."[86] A central figure is described as "older than she seems to be. She has been extraordinarily well preserved by the professional restorers."[87] A student is introduced in the following terms: "His dulness appears to be not congenital but acquired in the process of education."[88] As E.W. Thomson noted in letters to Macphail, who had sent him a draft, these nuances would be better conveyed through reading than performance, and it appears that the play was never produced.[89] A few months prior to Thomson's letters, Macphail had told MacMechan that he was working in a new medium and confessed that he found the material "very refractory";[90] the reference was almost certainly to the drama. Nonetheless, *The Land* remains rich in its revelation of the author's social assumptions.

That Macphail had more than stereotyped abstractions in mind is indicated by a short piece on farming as a way of life, significantly entitled "Prince Edward Island":

> The man who farms only for the money there is in it is a fool,
> because one who can make money out of farming can make a great
> deal more out of something else. But for the man who would live a
> quiet, interesting, reasonable and useful life there is no occupation
> which affords so favorable an opportunity. It demands the exercise of
> every faculty. Every moment of the day is full of surprise, and every

effort has its immediate reward either in success or in failure. For the finest minds it affords an outlet for activity; for the poorest it affords a living without the sordid accompaniament [*sic*] of poverty.

And Prince Edward Island presents a field the freest for all who would live this life.[91]

In spite of this, the Island was in a period of decline. But Macphail went on to express the opinion that the "weakness and cost of factory made goods is being exposed; and as the people discover that they can make those articles for themselves, they will be relieved of the enormous transportation charges which now they bear." He was confident that "as prices rise the exodus will be reversed, and Prince Edward Island and those who live in it will come into their own again."[92] In Macphail's writings of these years, "back to the land" became an incresingly frequent theme, and even his essays in *Canada and Its Provinces* ended on this note.[93]

Macphail also made it clear that he believed the businessman and the farmer were entirely different social types. His emphasis consistently bore on the limitations of the businessman's outlook and the contrasting breadth and versatility of the farmer: "Banking is easy and mixed farming is the most intricate business in the world. It cannot be learned. It must be born with one. It must be fostered in the experience of successive generations."[94] Businessmen were concerned only with narrow details in pursuit of money, the single unquestioned goal that justified any means. "To the farmer leisure is more precious than money, and the more prices advance the more leisurely he becomes, because it requires less to satisfy his needs."[95] Macphail believed that the relationship of the two types was akin to that of the parasite to the host, and he even challenged the contemporary usage of terms: "By a strange perversion the term 'business' has come to be restricted to secondary occupations, to stock-broking, money-lending, distributing goods, and making tools for meeting primary needs. The man who really does the business of the world is the original producer, the farmer, the fisherman, the miner, the artist."[96] The dichotomy was moral, intellectual, and rooted in the daily work of each type. One worked at a wide variety of tasks to meet the necessities of life and produced necessities; the other consumed necessities and worked mindlessly for the accumulation of treasure through the production of commodities of questionable value.

Were Macphail's feet planted firmly on the ground – figuratively speaking – or was he simply, as he has been described, an "urban intellectual

[who] did completely accept the agrarian myth"?[97] In fact, he was much
more than an armchair agrarian. He had intimate experience with both
town and country, and personally embodied qualities of each environment.
In Montreal and in the academic and journalistic worlds he was known
as the epitome of the busy man. He was deeply involved in innumerable
activities in addition to his duties associated with the *University Magazine*,
the *Canadian Medical Association Journal*, and McGill. He gave steady
encouragement to local theatre and played an instrumental role in arrang-
ing for leading companies to visit Montreal. At his own expense, he saw
Marjorie Pickthall's first volume of poetry through the press, bearing the
imprint of the *University Magazine*. He hoped to undertake more publishing ventures, "to remove the discredit which now rests upon us, that all
Canadian books of importance are made out of the country."[98] He participated with MacMechan, Leacock, and others in a temporarily successful
attempt to form a syndicate of Canadian writers to provide the periodicals
and newspapers of Canada with Canadian material. His friends frequently
expressed wonder at his stamina, versatility, and long hours. "You," wrote
MacMechan, "are almost as bad as an American Businessman in the absurd
value which you attach to Time, Time!"[99]

SUMMERS IN ORWELL

MacMechan knew Macphail equally well in his summer retreat at Orwell.
After a visit in 1910 he wrote:

> There is a hospitality in material things and there is a hospitality
> in the things of the spirit. You understand and practise both the
> commoner and the rarer virtue. And although you are not the kind
> of man who likes to be thanked or to have things spelt out, I feel
> that I must tell you how much I enjoyed the few days I spent under
> your "guest-friendly" roof-tree. I am not a great visitor, as the phrase
> goes; it is rarely that I feel completely at my ease, completely at home
> in any house but my own. So I must tell you what is literal fact, - I
> never enjoyed a visit anywhere as I did my days at Orwell. When I
> come to analyze that happiness, I find it composed of many elements.
> Nature has a large part in it. The open rolling country, the mysterious
> sky-line, the freshness, the clear colors, the friendly air, the seclusion
> that was not solitude or loneliness worked their charm upon the
> receptive spirit. Human nature had its part too. I liked your people

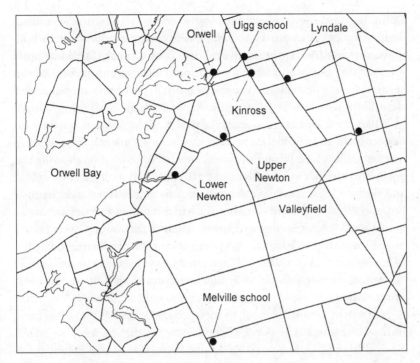

Southeastern Prince Edward Island: Macphail's bailiwick.

very much, by which I mean not only the family but the neighbors and friends. There was an atmosphere of quiet and peace about the place which was most grateful: and the men I came across in my fishing rambles were a new sort, which seemed at the same time as familiar as if I had always known it. I liked their soft low voices and their Highland courtesy ... Another proof [of] your wisdom and the characteristic flavor of your hospitality is the absolute sans-gêne. You should inscribe over your gates "Fay ce que vouldras." It was most delightful to be allowed to do as you pleased.[100]

Macphail did not lose touch with his Island roots. Between 1905 and 1914 he passed every summer at Orwell. Unlike the urban dwellers who "spend a few summer days in the country, but ... exist as isolated communities, disdainful and disdained,"[101] he and his brother Alexander took an active part in community affairs. When fire destroyed the home of a neighbour, a community meeting was held and a ways-and-means committee appointed with Alexander as chairman and Andrew as a member. Within six weeks the family had moved into a bigger and better house. The local press reported that the "Macphail brothers furnished the stone and finished the cellar, ordered the building material, engaged workmen, superintended the building of the house. The public responded generously."[102]

When at the end of the summer of 1909 Andrew donated a bell to the new church in Valleyfield, the district where his paternal grandfather was buried, a Prince Edward Island newspaper noted, "Though living the greatest part of his time in Montreal, in connection with McGill College and Editor of *The University Magazine*, still he prides himself on being a Provincialist and has always taken a lively interest in the welfare of his native land."[103] Another newspaper article stated that "he has never ceased to be identified as an Islander."[104] A poem honouring the donation, entitled "The Church Bell of Valleyfield," appeared in the press.[105] The author was "E.S.M.," who had published "A Tribute" – in prose – to William Macphail upon his death.[106]

More than hospitality and charity occupied the Macphail brothers in those summers. They were vitally concerned that farming on Prince Edward Island should be a viable occupation, and they extolled the benefits of scientific agriculture, crop rotation, and the development of new crops. But they also knew their audience and realized that the Island farmer had not only to be told but also to be shown; once he had seen with his own eyes, he would believe. Thus, beginning about 1908, Andrew and Alexander demonstrated how scientific methods in growing potatoes could dramatically increase the yield, initially growing an area of approximately fifteen acres. They bred new strains of potatoes, including a rectangular potato known as the "Orwell square," and according to Andrew's daughter, founded the local seed potato industry. Encouraged by their success, around 1911 they expanded their acreage in potatoes and ultimately grew between eight and ten varieties. A granddaughter recalled many years later that on a sort of notice board in the sun porch of the house in Orwell during the 1930s, there were many ribbons for the prizes their potatoes had won at the annual provincial exhibition.[107]

Around 1910, they pioneered the cultivation and curing of tobacco on the Island. The experiment was fruitful, and an informant who had worked as a servant in the house recalled in 1990 that the brothers had a large warehouse for their tobacco, some of which they gave to neighbours.[108] In 1911 Macphail sent a sample to Kipling, who smoked "a pipeful" and

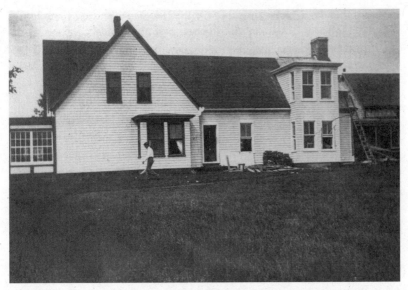

The east side of the Macphail Homestead as it appeared around the year 1912.

pronounced it "perfectly clean bright and good," though he added, "It's a bit full for my taste ... Maybe there will be something in it. After all the man who makes two blades etc. is *the* person."[109] Within a few years Andrew and Alexander, who had their own kiln, marketed a crop of about five hundred pounds, consisting of three varieties of tobacco. The product went on sale in stores in both Orwell and Charlottetown, packed in tins containing two ounces each.[110] The brothers' agricultural operations were sufficiently extensive that at times between five and ten men, as well as they themselves and their children, were at work. These activities attracted the attention of the Island press, and by 1912 the president of the provincial exhibition was writing to Andrew to solicit articles on potatoes and tobacco for the yearly report.[111]

With respect to potatoes, the intent was undoubtedly to improve what was already an important part of commercial agriculture on the Island. In the case of tobacco, a brief draft article or press release on the subject, almost certainly written by Macphail, probably in 1912, survived in his personal papers. It is slightly ambiguous on whether the primary purpose was to set in motion a new sector of commercial agriculture on the Island or to encourage individual farmers to grow for themselves what they would otherwise purchase as an import. Macphail wrote that "with a few hours' work" a smoker who spent twenty or more dollars a year – still a significant sum in 1912 – on tobacco could save that money for himself and the community. But his modest marketing operation was also setting an example, and he argued that although the product was not comparable to the finer grades of Virginia tobacco, "this experiment shows that tobacco can be grown on the Island of a better quality than ... [in] any other part of Canada."[112]

Gordy McCarville, a longtime researcher on the history of the tobacco industry on the Island, has found earlier instances of farmers growing it for their own consumption; by 1897 this was being reported in the Charlottetown press.[113] But documented cases of its growth on the Island for sale to the public before Macphail's efforts, even on a small scale, have not come to light. McCarville has discovered that Donald Nicholson, a tobacco manufacturer in Charlottetown since at least 1882, was ordering seeds in 1911, and there are pictures of him standing in a field of tobacco he had grown on the fringe of Charlottetown in the summer of 1912. As McCarville surmised, "it is certainly quite possible that Nicholson was inspired by Macphail's tobacco growing success."[114] But it was not until the 1960s that a significant tobacco-growing industry took root on the Island.[115]

Macphail's home was something of a local landmark, despite being on an otherwise obscure country road. One approached the house passing between two granite pillars, approximately thirteen feet in height, at the end of the lane. They had originally stood at the front entrance of the Macdonald Engineering Building on the McGill University campus. The structure had been destroyed in a catastrophic fire on 5 April 1907, and Macphail had had the pillars loaded onto a railway flatcar and taken to his home on the Island, where they were installed at the entrance to the property. The engineering building had been only fourteen years old, and Macphail's initiative could be seen as an act of salvage.[116] In Orwell, on the narrow country road, surrounded by trees, the pillars have excited the curiosity of generations of passers-by, Prince Edward Islanders, and others, as a unique feature of the local landscape. One other element made the property distinctive, although it was not visible from the road. Despite a five-year guarantee, the new bell that Macphail had given to the Valleyfield church cracked after five weeks of use and was replaced by the company that had made it. The cracked bell, weighing nearly a ton, is in the yard of Macphail's house in Orwell.[117]

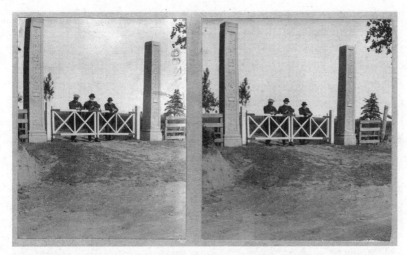

Macphail and friends at the pillars, Macphail Homestead. This stereoscopic slide shows Macphail, on the left, and two unidentified men, possibly neighbours, at the entrance to his property. The pillars had previously been at the front door of the Macdonald Engineering Building on the campus of McGill University. After that structure was destroyed by fire in 1907, Macphail moved the pillars to Orwell, where they became one of the most recognizable landmarks in rural Prince Edward Island.

As noted, the two brothers became widely known in their native province. Alexander was elected to the legislative assembly, and Andrew continued to be mentioned as a possible candidate for Ottawa. Yet it would be a mistake to infer that publicity or political opportunity were the governing motives in their activities during their summers on the Island. No one who reads the annual springtime correspondence between "Jim" and "John," as they continued to call each other, can doubt their genuine eagerness to renew contact with the Island soil. In 1909 Alexander, already in Orwell, wrote to Andrew in Montreal saying, "Planting [potatoes] was the only thing which for many months has given me release from the devil of indifference which has possessed me ... From my height your golf-playing sounds very trivial."[118]

It was the concrete experience of these summers, reinforcing the memories of his earlier years – not mere patrician nostalgia emanating from Montreal – that made Andrew Macphail the "agrarian" intellectual that

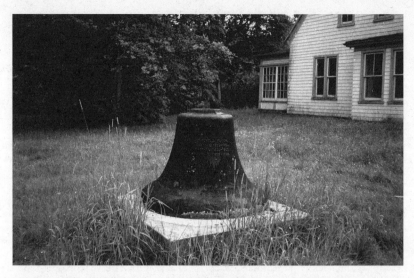

Bell from Valleyfield Church, Macphail Homestead. In 1909 this bell was purchased by Macphail for the new church in Valleyfield, the district where his paternal grandfather had attended church and where he was buried. It cracked in 1910, shortly after installation. The supplier replaced it, and Macphail moved the cracked bell to his property. The inscription reads "Vivos Voco Mortuos Plango [L: I call the living, I mourn for the dead] William Macphail 1802-1852   William Macphail 1830–1905   William Macphail 1859–1893."

he was. Orwell, or more broadly Prince Edward Island, its people, and its way of life were a part of him, and he could not bear to see industrial society encroaching on them and destroying their distinctive character. When telephones came to Orwell, rather than having his road widened and trees cut down, Macphail paid the extra expense to have the poles placed on the parallel Kinross Road and the lines run across to it from Orwell.[119] His own house of course had no telephone. Indeed, he made no concessions to modernity; there was no radio, no washer, or other modern convenience. The candles, the lamps, and the well, with its wooden bucket, remained in use. Everything was to stay as it had been, and nothing was to be unduly disturbed. When he did have occasion to have trees felled, it was always with the warning to "look out for my pet crow" or "watch out for my pet snake."[120] To this sanctuary, this remnant of the real Canada, he welcomed MacMechan, Thomson, Earl Grey, James Mavor, Tait McKenzie, the portraitist Alphonse Jongers, and other academic, artistic, journalistic, and political friends.[121] It is MacMechan, again, who portrayed the host in verse:

A close-lipped man; yea, somewhat saturnine;
A good deal of Mephisto in his air;
A red Satanic beard; cropt, scanty hair;
A forehead plowed by many a thoughtful line;
A Highland accent with a humorous whine;
A scholar's stoop; a disconcerting stare;
Inclined to stoutness (but he does not care);
And Highland legs to prop the whole design.
A Highland voice; and Highland courtesie;
A Highland welcome for the favoured guest,
Who visits him within his Island cell,
Embowered in lush potatoes, wild and free.
Mephisto – (may be!) – to advantage drest,
But Mr. Greatheart underneath the shell.[122]

He enclosed this untitled sonnet in a letter he sent to Macphail. Several years later, during Macphail's absence at war, it was published in the *University Magazine* with two minor changes.[123] Afterwards Thomson wrote to MacMechan, "Often I've mentally applauded your sonnet describing MacPhail [*sic*] – so accurate, so witty it was and is – simply bully."[124]

9

Military Service

How was Canada to return to the simpler way of life that Andrew Macphail remembered and relived each summer? Although an activist in his own way, by 1914 he had not much faith in the efficacy of exhortation. The only lights at the end of the tunnel had a curiously apocalyptic glow. When not predicting that the complexity and consequent vulnerability of urban life would prove its ultimate undoing, he tended to see redemptive qualities in the cultivation of the military virtues and even in the experience of war.

Thus, when the news of war shattered the calm of Orwell in early August 1914, Macphail was anything but dismayed. His nineteen-year-old son Jeffrey, who was to have spent the winter studying in Germany, enlisted immediately. His brother Alexander, age forty-four, belonged to the militia and did the same; he was to spend four years at the front and participate in every battle the Canadian forces fought. Andrew, almost fifty, virtually blind in his left eye, and never having worn a uniform, decided to volunteer as a medical officer. He did more than go through the motions of formally offering his services, for he was determined to be accepted. When rejected, he appealed to the prime minister in the following terms: "A man must save his soul at least, and this seems to be the way for me. One who does his part may await the issue with equanimity."[1] He also appears to have utilized the influence of Principal Peterson. These pressures were effective, and on 28 September Sir Robert Borden informed Macphail that his application was to be granted. Six days later he began the enlistment process in Toronto, where he took a course for newly commissioned officers in foot drill, tactics, and equitation. He was already an accomplished rider: "I remembered this old art as a compensation for advancing age ... For the trials, horses were brought in, and I gave the sergeant a dollar for the worst,

a procedure so reverse that it could not be called improper. He assigned
to me a horse called 'The Devil.' The name by the horse and the pay by the
sergeant were honestly earned. I gained the certificate."[2]

Macphail set his civilian affairs in order before departing for Halifax
on 16 April 1915. He left his Montreal home in the care of a housekeeper,
a secretary, and his seventeen-year-old daughter Dorothy. He took a leave
of absence from McGill and placed his two journals in the hands of com-
mittees. The April 1915 number of the *University Magazine* was the last he
prepared before his departure. He was too absorbed in military, personal,
and editorial matters over the winter to give much attention to his own
writing, but in mid-September he had outlined his initial responses to the
war. The cause was just: "It is a war of civilization; that is, to determine
whether the military or the civil method shall prevail. Our opinion is that
the human mind thrives best in a civil atmosphere. The German opinion is
that the way must be cleared by the sword."[3] The entire German nation was
infused with militarism, he asserted, and it was the role of the Allies to contain and destroy this spirit: "Professor and philosopher alike have extolled
war, not only as a means but as an end in itself, as 'the extreme felicity of
mankind'... They have taken the sword in their hands. Let them perish by
the sword."[4] The Germans were an "outlaw nation."[5]

Although Macphail did not place an intrinsic value in war, he claimed at
least an instrumental justification for it, which he expressed in quasitheo-
logical language:

It may be that, perhaps after all, God really does know what He is
about, and that war, as well as peace, forms a place in His universal
design. It is only now that one perceives how dreadful those days
of peace were: the whole world sunk in sensuality and sloth, where
only the feebler vices and the meaner virtues could thrive in the
stagnant and fetid atmosphere; the whole creation perishing in its
own exhalation, emanation, and excretion. For this corporate sin and
misery war is the only cure ... Already there are signs of an increasing
hardness of fibre, a sense of well being, a feeling of relief from
softness, and of deliverance from the adscititious and unessential.[6]

Macphail even wrote an article on the new camp at Valcartier, which he
had visited at the invitation of Alexander, celebrating the orderly, simple,
efficient, clean, and hard life of the soldier: "a world of youth, and strength,
and beauty." He contrasted these men with the racetrack crowd, wonder-
ing why the shrapnel should be for the soldiers and not for those "business

men in search of excitement, touts alert for money, panders and harlots in pursuit of their prey."[7] In the final analysis, the advantage of war was that it provided a reason for military training: "If half the money which is spent on public schools were spent on military camps, and attendance made compulsory, Canadian boys would be better mannered and better educated too."[8]

The war was to be more than a spiritual purgative for individuals. Macphail hoped it would lead to a regeneration of Canadian society.

For years we had struggled against an industrial and financial system which was making headway in spite of all resistance ... At the first breath of war the whole fabric of speculation came to the ground, and we are free once more. The parasite stands revealed ...

The fabric of that fictitious industry which we have been erecting so sedulously these thirty years past has also gone down. Factories are closing, some as a precaution against loss, some because their owners are already ruined. Industries native to the village and the country were torn up by the roots and transferred to the city. By encouraging we have destroyed. In the era of public poverty that is to come industry will be left to itself to find its proper habitat; and constituencies will be free to vote as they please, uninfluenced by the expenditure of public money. There will be no more contracts: therefore, no more corruption; and public life will be purified as by fire.

When this war is over our citizenship will be no longer an anomaly. We shall be British subjects, nothing less, nothing more.[9]

Already the crucial question of peace and war had been resolved: when the mother country was at war, Canada was at war.[10]

Macphail went to war in high spirits. Over the winter of 1914–15 he had grown impatient at the repeated delays in departure. He wrote to James Mavor in late March, "I am beginning to fear that the war will end too soon; that is, before we derive the full benefit of it in suffering."[11] On 9 January 1915, when he made his one appearance at the Pen and Pencil Club between its season-opening meeting of 3 October and his departure, he was in uniform.[12] He spent several months in England and reported to his daughter that the "conduct of the men is excellent ... Compared with them students are ruffians."[13] In making this comparison, he may have had in mind an incident that occurred on the ship conveying his unit overseas:

"The Engineers have ... a number of young officers from the Royal Military College, and in all my experience ... I have never encountered a dirtier set of young blackguards. Eight of us older men were sitting in the smoking-room when a party of them came in. After ten minutes we all got up and left."[14] But all in all he was highly pleased with his new environment, and he relished the austerity of military life. On 16 September 1915 he arrived in France and two days later heard for the first time heavy guns in serious action: "The sound was mellow and singularly musical. The notes were almost bell-like in their purity."[15]

AT AND NEAR THE FRONT

For more than twenty months Macphail was stationed at the front. Initially commissioned as a lieutenant, he was by then a captain. He served most of his time in France and Belgium with Field Ambulance No. 6 in the 2nd Canadian Division, treating casualties, including prisoners of war, and often dealing with large numbers of patients by himself.[16] He was also "transport officer" for his field ambulance, which meant, in effect, having to attend to logistical matters. These included not only coordinating movement of personnel, vehicles, and equipment but seeing to matters of care and maintenance. In the words of David Campbell, the historian of the division, he was "superlative" as transport officer. Part of his work involved responsibility for some fifty horses, and Lieutenant General E.A.H. Alderson, the British commander of the Canadian Corps, "judged Macphail's horse lines the best in the two Canadian divisions."[17] Alderson, according to historian J.M. Bourne, an authority on the British forces in the First World War, "was a master of everything connected with horses"[18] – consequently, a most competent judge. Thus, Macphail's early life on the farm in Orwell served him well in this respect.

During the war Macphail kept diaries. Entries were not made every day, and there might be a gap of several days; but sometimes there was more than one entry for a single day. His entries relate the horrors of the conditions in which the war was fought, the sense of uncertainty about the fate of one's daily companions (whether each meeting would be the last, for example), and the psychological impact on the men. "The effect of ... [trench] life is first to destroy the will, then to suppress the emotions," he wrote on 8 February 1916.[19] Just over eight months later, on 14 October, he wrote, "At last I am tired, as if I could do no more, as if two years were enough ... In the afternoon I slept for two hours, and wished I were dead on

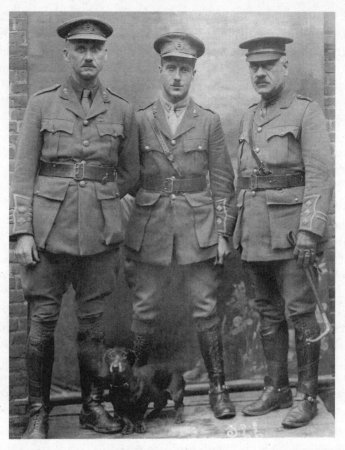

Andrew (*right*) with his son Jeffrey and brother Alexander during the First World War. At their feet is Macphail's dog Kemmel, which he had purchased in Paris in February 1916 and to which he was deeply attached. Kemmel's accidental death later in the year left Macphail overwhelmed with grief.

the Somme ... I see no end to the war."[20] The diaries also provide much trenchant commentary on the high command, on the politics that determined promotions, and the lack of congruence between the combatant officers in the field and the staff officers who planned in ignorance of all-important local conditions – an unfamiliarity with the facts on the ground which he believed obstructed the war effort.

Macphail had the comfort of knowing that Alexander and Jeffrey were sufficiently near for most of this time for regular visits to be possible. On 29

October 1915 Jeffrey celebrated his twenty-first birthday with his father. Yet Macphail was necessarily conscious of the danger that could strike them, and on 23 March 1916 he recorded in his diary that his brother believed "they" – and especially Alexander – might die during the coming summer.[21] Despite his surroundings, Macphail apparently felt very tranquil much of the time and took pleasure in observing the agricultural and domestic practices of the areas he passed through. The less mechanized the methods, the more he approved. He reported to Peterson, "All reading and writing have gone from me. I gave away my last book, 'The Tempest.'"[22] In a letter to a member of the Pen and Pencil Club, he added the following curious detail about the donation. He had given his copy of *The Tempest* to the daughter of the man in whose house he was billeted: "I apologised to her for not having offered to her the greatest compliment a man could offer to a woman and endeavoured to console her by explaining that this was a life of temperance, poverty and obedience, but when the war was over it would be different."[23]

When Macphail had his first leave in England, he visited Rudyard Kipling at Bateman's Burwash in Sussex, where at one time or another during the war, Alexander, Jeffrey, and Dorothy were also made welcome. During his visit Macphail made the acquaintance of Sir Max Aitken, the notorious Canadian financier, whom he had always regarded with distaste: "I could not refrain from a certain admiration of the man, as one who had beaten the financial crooks at their own game, the English at the social game, and the politicians at the political game." He noted that "after luncheon he went quite out of his way to be polite to me."[24] It was the beginning of a friendship that would blossom in the 1920s and 1930s. Back at the front, Macphail was visited by the novelist Ralph Connor (the pen name of the Reverend C.W. Gordon), who was serving as a Protestant chaplain. Gordon was one of the social gospellers whom Macphail may have had in mind when excoriating the movement in prewar days; he was also a "temperance advocate" and as such would have been a likely object of derision for Macphail and Stephen Leacock, among others, at meetings of the Pen and Pencil Club. But in his diary Macphail recorded, "I liked him well. He is quiet and reflective."[25]

Macphail spent fourteen months with Field Ambulance No. 6 before being posted to the office of the assistant director of medical services for the 2nd Canadian Division on 22 November 1916. Although now a staff officer, he remained within approximately six miles of the front line, and a week after taking up his new posting he was able to ride over to see his old field ambulance colleagues; the following month he ate Christmas dinner with them.[26] Yet there was a significant change in Macphail's perspective now that he was no longer at the front on a daily basis; his comments became much more favourable with regard to the work the staff did.[27] His role had changed, and with it his viewpoint. So had perceptions of him: in his diary entry for 1 January 1917 he acknowledged that he was coming to be looked on as being "of 'the Staff.'"[28] Nonetheless, an ambiguity remained in his attitude regarding the staff element within the army, as is evident from a certain grim pleasure he took at news of the burning of the Canadian Corps headquarters offices later that month.[29] And he continued to have occasional graphic reminders of the hardships men in the trenches experienced. On 16 March 1917, exactly eighteen months after his arrival in France, he wrote, "So long as I live the remembrance will be with me of the walk down Guillemot trench to Vistula, 1000 yards, each step to the knee, and it required all the strength of my arms to pull my foot out of the mud. Barrett [his batman] who was with me lost his rubber boots and socks. He came in bare-footed and bleeding."[30]

During Macphail's time at and near the front line, whatever exhilaration he had formerly felt disappeared; he was reminded of this when he encountered the enthusiasm of a new man. In its place was a mixture of resignation and disillusionment.[31] He found the society of many fellow officers trying: "The heaviest cross I have to bear is the company I have to endure."[32] The Mess was a particular trial, and he likened it to what one would face at a cheap hotel: "Those who do not care for the company take refuge in gloom and silence."[33] Part of his complaint was aesthetic; on 29 April 1917 he wrote in his diary of "the utter illiteracy of the men with whom I have to associate. Their poverty of mind discloses itself in the horrible jargon and worn out slang which they employ."[34] His sense of isolation became extreme after the death in September 1916 of a medical officer he had found particularly congenial – Lieutenant Colonel R.P. Campbell, a former demonstrator at McGill.[35]

The most objectionable aspect of military life was the officers' treatment of the men. By following the rules too closely, an officer "loses all sight of humanity," he wrote in his diary. "The inhumanity of the service is appalling to me. It is only under the most exceptional circumstances that one can do the slightest favour for a man without breaking some regulation."[36] Macphail's diaries reveal much more affection for the enlisted men than for his peers; indeed, he frequently acted as a "prisoner's friend" at disciplinary proceedings, with as much success as possible in such cases. His morale

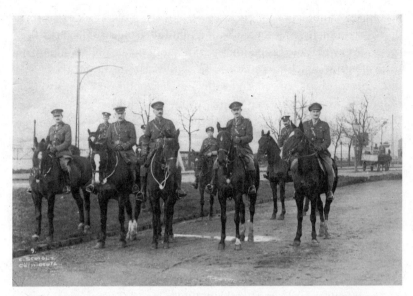

Soldiers on horseback. Macphail is pictured here (*third from the left*) with his brother Alexander (*next to him, on his left*) in Germany. He is riding Gypsy II, which he had selected in England. At the end of the war he purchased the horse and took her to Orwell.

reached perhaps its lowest point when he was assigned as the medical officer attending the execution on 29 October 1916 of one of the twenty-five Canadians who died by firing squad in the First World War. His distress was not owing to squeamishness, for as a young reporter he had witnessed several executions, and as a civilian pathologist he had performed thirteen autopsies on persons judicially hanged.[37]

The inhumanity of life in the army probably accounts in part for the intensity of his feelings for his dog Kemmel, a dachshund he had acquired when on leave in Paris during February 1916, and his horse Gypsy II. Of Kemmel, he wrote on 9 July 1916, "I cannot tell how grateful and how much I am indebted to this dog."[38] When Kemmel was run over and killed by a truck a few months later, Macphail was devastated: "All interest in my work, in my future, in the war has vanished, and a great desolation has come upon me … He was through the trenches with me at Ypres and in the horror of the Somme, yet always lovely and pleasant."[39] Macphail had obtained Gypsy II in 1915 when selecting horses in England for his field ambulance, as part of his duties as transport officer; he had named her after his mother's favourite horse, which he had acquired for her. At the end of the war he purchased the horse and took her to Orwell, where she lived for many years – among other things, teaching several children to walk by allowing them to use her foreleg for balance.[40]

TO HQ, RECOGNITION

In early 1917 Macphail wrote, "I have seen all of war that I desire to see. I know every move and operation. The interest is gone."[41] Thus, at the end of May, after having served on such fields as Ypres, the Somme, and Vimy, he accepted with some relief a transfer to Canadian Medical Services headquarters in London, where he remained until leaving for Canada in 1919. Once in London he had second thoughts, but he was persuaded by Alexander, who was still at the front, not to return. In June he received a promotion to the rank of major. That summer, for the first time, he and Dorothy visited the ancestral home at Inverairnie, Scotland.[42]

On 1 January 1918 Buckingham Palace announced that Macphail would be knighted early in the new year. He was pleased but could not resist commenting to Archibald MacMechan, "This mark of honour from 'the other King' I take as a sign that the 'Cause' is really lost, and we may now very well let bygones be bygones."[43] There seems to be no precise explanation for his knighthood, but reason suggests that the predominant element was his literary achievements. His military service as such was not greater than that of thousands of other Canadians; what made it exceptional was his peculiar circumstances in terms of age, disability, and public prominence, and consequently the example he was setting. One writer declared:

I would fain believe that this knighthood means recognition of Canadian letters. Of Macphail it might be said as of Goldsmith, he attempted almost every kind of writing. There are his three volumes of essays, the most brilliant and the most subtle ever produced in Canada, his novel, his play. He established a quarterly review which gave a new tone and new direction to Canadian thought; he edited with success a medical journal; he compiled an anthology, 'The Book of Sorrow' which attracted wide attention. He has written verse. Almost as valuable as his personal services is the encouragement he has given to Canadian writers.[44]

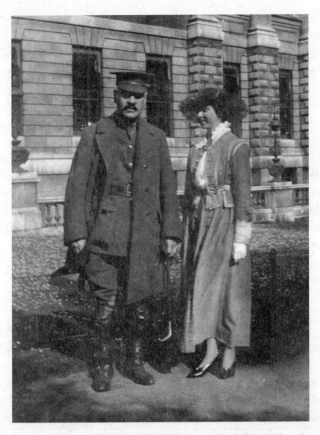

Andrew with his daughter Dorothy during the First World War. The photograph
was probably taken in London, where Dorothy had arrived on 8 May 1916;
Macphail was on leave there for several days in June. Dorothy worked for the Red
Cross during much of the war.

Macphail kept his literary talents in abeyance for much of the war. In
1916 his anthology of verse, *The Book of Sorrow*, which included two of his
own poems, appeared. He had compiled it many years earlier, following
the death of his wife, and the war simply provided an appropriate occasion for publication. It seemed "to have been born for such a time as this,"
MacMechan told him. "If you had never done anything but this, you had
done a great work. It is something which must come very near to many a
lacerated heart."[45] Macphail took unusual pride in the book and stated in

the preface that it "contains all that has been said, all, indeed, that can be said upon the theme of Sorrow."[46]

Unless one counts portions of letters that E.W. Thomson published in his newspaper columns, virtually nothing of an original nature came from Macphail until 22 June 1917, when he delivered the Cavendish Lecture to the West London Medico-Chirurgical Society. The lectureship, reserved for medical men, had been founded in memory of the physician and chemist Henry Cavendish. Macphail was only the second Canadian to receive this honour, and he spoke on the theme of "A Day's Work" – the taking of Vimy Ridge. The address was inspirational in tone and consisted of a vivid description of the work of a field ambulance in battle. He included some general observations on the scientific spirit, the defining characteristics of the English nation, and similar topics. He concluded with a reaffirmation of his belief in the value of war: "It restores simplicity to life ... This generation has been dominated by the machine ... that in future ... will have less power."[47]

RETREAT FROM CRITICISM

A notable feature of the Cavendish Lecture, coming as it did after the February revolution in Russia, was Macphail's attack on the "lesser intellectual breeds." He counselled his audience, "Mistrust your 'intelligentsia,' mere bores and busybodies, who seize the moment to put into effect their vagaries ... These are no times for experiments."[48] It was Macphail's most categorical condemnation to date of intellectuals as a group. The war was a time for deeds, not words, and with its advent he came to place more faith in men of action and less in men of letters. Even before leaving Canada he had urged wholesale enlistment on the university community: "A blank in the calendar for 1914–1915 would be much more significant than anything which can be said at Convocation next May."[49] He appears also to have seriously considered discontinuing the *University Magazine*.[50]

The wartime experience marks a watershed in Macphail's development as a social and political commentator. Never again would he be so uninhibited as he had been in assailing specific governments and parties, naming names, and so on. For the duration of the war, the cutting edge of his criticism was dulled. Although his diaries manifest considerable dissatisfaction with the conduct of the war effort, his disillusion was not made fully public until the end of the 1920s. Delay in speaking out is readily understandable in the context of his commitment to the war.

Yet even in peacetime, after Armageddon had become a memory, there was a new restraint in his dealing with the particulars of public life. In these later years Macphail oscillated between abstention from comment and condemnation in general terms. Although he sporadically resumed his critique of fundamental social tendencies, he blunted his articulation of dissatisfaction with the status quo when mentioning persons and groups in power. This "moderating" process had begun with prewar alarm at "theorists" and militant feminists. If he had to choose between those in authority and those who styled themselves radicals or revolutionaries, he would unequivocally stand with the former – which was a far cry from the days when he had read and admired Gustavus Myers's *History of Canadian Wealth*.[51]

Most of Macphail's articles in these years were straightforward descriptions of various aspects of his wartime experience. The titles of such pieces as "An Ambulance at Rest," "The War: A Wet Night," and "The Bridge-head" indicate their contents.[52] The precision and simplicity of military life are brought home to the reader through graphic narratives. The most ambitious essay Macphail composed overseas was also closely related to the war. Ninety-five pages in length, "John McCrae: An Essay in Character" constitutes the bulk of a book, *In Flanders Fields and Other Poems*, devoted to the memory of the Canadian poet, who had died early in 1918. McCrae had been a lecturer in pathology at McGill before enlisting in the medical services, and many of his twenty-nine poems accompanying the essay had first appeared in the *University Magazine*. Macphail, who had known McCrae since 1900 and had shared many Saturday evenings with him at the Pen and Pencil Club, appears to have been requested by the poet's family to undertake the task, which he completed on Armistice Day. The result was a sensitive portrait of his dead colleague and the effect the war had had on him. Discursive, personal, and interspersed with McCrae's letters, it displayed to the full the author's talents as an essayist. Sir Robert Falconer, president of the University of Toronto, wrote to Macphail that it was "well done, particularly as a revelation of yourself."[53]

Macphail's comments on the Canadian scene were necessarily limited by his absence. His only trip home was in November and December 1917. He had an audience with the prime minister in Ottawa and then proceeded to Prince Edward Island, where Borden had asked him to contest the constituency of Queens as a Unionist during the election to be held on 17 December. But Macphail decided not to do so when it became apparent that he would not be acclaimed. He also visited Halifax, Toronto, and of course Montreal, making eighteen speeches on contemporary themes. Although he delivered an address entitled "War and Business" to the Canadian Club of Toronto, Macphail let the opportunity pass without admonishing the businessmen present. He contented himself with an account of the accomplishments of the army and a plea to support the men at the front. He informed James Mavor that although he could not "speak at any 'political' meeting," he had "managed to say the things desirable to be said without infringing the technical regulations."[54] The Montreal *Gazette* recounted the delicacy with which this was accomplished on one occasion: "After giving his address, Major Macphail withdrew from the hall to fill other engagements, and the meeting at once resolved into a political assembly for the support of the Union Government ... and Sir Herbert Ames as the candidate of that Government."[55] A conscriptionist since 1914, Macphail described his purpose in a letter to Borden as "present[ing] the reasons why your government should be returned."[56]

Prior to the election, Macphail published an article entitled "In This Our Necessity." He began by stating that in early November he "came into this country with vision of a people united in heart and resolution. At the first touch of reality the vision faded, and there arose instead the spectre of a people divided in counsel, antagonistic in race, antipathetic in religion."[57] He noted that Canadians were indulging in the luxury of peacetime pursuits during a war, and warned the electorate that they would be voting "before God and the Army."[58] To drive this point home, he alluded to Oliver Cromwell. Nonetheless, in the election Borden's Unionists won only 3 of 65 seats in Quebec while taking 150 of 170 in the rest of Canada. The results, particularily the isolation of Quebec, were a profound disappointment to Macphail. He wrote to MacMechan, "The illusion of Confederation perished on Monday ... The French Canadians hate us: they always did."[59] Without enthusiasm he went back to London.

One cannot close this section of a study of Macphail's life without reflecting on the effect the war had had on him personally. It had seared him. He recognized the impact at a personal level on those around him. In a letter to Tait McKenzie on 12 June 1918 he had written regarding his son and his brother: "Jeffrey ... is old, haggard, dull. 40 months at the front has left an indelible mark. Jim [Alexander] is an old man."[60] About himself he was less forthcoming. But Kipling noticed, and wrote to Aitken as early as November 1916, that Macphail "has worked and suffered like a devil ... and lived in every Hell that your Armies have endured. *You* know what a Field Ambulance means. Now he is finished – used up – worn out."[61]

To the observer attempting to make sense as a whole of Macphail and his attitude to the war and his experiences in it, one of the most striking impressions is that of contradictions. His views on a number of matters oscillated from one pole to another. Before he joined the staff, first on the Continent and then in London he had been contemptuous of it; but once part of it, he was impressed by how hard the staff worked. He had previously seen the regulation of so many details of soldiers' lives as a bane, but he now understood the reasons for all of it. At the front he had been sympathetic to the psychological trauma of soldiers, and he had recognized the difficulty in finding a balance between fair treatment of the soldier and the just demands of the army; but in later published comments he was be utterly dismissive of "shell shock."[62] While some of his references to the enemy are of the conventionally stereotyped variety, there are occasions of real doubt about the dichotomy between "them" and "us." For example, on New Year's Day 1917 he wrote in his diary, "We took up arms against the 'Prussian spirit.' Now the spirit is entering into our own hearts."[63] Already in his diary he had noticed authoritarian, inhumane attitudes developing even in men with whom he felt a kinship, compared with his wartime colleagues as a whole: "This quality I understand to be the militarism which we ascribe to the Germans."[64]

The prevalence of self-contradiction and uncertainty about fundamentals in a person who was normally as consistent as Macphail probably reflects the intensity of the wartime experience, the extent to which he was driven to the limit of his capacity for endurance, and the gap between what he had expected of the war and his comrades and what the reality was.

The End of the *University Magazine*

When Andrew Macphail returned to Canada in March 1919 he faced a dispiriting situation. Many of his prewar and wartime friends, including John McCrae, Fayette Brown, R.P. Campbell, and his brother-in-law Jeffrey Burland, were dead. The *University Magazine* was faltering; Sir William Peterson and E.W Thomson were incapacitated; and the war years had taken their toll on his own health. Both he and his brother Alexander suffered great pain from neuritis – in the latter's case an aggravation of a prewar ailment. Andrew's eyes troubled him frequently, and he had been obliged to use eyedrops throughout the war. He contracted glaucoma and on 9 April 1919 entered hospital for treatment. For about seven weeks he was confined indoors and then was not permitted to use his eyes for reading until the autumn. On 20 April, with his formal discharge from the army, he resumed civilian status.[1]

RESUMPTION OF CIVILIAN LIFE

Macphail had gone to war in his fiftieth year with extravagant and, as events proved, misplaced expectations. Throughout the 1912–14 period his writing had been suffused with pessimism in the wake of the failure of reciprocity and imperial reorganization, the impairment of his eyesight, Alexander's disappointing venture into Island politics, the dispute with G.N. Morang over the *University Magazine* finances, and the rise of such movements as feminism and the social gospel. The guns of August 1914 had lifted the gloom. War was to be the cleanser. It was to purge the collective soul and clarify the politics of Canada. To a certain extent, war met Macphail's personal needs for a simpler, more ordered and predictable way of living. At the end of 1916 he could write in his diary that it had been "a happy year, the happiest I ever spent … All the years between 1885 and 1914 seem to have slipped away out of my life, and the ends to have closed together."[2] He remained convinced that military service improved the conduct of the individual soldier.[3] But the war had also reintroduced French-English divisions into domestic politics, weakened the imperial connection, and advanced industrialization, reinforcing the hold of the parasites. It had not brought deliverance.

The exhilaration Macphail had expressed at the prospect of war in 1914 raises the question of whether he can be accurately categorized as a militarist. The answer requires an understanding of his reasons for welcoming the war. At the base of his unaccustomed enthusiasm was a concept of character, which underpinned both his view of education and his conservatism in general. The military life, with its emphasis on discipline, humility, and austerity would instil in young Canadian men a disposition towards obedience. They would have well-defined roles and would act accordingly, with deference to those above and with due regard for the humanity of those below. The instrumental value of war was to perform the task that schools were neglecting. Indeed, Macphail would have been satisfied with much less than war, for, as he wrote in the autumn of 1914, the "advantage of war is that it provides a reason for military training."[4] In the prewar years he had not advocated military training for preparedness, much less for wars of conquest. His reasoning was exactly the reverse: the justification of war was the concomitant training, with its regenerative effects on the trainees and ultimately on society at large. Preparedness definitely took second place behind character building as a rationale for military training. Indeed, preparedness may even have taken third place, behind the potentially positive effects on the evolution of imperial relations because, Macphail hoped, the organization of military training would lead to closer integration of the empire for planning purposes and therefore a greater role for Canada within a politically reorganized empire. All this could happen without war.

Hence, if "militarist" means one who desires to foster both a strong military organization and the military spirit for essentially warlike purposes, Macphail does not meet the description. He did not desire that military institutions become dominant within society, and in later years, writing about the British soldier who had been chief of the Imperial General Staff in the First World War, he made his position on this point absolutely explicit, declaring that the "essence of the British Army is loyalty to the King, *support of His Majesty's Government*, fidelity to comrades, submission of self to the common good, resolution in the face of the enemy."[5] Macphail only praised the military spirit because he believed it would counteract the enfeebling effects of modern society. Yet in the end, war simply deepened his gloom about the direction of Canadian development and introduced new inhibitions into his writing. One of his last hopes had come to naught.

Macphail resumed writing and editing on a full-time basis in the autumn of 1919. As he had already relinquished the editorial chair of the *Canadian Medical Association Journal* to a McGill colleague, A.D. Blackader, he was able to devote his energies entirely to the *University Magazine*. In 1915 he had entrusted his duties to a four-person "local committee," of which Peterson was the driving force. The other members were drawn from the McGill faculty: Stephen Leacock, historian C.W. Colby, and Paul Lafleur, professor of English and of comparative literature. F.P. Walton was not involved, although his name remained on the editorial committee, as listed on the inside cover of each issue of the magazine, through December 1915. Walton had left Canada for Egypt (and had resigned as dean of law) by the spring of 1914, but Macphail, ever the diplomat in matters relating to the magazine, had allowed his name to remain because, as he explained to Peterson, academic people were often sensitive about such matters.[6]

Peterson had taken a deep interest in the journal since its inception; he had always proofread the entire magazine, and Macphail had consulted him regularly about contributions bearing on classics. After the April 1915 number, he had taken full command. The extent of his control was indicated by the fact that at one point he more or less refused to reprint an article by Macphail that had appeared in another journal. Peterson used his power to institute certain changes in the magazine's format. Issues began with about fifteen pages of "Topics of the Day," short commentaries on the war and other contemporary themes by individual editors or friends of the magazine. Of the "local committee," only Lafleur did not contribute to "Topics of the Day"; other writers, not members of the committee, who did contribute included the philosopher J.W.A. Hickson and the university administrator Walter Vaughan. In December 1915 Peterson introduced a second innovation, a book review section managed by S.B. Slack of the McGill Classics Department. The emphasis was to be upon works dealing with Canadian or imperial politics.[7]

Since Macphail was no longer present to meet deficits with his own money, Peterson decided to put greater effort into obtaining advertising revenue. As an economy measure, payment was to be promised only for articles commissioned by the editors. Payment of contributors became more

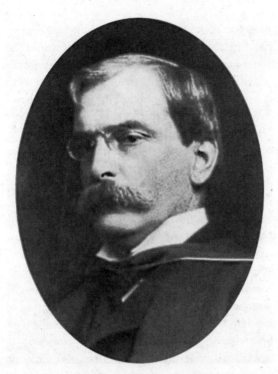

Sir William Peterson. Principal of McGill University from 1895 to 1919, Peterson was a distinguished classicist who supported Macphail's quarterly, the *University Magazine*, from the beginning, proofreading the entire copy. He was in control when Macphail was absent during the First World War, but despite his best efforts, it declined in quality and circulation.

and more infrequent throughout the four years of Macphail's absence. Consequently, by 1918 the *University Magazine* under Peterson had made a profit of $1,400 or $1,500, which was applied to the money owing Macphail. Another result was a decline in quality, since good articles became more difficult to obtain; as well, the journal actually shrank by about a hundred pages a year. Coupled with this tendency, and aggravating it, was an increasing flow of patriotic bombast concerning the war effort and the imperial connection. As the struggle dragged on, a bellicose chauvinism that did nothing for the reputation of the magazine became more evident in the editorial notes and some of the articles. Circulation, which for one reason or another had declined to 2,100 by early 1915, further decreased to 1,400 or 1,500 by March 1918.[8]

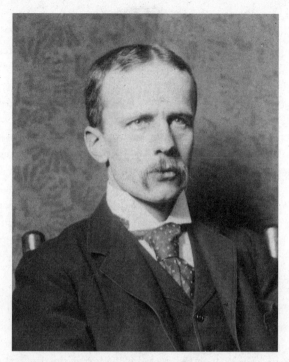

Paul T. Lafleur. A literature professor at McGill University, he was also a longtime active member of the Pen and Pencil Club. During Macphail's absence on military service, he played an important role in keeping the *University Magazine* publishing. He was legendary for his personal quirks.

Peterson had done his best to maintain the magazine at its previous level. But he lacked Macphail's leisure for the task and seems also to have lacked his extraordinary ability in handling people. Through a misunderstanding in 1916 with the prickly James Mavor, he lost the collaboration of both him and W.J. Alexander. In addition, relations with Pelham Edgar appear to have been periodically strained. Given these circumstances, Peterson, who had pledged his services only for a year, told Macphail in February 1918 that it was "absolutely necessary"[9] to reorganize the *University Magazine* completely. For some time he and Lafleur had been doing almost all the work; Leacock had resigned from the "local committee" in 1916, and Colby had been residing in New York City since 1917. The resignation of Leacock may have been linked to another personality conflict since, according to one source, he and Lafleur, although both among Macphail's closest friends at

McGill, simply did not get along.[10] Leacock described Lafleur as "touchy as a sensitive plant," and comments by John Macnaughton and Peterson in letters to Macphail seem to support this. Various anecdotes also testify to Lafleur's sharpness of tongue and irascibility, and hint at a sense of self-importance.[11]

In the face of all his difficulties, Peterson wanted a regular editor appointed, a vigorous drive for subscriptions begun, and new financial arrangements made. He proposed that a joint-stock company be organized, which would enable the new editor to solicit articles and pay contributors. When Macphail seemed ambivalent in his response, Peterson offered on 29 April to personally buy out his financial claim on the journal. The two met in London that summer and resolved their differences: Macphail gave Peterson a free hand and offered to put up $1,000 of the estimated $10,000 or $15,000 necessary for the magazine's reorganization. But the plans were never carried out; by November the war was over, and Peterson decided to leave things for Macphail to settle.[12]

When Macphail was still recovering from glaucoma in 1919 he inquired of President Falconer whether the University of Toronto would resume its former grant (raised to $1,000) for a period of two or three years. He indicated that he would be willing to let the editorial chair go to someone in Toronto, as had been suggested periodically during the war. Falconer, who along with Edgar had remained sympathetic to the undertaking and had in the previous year suggested a merger with the *Queen's Quarterly*, replied that there was no hope of financial aid. "When I send you such discouraging word it may be adding insult to injury to say that such a valuable magazine should not be allowed to disappear. The fact of its being edited in Toronto would not matter. Your own editorship would be accepted by everyone as being obviously the best."[13]

The prospects for the *University Magazine* were bleak. The subscription list had fallen to 1,400, and there was still a debt of some $3,000 on the operations over the past twelve years. Of the old editorial committee, only Edgar and Archibald MacMechan were functional; although Peterson's name remained on the inside cover, he had suffered a stroke in January 1919. The sole new member was Walton's successor as the dean of law at McGill, Robert Warden Lee, who had joined in 1918. Nonetheless, Macphail's enthusiasm returned, and in October the *University Magazine* appeared. His old policies were resumed: "Topics of the Day" and the book review section were eliminated, timely articles were sought, and contributors were again paid.[14]

In late 1919 and early 1920, through a series of articles and public addresses, Macphail expressed his disquiet about the peace settlement, the effect of the war on the British connection, the contemporary obsession with diplomatic "status," and the changing character of Canada itself. Although at the beginning of the war he had written of the prospect of spoils arising out of the "complete destruction" of Germany, he had long since taken a more moderate view of what constituted a desirable settlement. He was aware from his experience in France of the French desire for a Carthaginian peace, and in early January 1919 he had confided his apprehension to Rudyard Kipling. He feared Woodrow Wilson's "pre-occupation with laws, leagues, and legislation." Men such as Wilson had all the enthusiastic fervour of the amateur. By way of contrast he noted, "In all our previous wars we followed one principle: that we must continue to live in the same world with our enemies; ... the method worked." He appealed to Kipling: "You can do much to make wise and sane counsels to prevail in this awful moment, when our soul also is at stake, and you have a right, even better than mine, to speak. My fear is that the business will fall into the hands of lawyers, pedants, and traders who see only a victim to be destroyed with the sacrifice. We are not God."[15]

Macphail made no secret of his views, and at Mavor's suggestion he published his reflections on John Maynard Keynes's book, *The Economic Consequences of the Peace*. He agreed with Keynes in all the essentials of his case against the Treaty of Versailles and its authors, particularly Wilson:

> The only person in the transaction who was entirely sincere
> was President Wilson himself, as sincere as the young man from
> "Hickville" who comes to Wall Street with the model of an invention
> for producing perpetual motion, sincere as the madman who paces
> the corridor, believing and proclaiming that he is the saviour of the
> world. Such a situation is the stuff of all the comic books ...
>
> And the United States Senate is the only legislative body that was
> sincere – to continue to employ Mr. Keynes' term – in the discussion
> of the Treaty. They proceeded to examine very thoroughly this
> strange gift horse, and especially the teeth.[16]

Macphail was even more pessimistic than Keynes, for if the diagnosis was correct, "any remedy is too feeble and too late, but final sanction is given to the old judgement, that things are what they are, and the consequences of them will be what they will be."[17]

If the solemn commitments of the League of Nations meant anything, Macphail had a suggestion that would put the matter to a rigorous test. Article 19 stated that the assembly held the power to recommend reconsideration of treaties that had become outdated and whose continuance might threaten world peace. Conveniently discounting the Intercolonial and National Transcontinental railway routes, Macphail asserted that for five months of each year Canada, aside from the Maritimes, lacked a secure means of communication with the Atlantic Ocean: "All access to the ocean, even by the St. Lawrence, is under direct control of the United States, on account of the projection of the State of Maine to within 30 miles of the St. Lawrence. This one outpost dominates the life of Canada."[18] Such a situation, the result of an anachronistic treaty "drawn up far in advance of events,"[19] was obviously a latent danger to world peace. Accordingly, Macphail proposed that the United States turn over to Canada some 8,000 square miles of Maine.[20]

It is perhaps a measure of the times that this expression of views was apparently taken seriously in many quarters, particularly in the United States. During the U.S. Senate's debate on the Treaty of Versailles, a section protecting American boundaries was added to "Reservation Five." Sir Robert Borden appears to have been unsure how to respond to the proposal. When Macphail had first mentioned it to him in 1918, he had replied confidentially, "I should not have much expectation that [it] ... would succeed. The wishes of the population in the area mentioned would have to be taken into account and ... a favourable response could hardly be expected." He suggested that Macphail prepare a confidential memorandum.[21] Macphail did so, and when he presented it he gravely stated that he had designed it "with some care, as if it were to come under the eye of the President of the United States. My instinct," he told Borden, "is that the proposal would be instantly accepted by him, and by the people if the idea were slowly instilled into their minds."[22]

ON POSTWAR CANADA: CONSERVATISM, QUEBEC, WOMEN, AND DEMOCRACY

In a more serious vein, Macphail proclaimed his scorn for Canada's role in the making of the new international order: "Canada called a session of Parliament at the cost of a million dollars, and signed the Treaty without knowing what it meant, without considering its implications, without the slightest intention of carrying out its terms." In contrast, the "United

States Senate considered and reserved; it has been scrupulous to let the world know where it stands." If Canada had achieved a certain "status" by signing, it was "as another young man from the country achieves financial status when he puts his name on the back of a note already drawn up for the convenience of his signature."[23] A nation was not forged by signatures on meaningless treaties and membership in meaningless debating organizations. There were other considerations that Macphail believed would prove more important in the long term: he feared that Canada was being manoeuvred

> beyond the pale of Empire, her ancient heritage of loyalty to her
> King, veneration for the past, and love of the land from which she is
> sprung, all filched away and exchanged for a "status" ... If this is to be
> the end ... then of the dead it may well be confessed that they have
> died in vain ... Canada in a memorable debate was once likened to "a
> ripe apple ready to fall from the tree." What happens to a ripe apple
> when it falls to the ground is a matter of common knowledge.[24]

Macphail turned to the postwar domestic scene with equal denunciatory vigour. The net effect of the war had been to deepen, sharpen, and broaden his perspective. His first major pronouncement, "The Conservative," was a remarkable article, parts of which he delivered as addresses to Canadian Clubs in Montreal, Quebec, and Hamilton. He set out to identify explicitly the contemporary spirit in its various guises. He reiterated his belief that a conservative or a liberal was born as such.[25] The lines had become blurred in the Canada of his time, and both Liberal and Conservative parties had adopted "the low and interested ethics of business which is love of gain, and the root of all political evil." Yet there remained a mass constituency for a principled conservative movement: "Farmers everywhere are Conservative. They merely ask to be let alone ... Their theory of life is to take what they can get, be it much or little. The more they get the less they work. They do not love work for its own sake."[26]

The most striking aspect of Macphail's essay on "The Conservative" was the blossoming of his latent sympathy and admiration for French Canada: "Canada can only be saved by the Conservative spirit, and that spirit in organized form exists only in Quebec."[27] The French Canadian family, church, and school were all successful where their English Canadian counterparts were not: in inculcating a conservative cast of mind. Quebec women still bred, and their large families were instrumental in making farming a viable occupation. The schools of Quebec were reserved for an élite. Anyone with the required talent could start on the road to the professions, but those who were neither fitted nor motivated remained on the farm and learned the vocations of their fathers. Consequently, they were "the best farmers in Canada." They were also "the best craftsmen, and have never learned to rely upon the factory alone."[28]

The centre of this well-ordered and traditional way of life was the Roman Catholic Church. It guided the family and the educational system but abstained from the reformist political dabblings that were leading Protestant churches astray. Priests were not to be found at labour or prohibitionist meetings. "The spirit of Quebec is an ancient brooding spirit, and has made of that Province a haven for good sense, political wisdom, and personal freedom. If this spirit is left undisturbed Quebec will become the last refuge of civilization upon this continent."[29] In the month following publication of "The Conservative," the Pen and Pencil Club, with Macphail in the chair, passed a resolution (as already noted) explicitly declaring Quebec to have achieved this distinction already; it was in the context of a discussion of Prohibition.[30]

Quebec's most persistent disturber was Ontario, and Macphail left no doubt about where his preferences lay. He used Ontario's educational system as a foil in expounding the virtues of the Quebec approach: "Quebec believes in education. Ontario believes in schools."[31] In response to Ontarian sneers at the quality of Quebec French, he wrote that the "speech of the complete victim of the Ontario public school is scarcely intelligible. He has a language of his own."[32] Macphail admired the cultural achievements of Quebecers; they "have been *couronné* by the French Academy: Canada is ignorant of them, and that ignorance is made the ground for a charge of illiteracy against Quebec."[33] He rejoiced in the increasing use of French in Montreal, and unlike newspaper editor and author Robert Sellar, detected no tragedy in the advance of French Canadians into the Eastern Townships.[34] In his address to the Canadian Club of Montreal, Macphail was reported as advocating a return to "the old true French conservative spirit of pre-revolutionary days, the more so as the French of this province were the only true French, being unspoiled by that revolution, as it occurred after they had settled here."[35]

Yet Macphail was totally out of sympathy with the self-conscious and assertive *Nationalistes* of the day. The militant spirit was not conservative, and French Canadians, like everyone else, were more admirable when they recognized and accepted their place in society. He showed his annoyance by reproducing several pages of documents purporting to demonstrate that the language, laws, and religion of French Canada had no special legal status. The thrust of this section was quite out of keeping with the rest of the essay, and indeed was based on a wartime memorandum he had submitted to Borden. Perhaps ironically, he concluded with a somewhat sympathetic explanation of Quebec's rejection of conscription.[36]

Woman was another natural conservative. "Civilization has been created to protect her. When the system fails she is the first to suffer ... In all revolutions the record of this sudden degradation is the darkest page."[37] Civilization was a series of interdependent conventions that had been built up over time; womanly reticence, filial deference, and good manners were examples. "He who breaks one convention is guilty of all. The man who is late for dinner will lack in reticence towards the woman of the house." The conventions of civilized behaviour had brought a sense of form and an appreciation for art and beauty. "Religion itself ... is a series of closely knit conventional beliefs, any one of which can easily be made the object of destructive criticism to the peril of the whole."[38] The dislocation of one aspect of civilization risked the dislocation of all.[39]

In contrast to this orderly way of life stood democracy, which for Macphail had increasingly come to mean not the positive value of self-government but the destructive levelling of conventional forms and distinctions. An example was the newly granted franchise for women. It removed the wall that had formerly existed between women and public life, and it held the potential for dividing families along political lines. (Indeed, by 1916 Macphail's own mother appears to have been in favour of female suffrage.) "The individual and not the family is now the unit of the race,"[40] he wrote. The dismembering of the family was a regressive step. Democracy was a cancer on the body politic, for it strove "to destroy the organs and organization of society" and "to reduce races, nations, and families to an unorganized congeries of individual units." Macphail was emphatic that democracy was not a form of government. It was a "condition out of which some form of government may eventually arise." He likened this condition to savagery and stated that civilization had only evolved in the face of continual resistance from "democrats, liberals, radicals, anarchists, nihilists." He concluded: "When democracy has accomplished its perfect work we shall begin again the slow and painful Sisyphus task ... In the process we shall again pass through another slow age of darkness."[41] He carried this message even to Orwell. In an address there in the summer of 1920 he stated that "the progress of the world today is in the direction of anarchy and atheism."[42]

Macphail was profoundly pessimistic about the immediate future, for a "man in these days acquires political fame as he succeeds in destroying the customs and institutions under which we live ... Any system stands as a system." In revolutionary Russia he saw the fate of civilization as a whole, a regression to rule "by starvation, by the knout, and by murder." The root of the problem lay where it had always been – in the factory system. "The real solution is that every man will do his own work, and every woman hers." This had been the way in former times, and every aspect of contemporary life reinforced his conviction that "all that is good is old."[43]

FARMING

In early 1920 Macphail published "The Immigrant," the longest article he ever contributed to the *University Magazine*. He chose this title for the article because the "industrial life of America was built up by the immigrants ... Immigrants we must have if the system is to endure."[44] From this perspective, the immigrant was the keystone of the arch, for the native-born could not be made to do the "work" of industrial society, with its monotonous repetition, unpleasant environment, and lack of variety. But the real heart of the article and two addresses he delivered before the Canadian Club of Ottawa (also titled "The Immigrant") and the Empire Club of Canada ("The Farmer") was his elaboration on the ethic of farming:

> It is important to have clear ideas about farming also. Pictures of waving wheatfields with sixteen "binders" operating *en echelon* are not enough.
>
> Farming is a way of life. It is that and nothing else. It is not a business. If a man does not find his life's pleasure in his daily work, in the contact of his fields and the companionship of his animals; if he does not enjoy his labour in woods, by stream and sea; if he thinks less of his daily bread, of the provision for a serene and contented old age, and more of the profit he draws, he would be well advised to seek some other vocation. And yet the farmer is being recommended by all and sundry to convert himself into a "business man" ...
>
> The farmer has been sophisticated into an untenable position by those who have taken upon themselves the gratuitous task of his

education. They think in terms of the city. A farm to them is a factory, and a farmer is "labour." He must be persuaded, cajoled, "educated" to increase production, to lower prices, so that factories may be run at a profit, and let labour riot in the cities …

Next, the "business man" reprehends the farmer for his indisposition to purchase machines. Machinery is fatal to good farming. Worse still, it makes bad farming possible.[45]

Macphail's ideal was mixed farming, based on a fine network of interdependence among crops and animals. Both would be chosen with an eye to the soil, since "farming is an art … The soil must be learned as an artist learns his materials."[46] There would be useful work for both women and children. "On the farm the whole force of the family is directed towards the common end."[47] With such total mobilization there would be no need for hired labour. The non-agricultural needs of the family would be met by the craftsmanship of its members. Since machinery would be kept at a minimum, the amount of land used by each farmer would be modest. "If a man reaps his harvest with his own hand, he will concentrate his efforts … The land will support more people. They will live close and develop a society."[48] If one farmer had a gift in stonecutting he could exchange the products of his talent for those of his neighbour who was skilled perhaps in woodworking.[49] The life of the farm would not be centred on the production of "cash crops" to be exchanged in the marketplace for money to buy food and manufactured articles.

Government services, advancing technology, and universal public education were disrupting the fabric of the rural community. Rural mail delivery, whose advent in Orwell during wartime had been a source of much annoyance to the Macphails,[50] deprived the farmer of his pretext for going to the village. His telephone obviated the need for visiting neighbours. Laws making school attendance compulsory for up to ten years prevented his children from learning their vocations at an early age and convinced them that they were "too intelligent to work with their hands." The school was "the open door through which they escape[d] to the city over the 'good roads' that are now the fashion."[51] The source of all these evils was the city itself, always the inveterate enemy of the countryside. "A city justifies itself as a centre of intellectual and moral stimulus; but who ever heard of any intelligence proceeding from Toronto or morality emanating from Montreal?"[52] Everyday life in a city was excessively complicated and was vulnerable to sudden paralysis through such work stoppages as the Winnipeg General Strike. "One who lives in a city has given hostages because civic life has grown so vast and intricate ... He is too easily struck at. The situation too closely resembles slavery or civil war."[53]

Before the First World War, Macphail had advocated a return to the land, but by 1920 he recognized that this was no remedy for the evils he decried. The way of life he celebrated required human material of a very specific nature, and it was lacking.[54] Macphail had as scant hope for Canadian society as he did for the peace of Europe or the position of women in "democracy." He believed that "a great epoch has, as usual, ended in disaster, and that the first business of this generation is to observe the wreckage disappear."[55] The machine age had toppled the old social order and destroyed the "natural resources" of the planet. When these tasks had been completed, "the correction of hunger" would soon set in. Then mankind could start again. Macphail did not think the time was distant: "That is the measure of my optimism."[56]

Macphail's expression of these ideas coincided with the end of the *University Magazine*. The subscription list had not appreciably increased with his return. He would not consider raising the price, and with the persistent inflation in costs of production he began to doubt the wisdom and practicality of continuing. In December and again in February he published an appeal "To Readers." He categorically stated, "Neither the Magazine nor its contributors desire charity. All that is asked is that those who have been receiving the Magazine shall pay their accounts; and any other persons who feel qualified to read it will be welcome as subscribers." He calculated that one thousand new subscribers were necessary, and he reminded his readers that "to 'encourage Canadian literature' has been in every mouth. The only way to 'encourage' writers is to read, and pay for what they write."[57]

The response to Macphail's entreaty could not have been heartening, for at the end of September 1920 he decided to "suspend" publication of the journal. His sight was deteriorating again, the printing estimate was 65 percent in excess of the previous year, and there was no prospect of financial relief. Expenses had been steadily rising for several years. "I am sorry to see it perish after these 20 years," he wrote to Mavor, "but the detail of management has become too tiresome."[58]

In reflecting on the demise of the *University Magazine*, the editors of the new *Canadian Forum* declared that it had "maintained a higher standard of literary and material excellence than – it is safe to say – any of its predecessors."[59] They credited much of the success to Macphail and his policies, and were equally definite in stating that "the fundamental reason of its failure has been the apathy of the Canadian intellectual public ... There surely is a real need for such a journal ... and we hope that it will be able to resume publication in the very near future."[60] Macphail was convinced that his periodical had never been more needed, and at one time he had hoped to turn it over to Bernard K. Sandwell, then teaching economics at McGill and a member of the Pen and Pencil Club. Several contributors expressed their regrets, yet like Falconer the previous year, they had nothing more tangible to offer than appreciation and condolence. The *University Magazine* was not to be resuscitated. As Edgar remarked many years later, Macphail had been "its founder, its financial supporter, and the source from which its energy flowed."[61]

Macphail's last year with the *University Magazine* had been one of intense activity. The seriousness of his intent was indicated by the length of such articles as "The Conservative" and "The Immigrant"; his articles in the *University Magazine* ordinarily ran between ten and twenty pages, whereas the latter was thirty and the former twenty-six pages in length.[62] The seriousness was also apparent from the way in which he tended to come directly to the point rather than exercising the essayist's prerogative of meandering towards his central ideas at a leisurely pace. In 1919 and 1920 Macphail saw no reason to be coy. The truth required telling, and perhaps sensing that the end was coming for his journal, he seemed to be holding nothing back.

The pessimism Macphail expressed about the state of society must have been intensified when he considered the parts of the world close at hand. His journal was in its death throes. Of his own university, he wrote to his brother Alexander in 1920, "McGill has now less meaning than the grammar school at Orwell in our time. It is given up to the teaching of trades, and teaches them very badly."[63] In Orwell itself values were changing. Macphail had hoped to resume his agricultural experiments and had planned to put some 300 acres under cultivation in 1919 - "to begin life again," as he put it in a letter to Tait McKenzie dated ten days after the Armistice. But the four or five young men he had hired for the task abruptly left when they learned of a drastic reduction in the railway fare to Winnipeg. Macphail abandoned his plans.[64] In all respects times had changed, and as a conservative might have expected, the change was for the worse. There would undoubtedly be, over the years, an element of humorous overstatement in the way he expressed himself about such matters among his peers in

Montreal. Leacock captured this with characteristic deftness, remarking that in Macphail's early years of school and farm life,

> rural Canada offered little more than a pioneer life with few
> alleviations … This, to people lucky enough to get out of it, as both
> Andrew and I had been, was coloured with the mellow hues of
> retrospect … And for people like Andrew and myself our country
> upbringing became a source of pride and a bond of sympathy and,
> as the years drew on, something of an affectation. Andrew … could
> push reality hard, much harder than I ever could. He could speak of
> buttermilk (over a glass of whiskey and soda) with wistful relish,[65]
> and talk of long drinks of maple sap out of its wooden trough, – a
> beverage little better in reality than a solution of sawdust and dead
> flies. It became with Andrew a sort of whimsical make-believe that
> everything in the country was right, and everything in the city wrong.
> The only real boots were made by country cobblers: homespun
> clothes fitted better than the tailored product of the city: and so forth,
> till the thing verged on burlesque and Andrew himself would start to
> laugh at it.[66]

Yet the drollery should not be allowed to obscure Macphail's serious-ness. Behind every coherent body of social criticism, and certainly his, lies a conception of the good society – certain assumptions about the proper ordering of social relationships. The primary importance of Macphail's last year as editor of the *University Magazine* lies not in the number of people he reached but in the fullness with which he articulated the positive social vision implicit in his critique. As he looked around and considered what he objected to in modern Canadian society, the affirmative side of his convic-tions became clearer, probably to himself as well as to his readers. The ideal way of life was mixed farming, primarily oriented towards meeting basic needs within the family rather than producing for the marketplace. The farm would be operated by a fully employed family without hired labour and with a minimum of machinery. These requirements form the founda-tions for Macphail's "good society"; the defining characteristic would be the predominance of such a mode of production.

Military Historical Writing and Socialism

MACPHAIL IN THE 1920S AND 1930S: INTRODUCTION

Andrew Macphail continued to write in the 1920s and 1930s. But there were changes. The unity of purpose evident in his essays and books published from 1907 to 1920 was lacking. With the termination of the *University Magazine*, that phase of his career in which his concerns were primarily political, in the broadest sense of the word, also came to an end. Although he continued to hold to his traditionalist point of view, he seems to have decided to renounce direct involvement in day-to-day issues, the events that generated newspaper headlines and debates in Parliament. As an example, he let the King-Byng affair of 1926 pass without serious comment, which would have been unthinkable for him in the prewar years.[1] It was also rare in the twenties and thirties for him to write about the social problems arising from the development of Canada. His causes had been decisively defeated, and he consequently displayed little interest in immersing himself in current debates.

When articulating his stern brand of conservatism in 1919–20, Macphail had on occasion betrayed a certain self-consciousness and even, in his correspondence with James Mavor, self-doubt. In late 1919, when accepting an invitation to address a University of Toronto audience on "Women in Democracy," Macphail had confessed to a fear "that I am beginning to speak foolishly."[2] Thus it is unsurprising that in the 1920s he did not, by and large, raise what he considered to be the fundamental political and social issues. He was too much out of step with the times. As he wrote, again to Mavor, in 1925, "There is nothing to be said any more to any Canadian Club – except of the ruin impending over the country, and people are tired of that. I think for the future we will take refuge in things of the mind."[3] Like the good conservative of his imagination, he believed that the proper course was to accept the fate he saw overtaking civilization and simply hope that the task of reconstruction would soon be commenced. He made no positive response to a proposal in the mid-1920s to resurrect the *University Magazine*. He also discontinued his agricultural experiments during his summers on Prince Edward Island. Yet his house in Orwell remained unmodernized, a silent witness to his convictions and an indication of where his deepest commitments lay.[4]

Macphail was never again to be as central and as visible a part of Canadian intellectual life as when he had been regularly treating contemporary themes. His general level of activity decreased somewhat in the 1920s, and probably this would have happened even without his conclusions about the direction society was taking. He had been in his late fifties at the start of the decade and had just spent four and one-half physically arduous years in military service. His eyes continued to trouble him, periodically interrupting work in progress, and preventing reading and writing for weeks or months. This affliction, whose sole indication to his family and friends was a patch over his left eye, required at least two operations in the 1920s.[5]

There were additional misadventures and illnesses. In January 1921 Macphail broke his ankle; and, much more seriously, in the summer of 1931 he suffered such a severe attack of pneumonia and acute diabetes that he entered a sort of coma. He remained gravely ill for approximately three weeks, experiencing temperatures around 104°F and episodes of delirium, which brought him back – in his mind – to the time of his wife's death twenty-nine years earlier. He apparently mistook his daughter Dorothy, age thirty-four, for his wife, who had been thirty-two at the time of her death, and he misidentified a four-year-old granddaughter as "Dorothy"; Dorothy had been four years of age when her mother died. The diabetes had not been diagnosed previously, and the attending physician, Dr Wendell MacKenzie of Charlottetown, was about to give up and send to Montreal for a specialist when he tested Macphail for the disease for some reason unknown even to himself. Insulin revived Macphail within two to three hours. Reflecting on that experience almost forty years later, Dorothy Lindsay believed that Dr MacKenzie had "saved Dad's life."[6] Even then his recovery was not rapid; on 28 October he informed Lord Beaverbrook (the former Sir Max Aitken), "For three months I have been on my bed suffering from pneumonia." On 13 November he reported to Beaverbrook that his strength was increasing daily.[7]

But probably the closest Macphail came to death in these years was on 15 November 1921 when, at approximately 1:30 in the afternoon, a twenty-eight-year-old man entered his house at 216 Peel Street with a revolver and apparently attempted to kill him. According to a report in the *Montreal Star*, four shots were fired. The first wounded Macphail in the right shoulder – the newspaper mistakenly said it was the left – and the next two struck a door as Macphail backed from the hallway into the dining room; then his assailant shot himself in the head and "died almost immediately."[8] The background to this bizarre and harrowing occurrence, if there was relevant background, has remained largely a mystery. An obituary article published in the *Canadian Medical Association Journal* after Macphail's death stated, "Monomania, taking the form of a violent hallucination," was believed to have been the explanation.[9] In the story that appeared at the time in the *Montreal Star*, different members of the would-be assassin's family reported conflicting impressions of his mental state. According to Macphail, also as reported in the *Star*, they were nodding acquaintances, for the man's brother had a tailor shop at 212 Peel Street.[10] He subsequently wrote that the man, "who was growing progressively mad for a year, was in the habit of coming at times to my house to consult me about his troubles."[11] The report in the *Star* indicated that he believed stories were being spread about him. On the day of the incident he had come to Macphail and repeated this; Macphail had listened, and had shown him out, but then he had come back with a weapon.[12]

Macphail spent a month in hospital and never fully recovered his strength.[13] An operation to remove the bullet was not entirely successful. Almost five years later, when corresponding with Tait McKenzie, a close friend and fellow physician, he wrote, "A fragment that remained has chosen to wander into the brachial plexus [a network of blood vessels or nerves in the arm], and seems to be red-hot. They make beautiful pictures of it with their [x-ray] machine, but that does not help me much."[14] The consequences of the incident added to Macphail's level of disability resulting from the injury to his eyes in 1911, for he was right-handed. He commented in his letter to McKenzie, "I can read but little; and this [letter of fewer than 250 words] is all my writing for the day. Otherwise I am very well, and my sense of taste for food and drink is becoming extremely fine."[15]

Indeed, during the twenties and thirties Macphail became increasingly "social" in the more private circles of Montreal, thus somewhat redirecting his energy. Stephen Leacock wrote that his friend "seemed so different to other men that his presence seemed to lift an occasion out of the commonplace." He was particularly adept at entertaining celebrities, whom he "treated ... as a man used to horses treats a new one. It always seemed amazing to me that he could handle them so easily."[16] His spacious and comfortable house on Peel Street, situated conveniently between Montreal's downtown train stations and McGill University, served as "home" for many out-of-town scholars and savants. Known as a gourmet, every week or ten days he held formal dinner parties, usually attended only by men – typically professional men, about ten in number, although occasionally wives were also present. Described as "real social events" by a woman who had attended with her husband (who was Leacock's lawyer),[17] they were equally famous for the sparkling conversation and for the salads, prepared by himself. Macphail would cut up the vegetables at the table and, using a wooden bowl, rub the inside with a clove of garlic before mixing the ingredients. One informant who had worked for his daughter in the 1920s recalled many decades later that Macphail had asked her to come and pour the wine at these dinners. There was a different wine to complement each course, and Macphail paid her about ten dollars – a significant sum, for her monthly salary was forty-five dollars, although Macphail's daughter always gave her an extra fifteen.[18]

Macphail also seems to have had more time for travel in the 1920s and 1930s. Approximately every second spring he went on a trip, sometimes Caribbean cruises or fishing expeditions to Labrador. In 1922 he and three of his brothers visited Palestine and other places on the Mediterranean; eight years later he went to Poland; and in 1935 a cruise to the Baltic Sea took him to Soviet Russia. Perhaps his entertaining and travelling provided partial compensation for the loss of the *University Magazine* and its associated activities.[19]

Macphail's essays in the 1920s and 1930s covered a wide range of topics, including literature, medical history, religion, art, and military history. It was in the last-mentioned field that he produced his two most controversial books of these years: the *Official History of the Canadian Forces in the Great War, 1914-19: The Medical Services* (1925) and *Three Persons* (1929). He received the David literary prize from Quebec for the *Official History* (which carried with it a cheque for $700), and one year after the publication of *Three Persons* the Royal Society of Canada presented him with its Lorne Pierce Medal for distinguished contributions to Canadian literature.[20]

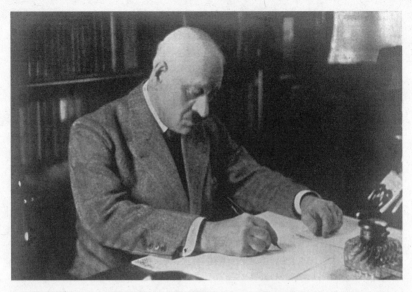

Macphail at his writing desk, interwar years. Writing could be physically challenging for Macphail in the final decades of his life. A bullet fragment that was lodged in his upper right arm, as the result of an apparent assassination attempt in 1921, periodically caused him great pain and prevented him from sustained use of the arm. Injury to his eyes in 1911 and subsequent glaucoma sometimes prevented any reading or writing for weeks or months.

WRITING ABOUT WAR: THE OFFICIAL HISTORY

"War being polemical," declared Macphail at the end of the 1920s, "writing about war must be polemical too. It is not intended to please."[21] Both the *Official History* and *Three Persons* had amply met this prescription. As early as 1919 Macphail had been approached about becoming official historian of the medical services, and he was commissioned on 7 October 1921. His qualifications were obvious: besides being an accomplished man of letters and holding the history of medicine chair in Canada's leading medical faculty, he was, one reviewer wrote, "probably the only senior physician to serve for any such period [14 months] with a field ambulance."[22] He spent some two hundred working days on the project over the next year, and the manuscript generated sufficient controversy at official levels that publication was held up for almost three years, even though he consented to several deletions. One recent historian has noted, "While the Cabinet had the option of not supporting the history, [Chief of General Staff J.H.] MacBrien warned that Macphail owned the intellectual rights and would publish it regardless, and probably in the original, unexpurgated form."[23]

Macphail made no secret of his interest in writing succeeding volumes, but he was not invited to do so. The project was to have run to eight volumes in addition to three more such specialized works as Macphail's. These were to have concerned the engineering, chaplain, and nursing services, and Alexander Macphail was to have been the author of the engineering volume.[24] Perhaps in part because of the nature of Macphail's book on the medical services – in his own words, "something less than eulogy"[25] – the only subsequent volume to appear was delayed until 1938, on the eve of Canada's next European war. Indeed, in the view of some Canadian military historians, Alexander's project specifically may have been undone by the controversy over his older brother's book, but there appears to be no definitive proof one way or the other.[26]

In addition to being a descriptive account of the subject, Macphail's *Official History* was a passionate defence, presented with his customary eloquence: "The Canadian medical service never failed; it never was embarrassed from any inherent cause, either when it operated in reliance upon itself alone or in those larger operations where it necessarily depended upon the co-operation of the British service."[27] He was definite in stating that of all branches of the Canadian army, the medical corps was best prepared for mobilization. Whatever "embarrassment" occurred arose out of confusion on the part of the minister of militia and defence, Sir Samuel Hughes, over the proper relations between civil and military authorities. "To provide the forces is a civil act," wrote Macphail, "to train and employ those forces to the proper end is the military business." Hughes's propensity for precipitate and ill-directed action "brought the Canadian medical service and the army itself to the verge of disaster; and wrenched the Canadian constitution so severely that it has not yet recovered from the strain."[28] Macphail believed that the medical services had been held responsible in the public mind for mismanagement not of their making, and he proposed to set the record straight. His volume can be seen as part of what has been referred to as a war of reputations that raged in Canada in the postwar years, principally over the abilities, character, and general standing of Hughes and General Sir Arthur Currie.[29]

The book was also notable for its strong emphasis on the need for operational unity among all branches of the army, its testimonial on the sexual purity of the soldiers compared with civilians, and its unsympathetic attitude to the psychiatric maladies grouped under the term "shell shock."[30] On the latter two points, the modern researcher must wonder about Macphail's candour. With respect to the issue of sexual self-denial, the military historian Desmond Morton reported in 1993 that venereal disease was "by far the largest single cause of hospitalization throughout the war."[31] Macphail could scarcely have been unaware of this fact; a combination of conformity to contemporary standards of prudery and a concern for the reputation of the soldiers once back in civilian life probably explains his published statement. His treatment of "shell shock" is peculiar in that his diaries demonstrate that when he had been at the front he had not been so certain in his disdain for those who suffered from the affliction.[32] This discrepancy between what he actually felt at the time and what he wrote years later was never explained. He reiterated his published opinion in 1929.[33]

With respect to undertaking the *Official History* project, Macphail was known to have remarked in later years, "I gave the matter serious consideration, and I decided that I would write the way history should be written; as though everyone who had played a part in it were dead. I have found that they were not dead."[34] Responses to the *Official History* were seldom neutral or half-hearted. Many critics extolled it as a model of its kind, setting a high standard for the rest of the planned series. The *Times* of London reviewer praised Macphail for his use of "apt historical reference and brief dissertations on the art of war which conform very closely with those of the great theorists," declaring that his book "might well become a text-book for Imperial politicians who desire to avoid error when war once again disturbs the Empire."[35] While several writers commended Macphail's objectivity, others took a very different position. The anonymous reviewer in the *Canada Lancet and Practitioner* denounced "Sir Andrew's so-called 'history'" as being "a melange of personal opinions, invariably prejudiced, and unsupported by proofs." He strenuously defended Hughes and his associate, Colonel Herbert A. Bruce, another of Macphail's targets, using as his main tactic innuendoes about Macphail's right to be called "official historian" and about the reasons for his being knighted.[36]

Taking an overview of the heated controversy, the influential *Manitoba Free Press* stated in early 1926 that the book "produced a storm all over Canada ... and evoked cries expressive of a variety of emotions. Only a book of real merit can ... compel attention and response to its challenge."[37] Perhaps the most searching and persuasive criticism came from E.S. Ryerson, a fellow veteran and an MD affiliated with the University of Toronto's Faculty of Medicine, writing in the *Canadian Historical Review*.

According to the university calendar for 1924–25, he was an "Associate in Clinical Surgery." He took exception to Macphail's remarks concerning "shell shock," and although conceding that the book's greatest strength was its treatment of the political crisis within the medical services in 1916, argued, "So much space has been allotted to the controversy, that the amount left for the drawing of a life-like picture of … the kind of work they [the medical services] did and the manner in which it was performed … is altogether too meagre."[38]

Modern historians have had their own perspectives, criteria, and interests to bring to discussion of Macphail's *Official History*. In 1983, writing in *The Oxford Companion to Canadian Literature*, J.M. Bumsted, in the course of locating Macphail as a significant figure in the transition from amateur to professional history writing in Canada, described the book as "a classic analysis of the non-combative aspects of modern war."[39] Another scholar, Mark Osborne Humphries, noted recently that Macphail was the first Canadian historian to write about the lethal influenza pandemic of 1918–19, an enormous catastrophe of the immediate postwar period, costing approximately an additional 50,000 lives. Humphries also noted that Macphail was the first to argue that it came to Canada via soldiers returning from overseas, an interpretation he disputes.[40] Jonathan F. Vance, in his book on Canadian memory and the Great War, published in 1997, referred to the *Official History* in passing as a "highly partisan volume"[41] and made no offsetting positive comment. Almost a decade later, in a volume on Canadian "military intellectual history" concerning the world wars, Tim Cook condemned Macphail's study as "a poor and confusing read."[42] In his characterization of its flaws, he relied to a degree on an unpublished paper presented to the Canadian Historical Association in 2002.

David Campbell, the author of that unpublished presentation, had subjected the text of the *Official History* to meticulous scrutiny, with the objective of determining how it measured up to the standards reasonably to be expected of an official history. He found essentially that the essayist and the editor of the *University Magazine* had been the father of the *Official History*. Macphail had footnoted the book only sparsely, which was in keeping with his prescription of broad accessibility for articles in the *University Magazine*. In an analysis that complemented Ryerson's criticism, Campbell examined Macphail's use of evidence concerning the aspects of his story that were not directly related to political and administrative matters or to the conduct of the Canadian war effort as a whole. He pointed out that in many instances when Macphail cited a wartime diarist with the medical services, in fact that diarist was himself; readers were given no warning that the various references were from one witness, let alone that the witness was Macphail. Campbell reported that "of some 44 quotations and anecdotes found between pages 41 and 101 of the official history, at least 27 can be identified as having been taken directly, or adapted from, entries in [his] own personal wartime diaries."[43] Most damning, he found that "in at least two instances … [Macphail] implies that more than one diarist authored several passages which are clearly traceable to his own diary."[44]

The scanty citation of sources and the reliance by Macphail on his own diary entries were in stark contrast to the copious use of documentation in the one later volume of the official history that was published. The author was A. Fortescue Duguid, the director of the army's Historical Section, whose entire approach was to emphasize carefully documented fact.[45] As Campbell noted, there were obvious problems of balance with Macphail's apparent assumption that his own experiences were representative of those of the medical services as a whole.[46] Considered as official history, Macphail's book was unconventional, and it was also at odds with Duguid's declared intent for the series.[47] Yet as Campbell stated, "It even could be argued that, given Macphail's literary track record, the government, the general staff, and the historical section should have anticipated from the beginning the kind of history Macphail would produce."[48] The author, after all, had always been more writer than researcher. As he remarked to Currie many years after the war in one of his characteristic epigrams, "Soldiers make wars, but historians make the history of them."[49]

PERCEIVING MILITARY FIGURES: *THREE PERSONS* AND OTHER ESSAYS

Three Persons was a collection of three critical essays on individuals who had emerged into public prominence in the course of the First World War: Sir Henry Wilson, Colonel E.M. House, and Colonel T.E. Lawrence (also known as Lawrence of Arabia). The book's distinctiveness lay in Macphail's method. For sources, he relied entirely on the published reminiscences of the subject, with the sole exception that in the case of Lawrence he dealt also with two books on him, which he presented as examples of misinterpretation: "If any Person, through his friends, were to protest that strong words are used in depicting his lineaments, the defence of *Electra* avails: You speak, not I; you do the deeds: your deeds find me the words."[50] The book appears to have grown out of a 37-page review essay in the *Quarterly*

Review of London, edited by Sir John Murray, whose publishing house also handled the finished volume. The article dealt at length with the *Life and Diaries* of Wilson, and it was to be Macphail's bare-knuckled treatment of the former chief of the Imperial General Staff that made *Three Persons* an immediate sensation in Britain.[51]

Macphail discovered in examining Wilson's diaries abundant evidence of the converse of what he had condemned so strongly in Hughes's conduct. Wilson, a military man, had interfered in what were properly civilian prerogatives, with disastrous consequences.[52] Macphail also found Wilson to have been an incompetent strategist and military planner whose advice, if taken, would have lost the war: "Sir Henry Wilson did much political harm during the War; he was powerless to do much military harm. Haig was too strong."[53] Wilson also emerged from the study as an untrustworthy sycophant and indefatigable intriguer – indeed, a man without redeeming qualities. Macphail wrote that Wilson "and the editor [of the diaries] have created a figure and not a man, an inhuman figure, calculating, callous, without a single generous sentiment or kind word; impersonal, with no suggestion of whom he loved, what scene of beauty he admired."[54] The evident lack of concern by Wilson and his peers for loss of life at the front led Macphail to state, "Had this book been in the hands of the soldiers during the war, it might well have caused despondency and despair."[55] At one point in *Three Persons* he even suggested that a mutiny would have given the British High Command some salutary instruction.[56]

Through all the manoeuvrings and betrayals of trust by Wilson, an Ulsterman, the "only coherency" Macphail could detect was hatred of Ireland: "It extended to all who refused to share that hatred with him ... The English are without hatred. For that reason he bewailed, 'the English are never serious about anything.'"[57] Wilson had been the official military adviser to the British government at the beginning and end of the war; in both periods he had been secretly intriguing with the opposition. His hatred of the government for its Irish policy had even led him to commit serious indiscretions in his dealings with the French. Macphail concluded that "he was a dangerous emissary; and that danger is proved by the confidences he gave as well as received."[58]

This devastating essay, with its rigorous argument and meticulous citation of evidence, was a masterpiece of its kind. Hence it is not surprising that it and the subsequent book created many ripples. Beaverbrook, who had for a long time taken a similar view of Wilson, wrote to Macphail saying, "For pure irony and invective I know of nothing in modern times to match it."[59] Kipling, on the other hand, thought Macphail had gone too far in his demolition of the former chief of staff.[60] The *New York Times* expressed the hope that "the interest aroused by this article may encourage other critics to deal more faithfully with books that call for censure."[61] The diaries had shaken Macphail's own faith in the process by which Britain had become committed to entering the war, and in the 1930s were to make him especially wary of any commitments to France.[62]

Summarizing the book's themes in a letter to Beaverbrook, Macphail wrote, "Wilson was the Play-boy; House the Comedian, and Lawrence the Artist of the War."[63] By comparison with the first essay, the pieces on House and Lawrence were restrained. He treated President Woodrow Wilson's adviser as "a revelation of the American mind,"[64] a Texan striving to find his way in the intricate world of European diplomacy, a task for which his background had not prepared him. House emerged as a somewhat comic and almost pathetically naïve figure; the portrait, although tinged with irony, was not unsympathetic. In character, House was portrayed as the antithesis of Sir Henry Wilson: "He never wilfully betrayed a confidence that was reposed in him ... In all of Colonel House's Intimate Papers there is not a single mean word or one mean thought ... He had no desire to advance his own interest or the interest of any friend to the detriment of the public good."[65] The second essay lacked the fierce passion that had gone into the dissection of the Wilson diaries and was not intensely controversial; it had the flavour of a well-executed academic exercise.

The final, and by far the shortest, section was devoted to Lawrence of Arabia. It stood apart from the other essays in that it was an appreciation and interpretation of an artist rather than an investigation of the daily comings and goings of a soldier or politician. After deftly disposing of attempts by Lowell Thomas and Robert Graves to penetrate the mystery surrounding Lawrence, Macphail developed his thesis that "Colonel Lawrence writes precisely as Shakespeare might have written had he chosen the more difficult mode [prose]."[66] To Macphail, his subject was much more than the successful "adviser, interpreter, liaison officer, and paymaster [of the Arabs] all in one."[67] With *Revolt in the Desert*, Lawrence had written

> a book that is worthy to rank with the best works in English prose ...
> The desert and all that it contains have been described a hundred
> times, but never so delicately or with so sure a touch. He describes
> not things themselves, but the inner beauty and meaning that lies
> in them ...

Colonel Lawrence had the capacity of the artist for entering into a situation and being the character he assumed. To the Arabs he became as an Arab ... He had one relentless purpose, to animate the Arabs with a national spirit and lead them in triumph into Damascus. The hardest task was the subjugation of his own spirit to their mood and to their way of life. But of this loathsome living he makes no complaint. He had subdued himself to his purpose. Over the foul details he casts, with the sure and delicate hand of the artist, a veil of beauty.[68]

Thus Macphail's essay was an attempt to rescue Lawrence's reputation from the aura of eccentricity and excessively romantic mythology that threatened to obscure his achievements. Macphail wrote that Lawrence was "a man of unusual courage, an artist in search of new emotions."[69] Indeed, his artistry and his ability to experience fully the alien had enhanced his practical work with the Arabs. Perhaps ironically, Macphail's only criticism was that Lawrence had come to accept and even practise the cruelties of warfare usually ascribed to the Turk but not to British officers.[70]

Three Persons, with its enormous variations in tone, was a *tour de force*, both by reason of the author's singular method and his skill in carrying it through. Although it was Macphail's most widely read book in his lifetime, its subject matter and appeal were more British than Canadian. It was Macphail's fourth collection of essays since 1905, and his acknowledged mastery of the genre underlined his comment to Beaverbrook that "the essay form ... is my trade."[71]

Among the large number of essays Macphail published in the 1930s were biographical sketches in the *Queen's Quarterly* of three other military figures: Currie, Paul von Hindenburg, and Robert E. Lee.[72] This continuing interest in military topics – also manifested in two brief reviews of books on military subjects, a short obituary of Currie and a published address entitled "Armistice Day, 1933" (which also largely concerns Currie)[73] – led Macphail's friend John A. Stevenson to write shortly after his death that he had "had an ingrained preference for the soldier over the politician."[74] This opinion is repeated uncritically by Carl Berger, the historian who has analysed the intellectual premises of Canadian imperialism; Berger also attributes to Macphail a preference for "the decisive and undebatable dictums of the military life" after the style of George T. Denison III.[75] Macphail in fact held an unflattering opinion of Denison, whom he regarded as something of a primitive.[76] A careful reading of what Macphail actually wrote does not bear out the implied undue admiration for soldiers and their values, as opposed to civilians and theirs. It is true that he had scant use for politicians, but his essays give little reason to suspect that he had much more for soldiers. He displayed no liking whatever for the harsh anti-intellectual atmosphere in which Hindenburg was trained to be an effective warrior; as a whole the article on him is notable for Macphail's spirit of detachment, as though the life of the single-minded professional soldier lacked sufficient interest to generate warmth in his writing. One senses Macphail's disappointment at the sterility of Hindenburg's life; and although there can be no doubt of the high regard in which Macphail held Currie as a person and as a soldier from the time of their first meeting at the front,[77] the thrust of the entire essay on him is to emphasize the limitations of even the best military men when applying their methods to other spheres. He irreverently remarked:

> The personal devotion of the troops to the heads of the higher command is a fiction of civilian minds ... [The] high ones would have been astonished had they heard the private opinions that were expressed and the general principles that were enunciated ... These were to them merely the authors of their present misery, and they the victims of the higher mistakes ... The apologias of these hierophants and the adulation of their biographers still create a feeling of nausea. The Life of Rawlinson, under whom the Canadians served so long, is the worst.[78]

The two soldiers for whom Macphail expressed the most undiluted admiration were praised primarily for their non-military qualities: Lawrence for his artistry, and Lee for his gentlemanly refinement. Although Lawrence's gifts were interpreted as making his military accomplishments possible, Lee, the kindly man incapable of hatred, was portrayed as "too gentle and generous"[79] for his role. Their characters, not their military achievements, captivated Macphail. In fact, the habits of the soldier carried over into civilian life were precisely what Macphail criticized in Currie's conduct as principal of McGill.[80] His partiality for the man of action over the man of letters or the man of civil disposition had been a comparatively brief wartime phenomenon.

Stevenson is also incorrect in asserting that "in war and military matters Sir Andrew had a perennial interest."[81] This interest began in middle age. There is no evidence of particular concern with war or military matters in themselves prior to 1914. Such articles as "The Navy and Politics," published the previous year, focused primarily on the constitutional implications of military policy; no articles or books in the prewar years take specifically military subjects as their themes, and Macphail's writings give no evidence of even academic knowledge of or interest in this field. His antebellum references to war were merely part of a general apocalypticism emerging from his assessment of the direction Canadian social and political development was taking. With the First World War all this changed. For the decade after the Armistice, military history and especially the history of the war he had just experienced dominated Macphail's reading and writing, a fact that is not surprising, given the trauma and the consequences of the conflict. In the 1930s his interest abated, perhaps because he had learned enough to be as thoroughly disenchanted with the allied military leadership as he was with the Peace of Versailles. There seemed little point in further investigations in this area, and when treating Currie he explicitly renounced any desire to deal with his military achievements; an evaluation of his work at McGill would be enough. Macphail was more concerned with making a contribution towards the prevention of another major war. Indeed this had been part of his reason for unmasking Sir Henry Wilson.[82]

The *Official History of ... The Medical Services* and *Three Persons*, apart from their intrinsic interest and merits, are important both for the controversy they generated and what they reveal about Macphail's values.

SOCIALISM AND THE SOVIET UNION

Macphail made a new departure in his attitude to socialism in the mid-1930s as the Great Depression wore on. This shift first became noticeable in 1934, with his lead article in the *University of Toronto Quarterly* entitled "Conservative – Liberal – Socialist." His intent was "to inquire into the pristine meaning of the terms Conservative and Liberal; and more strictly what the growing vitality of Socialism may in the future mean."[83] One of the most striking points in the essay was the link he perceived between conservatism and socialism. "Conservatives," he wrote, "have always contended that they were in reality socialists; but if they were going to fire a gun they would draw the trigger slowly."[84] This was a connection he had only once before come even close to acknowledging. Socialism to him, at least as he had expressed his views in writing, had been synonymous with confiscation, and the socialist had been portrayed as a particularly disorderly type of liberal. Yet under the impact of the Great Depression he was displaying an entirely new appreciation of the socialist, who, he elaborated, is the only one who yet has a principle ... Unless both parties [Liberals and Conservatives] return to their original discipline, the Socialists will be free to persuade and convince us that they are competent to assume command.

Ten years ago, Mr. Ramsay MacDonald described the real Socialist as the true evolutionist, who seeks to transform society by the processes proper to an organized living being; he does not stop life to try experiments or institute a new system. He is less concerned with immediate results than with the purpose which governs his actions; he is ruled by ideals; he makes no violent breaks with the old; he rejects revolution, convinced that when the convulsion spreads itself, he must begin all over again. Strikes, sabotage, limitation of output, violence, and doles are contrary to his ideals of unstinted service in return for a reasonable reward; these are contrary to his spirit, immoral, uneconomic, and sure to lead to disaster. This is what we require to be told.[85]

Macphail even had some friendly advice for contemporary Canadian social-ists: "If the Canadian Socialist would succeed, he must employ terms that are familiar to us, terms that have arisen out of our own experience, not from European conditions. The word in every Socialist mouth to describe us common people is *proletarians*."[86]

Despite his new friendliness towards socialism, Macphail still thought its exponents assumed too much about the potential of human nature, and he denied that any warrant for their vision could be found in Christianity. Drawing upon José Ortega y Gasset, he asked the Canadian socialist whether

he is quite sure that his Socialism will stop at the ideal mark within the spiritual bounds he has set ... Socialism may become statism, the people fuel for the machine; ... a new barbarism may arise from within ... This attempt at a transition to a new and different world may be a catastrophe to humanity. By a single mistake our civilization, such as it is, may disappear, and man may find himself once more a primitive being, a mere unit in an unorganized multitude, part of a mass, all of the same mental texture, making no effort toward intellectual, artistic, or any other kind of perfection, with life nothing more than a satisfaction of animal needs. The good gift will then have turned to evil, by a rebellion against destiny.[87]

In any event, to Macphail the basic issue was still that of town and country; he remained convinced of the inability of urban Canadians in the 1930s to make a successful return to the land. Neither liberals nor conservatives, and not even socialists, had any solution to this problem.[88]

Macphail visited the era's most deliberate attempt at "a new and different world" in 1935. It is not entirely clear why he went to the Soviet Union, but the explanation may be quite simple and divorced from politics. On 5 June he had written to McKenzie: "A passion for the sea has come upon me. I *propose*, on June 20th, going into the Baltic, as far as a ship will go, namely to St. Petersburg, as we used to call it."[89] During this trip he saw the Soviet Union – or at least part of it – for himself and, to his surprise, liked it. When he returned, he wrote in *Saturday Night*, "I went to Russia as one might have gone to Paris fifteen years after 'The Terror,' expecting to see signs of destruction ... there were none. Every public building is intact and beautified ... There was not a policeman in sight."[90] He confessed that in touring the museums and galleries he was less interested in Russian art – "even if John Ruskin were to be our guide" – than "in studying the groups of Russian workmen listening to similar lectures; they were as patient as University students under a similar ordeal." He was travelling with a thirteen-year-old grandson: "For three days we had driven over this compact city [Moscow]. We saw whole streets and large areas completely rebuilt with handsome modern dwellings for workmen and not a sign of slums. These things were not an illusion created for our deception." He was emphatic in stating that they had been left free to wander and explore as they wished.[91]

In Leningrad, too, Macphail sought out the churches that in earlier years he had assumed would be desecrated in any revolutionary upheaval (even in Montreal he had complained about churches being destroyed for commercial purposes):

> I went first to St. Isaac's, one of the four major cathedrals of the
> world. There it stood in all its old magnificence ... The Church
> was crowded with working people who had come to wonder if
> not to worship. They were provided with cotton slippers to protect
> the delicate floors against their heavy boots. I had read that it was
> converted into a museum. There were some trivial photographs and
> posters on frames, some models of inventions, a cogged wheel, and
> only one secular statue, whereas Westminster Abbey and St. Paul's are
> crowded with them ... We drove to the other churches familiar from

the guide-books; the result was the same. They were intact; but no
religious services, she [their guide] said, were performed in them.[92]

He seemed more amused than aggrieved by his guide's lack of religious
knowledge; for her part, she was "astonished" by his interest in the subject.[93] Above all, Macphail was impressed with the efforts of the regime to
raise the level of popular culture. He enthusiastically reported that in 1934
the Soviet press had published thirty-five times the number of books produced in any previous year, including an eighteen-volume edition of Guy
de Maupassant.[94]

There can be no doubt that Macphail's admiration was deep and genuine. He had been even less reserved in his private letters. To a friend in
Montreal he wrote, "One who fears ideas had better not come to Russia ...
In comparison the United States and our own West seem like a place of savagery. We have not faced our problems: these people have."[95] After leaving
the Soviet Union, he praised the regime in a series of interviews in London
and Montreal. He conceded that "ruthless measures" were still being used
to root out any traces of the old aristocracy but did not believe that the
primary fault lay with the Russians: "This cruelty will only cease when
the outside world recognizes the Revolution as an accomplished fact and
accepts Russia completely within the comity of nations."[96]

Back in Montreal, he had at least some contact with the organization known as "The Friends of Soviet Russia," for that autumn Norman
Bethune reported to a friend that the executive committee had offered him
the chairmanship for the coming year and that apparently his name had
been suggested by Macphail.[97] It is possible that the body had approached
Macphail, as a prestigious and well-known conservative who had made
positive comments about the Soviet Union, and that he declined and in the
course of doing so suggested Bethune. This is pure speculation, but otherwise it is difficult to envisage such a group and Macphail being in a situation in which he would be offering advice on its choice of officers. Within
his own profession Macphail expressed admiration for some Soviet medical practices, which he suggested Canada could do well to emulate.[98]

Macphail's tentative sympathies with socialism, as expressed in his
University of Toronto Quarterly essay, had taken a qualitative leap. Although
he had read a book favourable to the Soviet Union as early as 1931, nothing in his previous recorded references to the revolution would suggest
approval, let alone such rapture. He had accepted many of the early myths
propagated by the western press, such as the degradation of women and

atrocities by oriental guardsmen alleged to surround Lenin. Once in Russia, his method of observation was simple. The visitor who "goes with a free mind … can see much in a very few days even with one eye," he observed. "But he must confine himself to the things that can be seen, leaving aside what he has read, and judging what he hears by the usual caution and rules of evidence."[99] He retained his keen eye for warts, recognizing, for example, the danger that a cult of Lenin might arise. But by following his own precepts and precautions he concluded that the "creation of this new Russia is one of the major phenomena of history."[100] A year later he remarked in a public address, "Everything I had previously heard about Russia appeared to me to be false."[101]

Those who were completely surprised by Macphail's admiration for the Soviet regime perhaps should not have been. For a generation he had been denouncing ugliness, vulgarity, public rudeness, the desecration of holy places, the extremes of rich and poor, and the "abyss of unemployment" as he perceived them in Canada. On his trip he saw, or thought he saw, an orderly society that seemed to be industrializing without the flaws of which he had been complaining. The Russians appeared to be transcending their secular and religious past without obliterating its memory and its monuments; they were preserving and extending high culture; they were building factories without slums; and there was no evidence of destitution or unemployment. He even praised the Soviet leadership as an "aristocracy of intellect [which] remembers what the old aristocracy forgot … that those outside must be well cared for and kept content."[102] Such comments suggest that Macphail's response to Soviet Russia indicates more about his own conception of the ideal society than about the "new and different world" itself. His brother Alexander shrewdly commented — perhaps with a touch of irony — that the account of Russia put him in mind of "the State of Malpeque in the old days."[103]

Many writers have asserted that there is common ground between conservatism and socialism. When both ideologies have legitimacy within a political culture, a hybrid known as the "red tory" may emerge.[104] An obvious Canadian example would be Stephen Leacock. With the publication of *The Unsolved Riddle of Social Justice* in 1920, Leacock rejected both utopian socialism and laissez-faire liberalism, simultaneously advocating a remarkably comprehensive welfare state. In this respect, he was considerably ahead of his time; the state was to act as the paternalistic guarantor of the rights of all, rather than simply as the mediator among interests sufficiently powerful to enforce their right to be heard at the bargaining table. The latter concept of the state, combined with a loosely defined sense of responsibility to the community as a whole, was as far as a contemporary liberal reformer, William Lyon Mackenzie King, would go in his writings.[105]

One author has asserted that Macphail "did, in defence of his agrarian bias, eventually reach a 'Red Tory' position."[106] Yet he presents no evidence of substance, and he does not appear to appreciate that Macphail's comments, particularly when considered in the context of his other writings even in the 1930s, were a measure of his rejection of North American society, not an affirmation of a reform program that might fit a satisfactory definition of "red toryism." Consequently, in spite of Macphail's articles on socialism and Russia, he cannot be placed in the "red tory" tradition. At most, he had but a minimal tinge of socialism. He wrote no *Unsolved Riddle* or anything remotely resembling it. With few exceptions he was an antistatist; in his view the state was divorced from society. Its control over education had done nothing for the family, and the extension of its activities would not be likely to improve matters. Through the 1930s he remained hostile even to the American New Deal.[107]

Macphail appears to have had no idea of how to come to grips constructively and consistently with the problems of industrialism and urbanism to conserve what he considered the essentials of the good society. He had only one model of such a society, and it was a thing of the past. In this sense he was a more "radical" conservative than Leacock; his rootedness as a thinker in a society with fundamentally different assumptions produced an unbridgeable gulf between him and "red toryism." Hence there was — indeed, there could be — no substantial follow-up in later years to his writings of 1934 and 1935.

Like many others, Andrew Macphail had been profoundly shaken by the Great Depression. He had attempted to reconsider his attitudes — previously little more than prejudices — towards socialism and had even gone to the Soviet Union. He found much that was attractive there, and these positive impressions underlined the nature of his discontent with developed capitalist society. But he was unable to integrate his new experience with his deepest convictions in order to arrive at a new synthesis. It is only fair to state that such a feat was impossible. His "radical" conservatism went too deep for "red toryism." Perhaps Leacock should be allowed the last word: "Andrew would have made a fine radical if he hadn't hated radicalism."[108]

The Arts and Criticism, 1919–1938

PEN AND PENCIL CLUB

Andrew Macphail played an active role in literary and other circles in Montreal after his return from Europe. He continued to enjoy exceptional stature as a man with recognized leadership qualities. This was well illustrated by two incidents at the Pen and Pencil Club, where he had been a prominent if not dominant figure for many years before the First World War.

The club had its ups and downs. The best-attended meetings were in periods when, among active members, there was an approximate numerical balance between artists and writers. When there was an imbalance, artists usually predominated, and sometimes in this situation the rivalries or quarrels among different groups or schools of Montreal artists undermined the vitality of the club. On such occasions, comments, as recorded in the minutes, could become unnecessarily pointed and dismissive regarding entire artistic tendencies, reflecting, for example, the particular views of Edmond Dyonnet. Rebecca Sisler, in her history of the Royal Canadian Academy of Arts, of which Dyonnet was secretary for decades, introduces him thus: "He was warmly regarded by his contemporaries as a totally dedicated painter and teacher and a delightful if slightly irascible man. He was also ... an obdurate traditionalist."[1] The Arts Club, founded in 1912, and the much older Art Association of Montreal appear to have been seen as representing "the other," and resentment was evident in the minutes more than once.[2] The Group of Seven was a target.[3] Although the tendency to indulge in vituperation was not healthy, it seemed to surface when writers left the Pen and Pencil Club to artists.

In November 1919, at a time when art was dominant over literature within the club, Macphail, back from the war in Europe, was elected president. During his second meeting as such, he called on members to contribute with their former vigour. The minutes record that he reminded them of "the many contributions that had been put to the critical test by members of the Pen and Pencil Club in former years … [and] called on members in the order in which they were seated, for contributions in their several lines. Those failing to respond met with Presidential rebuke."[4] Judging from the decades of minutes stretching from the 1890s to the 1960s, this seems to have been an unparalleled attempt to energize members. Furthermore, it is likely that only someone of Macphail's prestige could have made such an appeal without facing a revolt: putting individual members on the spot, like children in a classroom being interrogated about their undone homework and their plans to do it. There followed a surge of activity. Macphail personally made a practical contribution to the cause by delivering unusually provocative papers on the history of education and the Peace of Versailles.[5] But the revival of energy did not last; by the spring of 1921 and certainly by 1922, attendance had declined and artists were overwhelmingly predominant.

In the spring of 1921, Macphail ceased attending frequently, frustrated by the lack of "critical" commentary by members. This was a major concern of his over many years, and the minutes record that he brought up the issue twice in February 1927, when he blamed the lack of bite in the club's discussions for the reduction in the flow of contributions.[6] Almost a decade later he was writing to a struggling young author on the Prairies, later to become famous – Sinclair Ross – telling him that "what we lack most in Canada is criticism."[7]

Macphail did not appear at the Pen and Pencil Club often after February 1921, and in the minutes for the 1930s he is listed as present only once. But there was an incident that appears to have been unique in the club's history that did bring him out. It had been a custom at the Annual Festival in the spring for the artists to produce illustrated menu cards. Some of these survive in repositories in Montreal, Ottawa, Charlottetown, and probably other places as well. They often featured caricatures of members sitting around a table with wine bottles, whisky glasses, cigars, et cetera, or in other situations. On 3 May 1924 there was a special meeting of the club one week after the Annual Festival because two menu cards had caused offence.[8] Percy Nobbs, who was an outspoken man known to have a short temper and to be subject to outbreaks of "explosive profanity," had raised

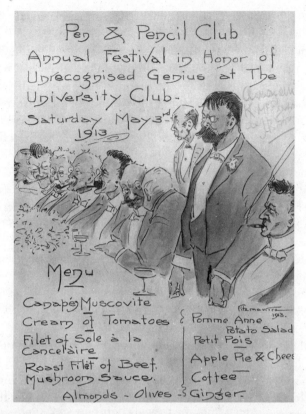

Pen and Pencil Club menu card for 1913. J.B. Fitzmaurice produced this card, which is signed "A mon ami K. Macpherson de J.B. Fitzmaurice." The toast "in Honor of Unrecognised Genius" was made to the most junior member, who was expected to respond with wit. The studio of Kenneth R. Macpherson, KC, a member since 1892, was the home of the club at this time. Fitzmaurice had joined in 1912.

the issue.[9] Apparently as a consequence, Randolph S. Hewton, an artist who had been a member only since 1922, eventually resigned formally from the club, and René du Roure, a professor of French at McGill, resigned because he believed that the artist had been censured. Such a meeting – shortly after the Annual Festival – was extremely rare if not unheard of, since the festival was, by definition, the last meeting of the season, after which the club closed down for five or six months. Moreover, such issues as the taking of offence and the matter of whether Hewton had been censured went to the very heart of a central component of the club's declared raison d'être: social enjoyment.[10]

At that special meeting Macphail was present, although he had not attended the Annual Festival a week earlier and indeed had not been attending regularly for years. In the circumstances, it is highly probable that he had been called in because of the difficulty of the situation, as part of an effort to limit the damage to the venerable club. Macphail's stature was clear, as was his standing within the organization; his proved ability, from his years as editor of the *University Magazine* and two medical journals, in dealing diplomatically with difficult people who had a sense of their own importance was probably the key. No one else emerges from the records of the Pen and Pencil Club in quite the same way as Macphail: he served as prominent contributor, admonisher of the inactive, and even, it seems, peacemaker. The Pen and Pencil Club material indicates a person who made a powerful impression on his peers and exercised a strong influence on them.

ESSAYS ON THE BIBLE AND LITERARY MATTERS

Macphail continued to write essays, short pieces, and reviews on a wide range of topics. In his most familiar genre, the essay, he treated (in addition to his usual diversity of subjects) architecture, chemistry, anthropology, and biology.[11] With respect to the majority of his writings in the 1920s and 1930s, there is no justification for extended treatment. His review of Sir William Van Horne's biography or his essay on Sir Sandford Fleming, while splendid evocations of personality, appear more as exercises in fine writing than as disclosures of the author's thoughts.[12]

The *Quarterly Review* was one of the periodicals to which Macphail contributed frequently. In 1931 he published an essay there, "The Bible in Scotland," which formed the basis for a short book of the same title that appeared later that year. Macphail had begun by reviewing *A Syllabus of Religious Instruction for use in Scottish Schools, approved by and issued by authority of the General Assembly of the Church of Scotland and the Educational Institute of Scotland*. Stephen Leacock once wrote, "If there had been no Westminster Catechism, Andrew would have invented it for himself."[13] Macphail described his study as "a polemic, an apologia, and a final defence of the Christian religion."[14] He criticized the biblical literalism of the text and claimed that the result would be to obscure "the essential Jesus ... The Syllabus is another stone placed at the mouth of the tomb ... It is the most studious of this scheme who will have the most to unlearn."[15] The book did not evoke the controversy he anticipated and did not reach a readership at all comparable to that of *Three Persons*. The subject matter lacked the broad appeal of "The Fallacy in Theology," which he had published twenty-one years earlier, and the book fell far short of paying for itself. Yet Macphail was not totally discouraged. Both Scotland and the Bible were lifelong interests of his, and the tract had been a labour of love. "It is a good book, one I always wanted to write."[16]

One of Macphail's favourites among his writings from this period was a review essay entitled "Johnson's Life of Boswell," which he had also produced for the *Quarterly Review*. When asked in 1929 to choose his "Best Work and Why," he ranked it with "Sir Henry Wilson," another review essay, "in purpose, in method, in expression, and in result."[17] As the title suggests, the intent was revisionist; but the thrust was towards rehabilitation rather than debunking: "Justice is due to the dead, even more than to the living. James Boswell ... remains the victim of current calumny ... [Dr Samuel] Johnson was never deceived by a man; he could penetrate to the heart of him; he had words adequate for judgment. The two were intimate friends ... and ... Johnson reproached Boswell only twice, once in temper and once in jest."[18] The anti-Boswell sentiment had originated with those of Johnson's clique who were jealous of his regard for the young Scotsman who had the remarkable capacity to become the intimate of great men. "To make matters worse, Boswell had an instant success in their own field. His 'Account of Corsica' sold for 100 guineas ... That was hard for his rivals to bear, and they took their vengeance upon 'the green goose from the country.'"[19] The conventional estimate of Boswell had been fixed since 1831 – for almost an entire century – with the appearance in the *Edinburgh Review* of an unsigned article by T.B. Macaulay, whose methods Macphail described as "dishonest."[20] Thomas Carlyle had accepted Macaulay's position "and expressed it in grosser terms."[21] Quoting liberally from the published correspondence between Johnson and Boswell, Macphail argued that the biographer was a figure of interest in his own right, that he was anything but servile in his attitude to his subject, and that his talents were well developed before he met Johnson at age twenty-three. In summation, he wrote that the Scottish lawyer and man of letters was a thoroughly admirable character by virtue of his literary achievements, his integrity, his qualities as a friend, and his family relationships.[22]

In such an essay as "Johnson's Life of Boswell" and in much of Macphail's other work on literary themes, he was relying for his assessments on the polemical and expository talents he had developed in writing on political, religious, and social questions. Thus he remained an essayist, writing from a strong and even idiosyncratic point of view, and was not writing as a literary critic. His friend Pelham Edgar once stated, "Although his interest in literature was keen he left nothing substantial in the way of literary criticism. He knew what appealed to him in poetry and prose; but as he needed no external guidance in the matter of his likings or dislikings he was not fatuous enough to suppose that his personal preferences or the reverse could be imposed upon other people. Here, in a negative way at least, we have a philosophical theory of aesthetics."[23] Edgar went on to support his judgment by describing Macphail's essay on John McCrae as "not literary criticism, but a tender personal tribute."[24]

Yet this lack of a systematic critical approach to literature did not prevent Macphail from taking an unmistakably clear position on the question of developing a specifically "Canadian" literature. He remained as suspicious of such enterprises as he had been in his student days when writing for the Montreal *Gazette*. In the early 1920s he stated that it was "even possible that this preoccupation with a literature which must be 'Canadian' will prove fatal to a literature of any kind, for a literature that is segregated from the general literature of the world is not literature at all."[25] On several occasions he affirmed that good Canadian writing did not require "a single mounted policeman, a vagrant miner, or a hairy lumberjack."[26] These remarks should of course be understood as a rejection of reliance on hoary stereotypes, not as a dismissal of the need for literature written by Canadians or set in Canada; its development would be a mark of the maturing of the country.

THEATRE AND SHORT STORIES

As well as essays, books, and addresses, Macphail experimented in other modes of artistic expression during his later years. According to his daughter, he never ceased attempting to compose poetry.[27] He wrote many dramas, some of which were published in whole or in part. At least one, "Good Theatre," a one-act satire on the Montreal Repertory Theatre, was performed in 1931 by that company; and it appears that the same company staged "Ingratitude," Act 1 of "Outland," a three-act drama, in May 1932.[28] Macphail's plays frequently had some basis in his own or his family's experience. For example, in Act 1 of "The Last Rising," published in the *Queen's Quarterly*, the main characters have much in common with his mother, his children, and his brother Alexander. The setting is somewhere in Canada on 4 August 1914, and what transpires is strikingly similar to what happened at Macphail's home in Orwell on that day.[29] Although one of the wittiest of these plays, "A Canadian Tragedy," is a straightforward satire on "Canadian content" in contemporary drama, as a general rule the later plays lack the didacticism of *The Land: A Play of Character, in One Act with Five Scenes* (1914). Their purpose was more to entertain than to instruct, but they do share the earlier play's paucity of action and reliance on dialogue.[30]

The short story proved to be a more congenial medium for Macphail, and in the 1930s he published several that attained modest success. Most of these were written in the first person singular and were destined to form part of his semi-autobiographical book, *The Master's Wife*.[31] An exception was "The Graduate," which appeared in the *Queen's Quarterly*; it concerned the tortuous struggles of a reformed alcoholic.[32]

These plays and short stories are primarily significant as evidence of the remarkable range of Macphail's interests and talents. As a eulogist had remarked at the time of his knighthood, Macphail tried his hand at almost every type of literary activity. The comment became even more fitting as the years wore on; this period, when pressing his social and political views seemed unlikely to be productive, was the time he chose for experimentation.

THE CRAFTS, ART, MODERN TECHNOLOGY

Occasionally, especially in the 1920s, Macphail published writings that were of a piece with the strong views he had expressed in 1919-20. Two brief essays in the *Dalhousie Review* were such statements. "The Hand or the Book" was the transcription of an address he delivered in 1926 before the Arts and Handicraft Guild of Montreal. He began by reiterating his criticism of universal schooling and his belief that "to most persons education must come mainly by work done with the hands."[33] He again endorsed the sensible attitudes of French Quebecers, and emphasized that the "boy who is to practise a craft ... must begin early ... and qualify himself not for one work but for all work. Then he will perform all his tasks with creative joy."[34] He praised the guild for insisting that work could be informed by a sense of beauty and told the members that they had a further task: "to subdue the machine ... that threatens to enslave men's minds, that denies them the joy of creation, and dulls their sense of beauty."[35] He could scarcely contain himself seven years later when, as he wrote to Tait McKenzie, "The Handicrafts have moved into a place opposite to mine [on Peel Street]. They operate a complete school of weaving – from raw wooll [sic] to the finished cloth." He appears to have asked his daughter for information and perhaps to scout it out, and he added, "P.S. I went to the school, it is perfect for the purpose, from the sheep to your own back."[36]

The sense of beauty and its fate in "democracy" had been central to an earlier article by Macphail in the *Dalhousie Review*, "Art in Democracy," which was really an elaboration on the themes developed in his essay "Women in Democracy," which was published in the penultimate issue of the *University Magazine*. He believed that art was the last and highest product of civilization and depended upon it for sustenance. Art required "a civilized aristocracy secure in its foundation, superior to base clamour, interested only in itself, curious about the mind, with a passion for ideas; willing to build, paint, sing, fight, and love from habit alone and not for ulterior gain."[37]

Democracy, by which Macphail meant the breaking down of conventions, the family, and deference, was the negation of civilization; it followed that art could not thrive in a democratic setting. Just as when he had been a critic for the Montreal *Gazette* in the late 1880s, Macphail identified the true artistic sensibility with a feeling for beauty and illusion – "the desire to escape from the reality of things." The artist's task was clear: "He suppresses the ugly, the mean, the sordid, so that the beautiful may be revealed." In contrast, Macphail detected "in this generation … the passion for ugliness,"[38] and he proceeded to denounce modern poetry, dancing, and music. The cause of this malaise was that mankind was passing through a revolutionary age. Democracy was integral to the problem; it "is fatal to the artist because it measures all human effort by the same human standard, and offers only the same reward … [which] is always mercenary."[39] Macphail had objected to the abolition of the honours system in Canada, which approximately coincided with such democratic advances as female suffrage, on similar grounds – that the ultimate result would be the reduction of everything to the pecuniary level.[40] In such an atmosphere, art was encouraged to appeal to the coarser senses, "and art put to base uses becomes itself debased." Motion pictures were a case in point: the "vast and facile pictures on the screen are ignorant of colour, and in their distortion destroy any sense of form or delicacy in line." Macphail held little hope for a restoration of artistic standards:

Art thrives only in an atmosphere of freedom; but democracy
and freedom are not at all identical. As democracy grows, liberty
disappears ... We in our time escaped from the Scylla of German
domination only to fall upon the Charybdis of democracy. It is a base
slander upon those who are fallen to say that they fought to make the
world safe for democracy. They fell in an attempt to make the world
safe for themselves ...

For the large freedom of the early nineteenth century we have
exchanged the numerous and hidden tyrannies of this. The modern
industrial system is a form of servitude none the less real because it
appears to be voluntary.[41]

Although in Macphail's later years he wrote little directly related to
contemporary Canadian political and social questions, there is no reason
to suppose that he had substantially altered his views. He frequently reiterated his opinions informally, particularly on the fate of the handicrafts.
As late as the summer of 1938, an interview appeared in a Prince Edward
Island newspaper in which he declared, "To teach craftsmanship is the one
fruitful task of any government; to practise trades at home, and supply
the needs of the community is the one safe refuge of every young man on
this Island. The professions are finished for all but the very elect."[42] He was
entirely serious in his concern, and in earlier years had had his son taught
blacksmithing, and his daughter taught to spin and weave.[43] Around 1927
his daughter gave an address on weaving to the Women's Institute in
Orwell. She stated her belief that "we are no longer wholly content with
factory-made materials," and made this plea: "Let us create and not be
oppressed mentally and spiritually by the power of machinery."[44] In a letter
written in 1979, she recalled that her father "said what was the use of his
trying to get the crafts going again unless he started with his own family."[45]
But at some juncture in the 1920s Macphail seems to have concluded that
the madness of the age was best left to run its course; in the meantime, he
would occupy himself with tasks other than exhortation.

In one brief piece, "Our Canadian Speech," Macphail elaborated on
the impact of technology. This was the first occasion on which he dealt
with the implications of radios and phonographs: "In both, the overtones
are lost; and we are becoming tone-deaf, incapable of hearing the subtle
and rhythmic beauty either of words or of music."[46] Perhaps ironically,
Macphail initially expressed these views to the public in November 1932

during a radio address, although they were later published in the *McGill News*, an alumni magazine, and, slightly revised, in *Saturday Night*.[47] They represented a logical extension of what he had said many times before about the impact of modern technology on older and better ways of doing things. What others welcomed as progress made Macphail apprehensive. Several years earlier he had written, "Speech was the last faculty to come; it is the first to go. Gesture, pantomime, pictures were much earlier. Gesture, pantomime, pictures are coming into their own again."[48] In preparing another radio address, broadcast in November 1933, he wrote, "All the modern mechanism for the transmission of sound and the display of pictures is designed as an appeal to the senses and a relief to the mind from the pain of thinking. To listen to the spoken word is easier … than reading the printed page."[49]

MARIA CHAPDELAINE, MODERN QUEBEC

In all the turmoil of the early postwar period, one artistic creation had caught Macphail's eye: Louis Hémon's *Maria Chapdelaine*. After reading the novel in Orwell during the summer of 1920, Macphail had decided that all English Canadians should have access to this "most perfect example of the literary art."[50] He began to prepare a translation, although his spoken French was less than fluent.[51] On 8 January 1921 he read his translation of a chapter to the Pen and Pencil Club. This was chapter 14, which emphasizes – indeed, celebrates – religious faith and family solidarity in the face of death and a harsh landscape.[52] On the same day, he wrote to Archibald MacMechan telling him that it was "the book that has interested me most in all my lifetime."[53] The reasons are not difficult to discern. As well as portraying the arduous and simple daily existence of the colonists of northern Quebec, their warm family life, and their spirit of submission to nature and the church, the book had a moral that was congenial to Macphail. The heroine, Maria, is confronted with a choice between two suitors – one embodying the values of urban life and the other the way of life of her ancestors. After being tempted by the prospect of comparative ease in Boston, Maria responds to the call of the land and the traditions of her people. She makes the correct decision after hearing "the voice of the country of Quebec, which was half a song of women and half a sermon of the priest."[54] The book had great symbolic meaning for Macphail, and so did the death of its author. Hémon "was killed in a railway accident in Ontario. The cause and place is an allegory."[55]

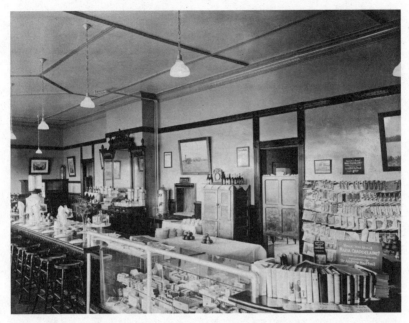

Advertising *Maria Chapdelaine* in Smiths Falls, Ontario. This Canadian Pacific Railway station included a lunch counter and newsstand, which in March 1922 prominently displayed at least two advertisements reading as follows: "Have you read Maria Chapdelaine? A Romance of French Canada. Translation by Sir Andrew Macphail. Price $1.00." The notices were apparently part of a broad campaign promoting the book in CPR stations.

In the autumn of 1920, after returning from Prince Edward Island to Montreal, Macphail learned that William Hume Blake, whom he had known since 1901 and who shared a commitment to a traditionalist view of rural Quebec society, was also planning a translation.[56] The two attempted a collaboration but eventually decided that their styles of rendering Hémon's French into English were incompatible. They then proceeded separately, and each published a version in 1921. Macphail's featured the beautiful drawings by the French Canadian artist, Marc-Aurèle de Foy Suzor-Coté, which had illustrated the original French-language edition five years earlier.[57] There also appears to have been a widespread promotional campaign in partnership with the Canadian Pacific Railway. Surviving photographs show advertisements prominently placed in waiting rooms, lunch counters, and the like within CPR stations, sometimes situated near a cash register.[58] Macphail's translation went through three printings, yet

Blake's, which appeared later in the year, became the standard version.[59] When informing Beaverbrook of his discovery, Macphail wrote, "Maria Chapdelaine ... is the epic of French Canada, as 'Evangeline' is of Acadia ... Louis Hémon, the author, is as new as Kipling was 30 years ago."[60] He gave his translation the subtitle "A Romance of French Canada," whereas Blake chose "A Tale of the Lake St. John Country" – more geographically specific and also more fitting, because the life of the *colons* was scarcely typical of rural Quebec.

Nor was *Maria Chapdelaine* representative of the Quebec Macphail encountered on a daily basis. Montreal had been rapidly changing during his decades in the city. The symbols were everywhere. One could see them, for example, in Place d'Armes, formerly the centre of the French and Roman Catholic town. The Church of Notre Dame, constructed there in the 1820s, had clearly been intended as a significant symbolic statement. According to one architectural historian, "Everything about [it] marked a first in the history of building in Canada. It was the highest building, it had the widest clear span, and it encompassed the greatest interior volume of any construction in Canada."[61] Moreover, for fifty years it stood as the largest church in Canada or the United States.

By the middle of the nineteenth century, important commercial buildings had begun to appear on Place d'Armes, particularly the headquarters of the Bank of Montreal, a very British Canadian institution, which faced Notre Dame. By the end of the 1880s, the church was no longer the clearly dominant edifice on the square.[62] A worshipper or a visitor emerging from it in 1888 and looking to the right saw that on the same square the New York Life Insurance Company had built the city's first "tall building." The tower on top of its eight storeys made it taller than the church. Yet the changes in the appearance of Montreal were only beginning. The characteristic built symbol of the majority culture in Quebec, the church spire, was becoming a secondary architectural feature in the metropolis, a trend that continued unabated decade after decade and was surely a metaphor for society at large.

Another architectural current, which challenged both English- and French-speaking Canadians, became evident in the city during the years 1880–1930, a period that has been described as a "golden age," and during which the population mushroomed from 140,000 to a million.[63] In the late 1990s the curators of an exhibition on the growth of Montreal as a metropolis in this era remarked that "the architecture of Montreal ... [previously] determined by French traditions in the eighteenth century and by British ones in the nineteenth, became Americanized."[64] As Macphail waxed eloquent regarding *Maria Chapdelaine* and what it said about Quebec, this was happening in front of him.[65] Possibly such changes provoked his enthusiasm for Hémon's novel, and it may even have contributed to his reflections on Americanization in other fields as well.

CRITICISM: "AMERICAN METHODS IN MEDICAL EDUCATION" AND MCGILL

Macphail remained a formidable figure and willing to speak his mind even when his views were almost certain to be controversial among persons and within institutions close to him. One address, eventually published as an article, that did not disappoint any expectations of controversy was "American Methods in Medical Education." On 29 October 1926 he delivered the paper to the Congress of the American College of Surgeons, which was meeting in Montreal. Perhaps pointedly, he commenced in French and did not provide a translation. Canadian hospitals and medical schools had been subjected in the years following 1910 to periodic inspection and grading by a number of American medical bodies, and Macphail took as his theme the distortions and rigidities that had been introduced into Canadian curricula to make them conform to standard American practices. He did not doubt that there had been a need for improvement of medical education in the United States; after all, Americans had cut themselves off from the mainstream of civilization in 1776. But the remedy that was being implemented reflected dominant American mores. The "American method in surgery," he declared, "is an application of the American method in business – uniformity, a single standard, mass production. The desired end is 'efficiency.'" Macphail did not quarrel with the aim but believed that "this mechanical method would be, and now is, fatal to us. In the end it will prove fatal to surgery in the United States as well."[66] He declared, that "Under this inhuman system a new kind of physician and a new kind of surgeon have been developed. The physician studies only a part of the patient; the patient is to him nothing more than a series of microscopic slides or chemical solutions. The surgeon knows the patient merely as an arrangement of typewritten cards. He sees him for the first time unconscious on the table, when he comes like a masked executioner to complete the sentence of the judge."[67]

The mechanical approach, operating through "inspectors of our hospitals ... [who] have never taught, never operated, never come into living contact with the sick,"[68] was supplanting a Canadian tradition that had always had the benefit of nourishment from Europe. Macphail argued that not only was the change harmful from his traditionalist point of view, but it was absurd for American professional bodies, given their own standards of judgment, to impose their procedures on Canadian medicine. In 1910 the Carnegie Foundation's initial survey of North American medical schools, popularly known as the Flexner Report, had placed McGill and Toronto in the first rank. "Our medical teaching and practice, English and French, is, and has been for a hundred years, equal to the best in the world. We never descended to the degradation of issuing diplomas for money. Those who desired such were compelled to go to the United States."[69]

Macphail believed that the American inspectors' criticism of the Dalhousie medical faculty and its affiliated Halifax Medical College in 1910 had arisen simply from an American tendency to be impressed by the size of physical "plant"; Dalhousie was small, and hence was given a low rating.[70] He rejected this reasoning. A few weeks after the congress, he delivered an address to the Kingston-Frontenac Medical Society on "The Small School." Speaking "under the auspices of Queen's University," at a meeting chaired by J.C. Connell, the dean of medicine at Queen's, he praised small medical schools for their effectiveness in turning out the practising physician, which he attributed to their emphasis on the teaching of basic principles, as opposed to the method of experiment repetition; consequently, the small school left more scope for excellent teaching. According to the Kingston *Standard*, "The large school, he said, was a product of the American mind which found 'efficiency' only in mass production by standardized methods."[71] Although Macphail may have been swimming against the stream, one cannot dismiss him as an incorrigible sentimentalist on this matter, for two decades earlier he had recommended the cessation of operations by his own medical school, Bishop's, largely on the grounds of lack of facilities. His record suggests that he did not believe that size itself, large or small, was the key to quality.

Close to the end of Macphail's address to the congress, he noted that he had delivered his message "without the anaesthesia of flattery." He then went on to compare the American enthusiasm to pressure others to accept their methods and standards to "the fatal error into which the Germans fell – a lack of sensibility to the feelings, emotions, beliefs, and prejudices of other peoples – they themselves being like you, so naive, so amiable, so ingenuous, so convinced, and sincere."[72] His plea was that American medical institutions confine their supervision within their national boundaries.[73]

Macphail's major problems over the content of his paper did not come from his audience but from the editors of the *Canadian Medical Association Journal*, to whom he submitted the address for publication. Alexander D. Blackader, who had succeeded him as editor, and Charles F. Martin, McGill's dean of medicine, feared offending their American readers. Correspondence and discussions between Macphail, Blackader, Martin, and others associated with the journal extended from early November until March 1927. In the course of these exchanges Macphail stated bluntly to Martin, "I am convinced that American methods are malign, that they have invaded us, and will destroy our whole medical fabric and their own as well … Quite seriously, the feeling in the profession against the American invasion is rising. At the proper time I shall do what I can to resist that invasion. The Medical Faculty of McGill is becoming too closely identified with American medical interests. They should be disentangled."[74] Finally, the editorial board offered to sponsor publication of the address as a pamphlet, believing, in Blackader's words, that "it would not be wise to have some of its statements published officially in the Association Journal. Its clever satire might not appeal favorably to some of our confrères in the U.S.A."[75] Macphail declined, and his wartime friend Sir Dawson Williams, editor of the *British Medical Journal*, published it in his periodical – although he, too, felt contrary pressure from colleagues. Once the article finally appeared in September 1927, Macphail received a remarkable volume of congratulatory mail, largely from Canadians. John A. Mathieson, former premier and then chief justice of Prince Edward Island, wrote, "Your reasoning applies with equal force to our whole system of education which is being debased by the application of American business standards."[76]

It is difficult to know exactly how the administration of McGill University regarded Macphail. McGill's official historian, Stanley B. Frost, a divinity professor who was an academic administrator at the university in the generation following Macphail's death, placed him as part of "a respectable minority on campus," in reference to his "arch-conservative" views on academic developments.[77] There is also some impatience, even a hint of irritation, evident in his discounting Macphail's criticism of the postwar principalship of Sir Arthur Currie as being "at fault in many of its facts, and perversely anachronistic in its opinions."[78] Yet he acknowledged that Macphail was a significant presence within the university, not least for his being, like Leacock, "another personality of national dimension."[79] Thus Macphail was an asset, though not entirely unalloyed. The McGill University Archives reveal that Dean Martin kept Currie, the principal, informed of the correspondence over publication of "American Methods in Medical Education," a sign that this matter was of more than academic interest to the Faculty of Medicine and to the university administration.[80]

A few months after Currie died on 30 November 1933, Macphail published in the *Queen's Quarterly* an article about him as principal at McGill. Along with some shrewd observations on such matters as the impact of Currie's particular administrative style on university governance at the level of the faculties, there was criticism of the academic directions the institution had taken during his regime, and of the financial situation at the time of Currie's death, with the implication that he was in some way responsible. There was also sarcasm, which extended to the choice of a subtitle, "The Value of a Degree," for Currie had had no degree.[81] Shortly after the article appeared in print, Macphail was confronted with a rebuttal from a possibly unexpected source: Dorothy McMurray, who was in the early stages of what was to be a lengthy career as secretary to several McGill principals. Able, remarkably strong-willed, and intensely loyal, she believed Currie "would have resented [the article] most keenly."[82] She took it upon herself to write a forceful and detailed memorandum, fourteen pages in length, refuting Macphail's comments on the substantive issues of academic developments and finances during the Currie years.[83]

McMurray reported in a letter that she spent two hours with Macphail on the afternoon of Saturday, 21 April 1934, arguing her case. Apparently Macphail had learned that she had written a critique and wanted to discuss it with her: "Sir Andrew would not take 'no' about my going over the article with him." No version of Macphail's view of the encounter is known to survive, but McMurray wrote in her letter, "He seemed quite defenceless as I pointed out wherein it seemed to many people he had done the late principal an injustice."[84] On the following Monday she wrote to Macphail with "one or two more things which I did not have time to mention."[85] In McMurray's fourteen-page memorandum, she stated that she had been motivated by a desire to remove any apparent stain from Currie's record, for she feared that Macphail's account would influence future writers.[86] Indeed, fifty years later, Frost referred to Macphail as Currie's "foremost critic."[87]

Frost stated that McMurray's memorandum "seems not to have been circulated,"[88] but in fact McMurray was not writing solely for posterity. Surviving correspondence in the university archives indicates that in April 1934 she was in touch with several leading members of the McGill board of governors over this issue. For their own sakes, they, as the financial stewards of the university, were doubtless interested in seeing Macphail contradicted. Certainly they passed McMurray's memorandum around among themselves; there were twenty-three board members.[89] Governor George C. McDonald, a prominent accountant, wrote to McMurray that reading the memorandum "afforded me considerable interest and satisfaction."[90] Furthermore, it is probable that the governors were not amused by Macphail's comment concerning them in the article, published during the depths of the Great Depression: "They are all business men; although it must be admitted that in recent years the 'business man,' like Samson Agonistes, 'is going somewhat crest-fallen, stalking with less unconscionable strides.'"[91] The *Canadian Forum*, for its part, advised its readers that they would find Macphail's article on Currie "very suggestive" regarding the power of the McGill board of governors, which he had portrayed as absolute.[92]

In the spring of 1938 Macphail, who had retired from the university the previous year,[93] sent the new principal of McGill, Lewis W. Douglas, an American, a copy of the most recent issue of the *Queen's Quarterly*, containing a piece he had written on Robert E. Lee. Douglas congratulated Macphail on "the clarity and penetration of your article." Next to the copy of the letter from Douglas in the "McGill Principals' Papers" at the university archives is an unsigned, typewritten comment, which agreed with the complimentary nouns but singled out a passage as "an example, I think, of how Sir Andrew mars his great literary gifts by a quality which is hard to name, but which runs through everything he does."[94] The writer was almost certainly someone at McGill who knew Macphail well, had known him for quite a long time, and was wary of him. It appears that Macphail, the condemner of American methods, critic of former administrators, and sometime friend of the Soviet Union was a person about whom new principals were warned – as someone associated with controversy who might embarrass the university, irritate the governors, and be very unrepentant about it. As for Macphail and the governors, Leacock's comment after his death seems apt: "Andrew, though frequenting the rich in his daily walk of life, was never quite satisfied of their right to be. Towards plutocrats, bankers, manufacturers and such, he felt a little bit as a rough country dog feels towards a city cat. He didn't quite accept them."[95] This may have been one reason that, according to another obituary writer, "after the site of his house on Peel St. became very valuable for business purposes he steadfastly declined all offers for its purchase."[96]

MACPHAIL IN THE POSTWAR ERA: CONCLUSION

In an interview conducted in 1990, a Prince Edward Island clergyman recalled hearing from a member of his church who worked for Macphail as a housekeeper in his home at 216 Peel Street that one day she noticed him peering into a mirror and saying, "You're getting old, you old bugger, you're getting old."[97] Yet in the final two decades of his life Macphail was more than an aging curmudgeon. In addition to his own work – and his trenchant critiques of Americanization, modern technology, utilitarian education, and other ills of the period – he was a patron of the arts and actively encouraged new talent. This was manifest at both an individual and an institutional level. During the Great Depression he took in and housed, apparently for an extended period, at least one artist who had fallen on hard times, a man he had known for decades; while living at 216 Peel the artist used it as a studio.[98] Macphail was particularly supportive of the Montreal Repertory Theatre, served as vice-president at its foundation in 1930, and was known as an enthusiastic first-nighter. At the time of his death he was still vice-president, and Samuel Morgan-Powell, the longtime drama and literary critic for the *Montreal Star*, stated, "Many a time, sitting with him in his quiet home, I have wondered at the intensity of feeling he displayed over everything that affected the Repertory Theatre, how anxiously he would ponder over its progress, and how earnest he was in his determination that it should go forward. He would shake his leonine head with emphasis and declare that there simply must be no question of a retrograde movement."[99] In a memoir written six decades later, Herbert Whittaker, who had been a designer for amateur theatre productions in Montreal during the 1930s, singled him out as having been "a very handsome benefactor" of the company.[100]

Macphail was especially pleased that the troupe cut across traditional lines, involving French speakers as well as English speakers. This was far more than a token gesture, for, according to Whittaker, "A concerted effort to appeal to both French and English communities continued through the 1930s." Many plays, including original French Canadian works, were produced in French.[101] Whittaker also noted that in 1920 Macphail had signed the founding manifesto of the predecessor group, the Montreal Community Players, which stated that its purpose was "to facilitate the production of plays dealing with Canadian life or written by Canadian authors," explaining, "Up to the present time, such plays have had practically no chance for production in the Dominion."[102] All of this sounds much like so many of Macphail's earlier endeavours, providing Canadian venues for Canadians in the arts, and, as with the Bishop's medical faculty in the 1890s and the Pen and Pencil Club in the 1900s, attempting to reach out to French speakers.

The letters Macphail sent in 1936 to Sinclair Ross, who was then in his late twenties and virtually unknown, reveal the extent to which he would go out of his way to nurture a new talent. After reading in the *Queen's Quarterly* two of Ross's gritty short stories about farm families struggling within themselves and against the forces of nature on the Canadian Prairies, he wrote to him saying, "Kipling could not have done better. My hope is that you will continue." He also made an editing suggestion and explained his rationale.[103] Ross replied to him and evidently indicated that he had experienced some setbacks in his attempts to have his work published; one of the *Queen's Quarterly* stories had been the first of his to appear in a Canadian periodical. Macphail wrote, "Let not your breast be troubled. If you receive 'rejection slips,' it is because you send to the wrong market." He closed by stating, "I shall look for your work with confidence."[104]

Macphail's surviving papers indicate that he was more than willing to participate in projects attempting to create a greater awareness among the public of the existing Canadian literary canon. In the first half of the 1920s he prepared to contribute to two ambitious series which, in the end, were not to be completed. He produced an introduction to a planned reprint of Sir Gilbert Parker's *Pierre and His People*, which was to be part of a twenty-five-volume series edited by John W. Garvin and entitled "The Master Works of Canadian Authors."[105] The volume for which Macphail prepared his essay on Parker was never published, and Lorne Pierce read it to the Royal Society of Canada on his behalf the year after he died.[106] Macphail also wrote an introduction to an anthology of works by Norman Duncan, to be included in a series of thirty or more volumes on "Makers of Canadian Literature," a project of Pierce. The Duncan piece has never been published, although two drafts survive in the Macphail Papers, the second more appreciative than the first, after urging from Pierce.[107]

Macphail was stricken by heart attacks in May 1937 and August 1938. Despite his illness he remained characteristically uncomplaining and self-contained. After the second and more severe attack he wrote from Orwell to Charles Martin, his former medical colleague at McGill, "For six weeks I have been looking upon the same beauty; and the world becomes more beautiful as the time for leaving it comes near." He would soon be back on Peel Street "and so escape the 'slow despair of summer on the wane.'"[108] But when he returned to Montreal it was to the Royal Victoria Hospital. He died there on 23 September 1938 and was buried beside his wife in Mount Royal Cemetery.[109] Leacock wrote: "Andrew Macphail's death came to those of us who were his friends with the shock as of something that could not be. It had not seemed that he could die. Always he had kept his sorrows and his ailments to himself ... To most of us the news of his death came, sudden and unbelievable, for the moment holding even sorrow numb. Even now it is hard to think that he is gone."[110] He had remained active almost until the end. In his daughter's words, many years later, he had led "a very full life, but not an easy one."[111] No doubt she had in mind, with her emphasis, the loss of his wife in 1902, the loss of much of his eyesight in 1911, his military service in his fifties, and the shooting in 1921 whose effects he lived with for the rest of his life.

The Master's Wife, Macphail, and the Island

Andrew Macphail's most enduring work was published posthumously, and it has been absolutely central to making him an iconic figure in Prince Edward Island. This was *The Master's Wife*, a semi-autobiographical portrait of life as he had experienced it growing up in the Scottish Canadian rural community of Orwell in the latter part of the nineteenth century. The master of the title is Andrew's father, William Macphail, and the master's wife is Andrew's mother, Catherine Smith. The perspective is that of a child.

THE MASTER'S WIFE

The Master's Wife is, in the first instance, a successful penetration into the inner life of a particular type of Scottish Canadian community and is a fund of information on its practices and world view. There are detailed accounts of the activities of the people and their families, be they spar-makers or homemakers. Their passions are recounted, whether for religion and quoting scripture, for books, for tea (the women), or for liquor (some men). Their ambivalent relationship with domestic animals, to which they became attached but which they eventually slaughtered for food, is sensitively portrayed. Referring to an occasion when, "as a very young child," he and his father came upon nine animals of three species that five Smith grand-uncles had just dispatched in preparation for winter, Macphail writes, "These animals for years had been loving friends, and now they made a cheerful sacrifice for human need."[1] He elaborates:

Life is not life where there is no tragedy. That little world was a
world of death – a wild animal caught in a trap, a partridge slain by
a hawk, a cow submerged in the marsh, a dog whose time had come;
and always the mild-eyed creatures that must be killed for food.
Indeed, a boy himself must learn to take part in that ceremonial, and
finally to conduct the sacrifice. Thereafter, he was never the same. It
was not uncommon to see a boy in tears before the bound animal.[2]

Macphail himself felt this closeness to animals, which he carried into
later life and took to unusual lengths. In *The Master's Wife* he relates an
encounter while near a Quebec resort, waiting for a train: "In a field was a
small black Canadian pony, and a profitable hour was spent in talking with
her."[3] Someone who had worked as a server in Macphail's house in Orwell
during the early postwar years remembered in an interview in 1990 that
the tail of a favourite horse was in the dining room, possibly hanging next
to the fireplace.[4] A granddaughter recalled from the 1930s that his dachshund Lisl "went everywhere with him" and would be leashed and on the
tablecloth as Macphail ate; the leash was tied to a hook on the table. A "very
lovable" dog, Lisl caused no fuss, never touched the food or the dishes, and
never begged for food.[5]

The Master's Wife was written as a celebration of the traditional way of
life Macphail had known, a tribute to his people and his place in their time.
Through skilful characterization and use of anecdote, all viewed through
the prism of an observant child, Macphail conveys an appreciation of what
it was like to be born and raised in such an atmosphere. The closeness
of the family circle was cemented by the interdependent duties of each
member, all performed on the same farm. There was pleasure in learning
the many skills in which farm children had to become proficient. Hovering
over everything, it seemed, was the omnipresence of religious sanctions. By
far the lengthiest of twenty-two chapters, at twenty-seven pages (compared
with an average of less than eleven pages per chapter for the others), was
one entitled "The World of Religion." The long Sabbaths could be broken
only by going to a field with a hidden book, under the pretence of tending
grazing cattle. The emphasis within the community on a specific variety
of religion bound up with self-denial manifested itself in such ways as fear
of the temptations presented by musical instruments: "One young man
who performed very well on the bag-pipes abandoned the practice at the
time of his conversion; and to prove his sincerity destroyed the instrument which he had created with his own hands. The violin was unknown,

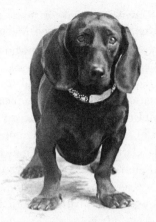

Lisl. This dog went everywhere with Macphail in the interwar years, even accompanying him to the Ritz-Carlton Hotel, where it was treated to ice cream. When at home, while Macphail was eating his meals Lisl kept him company, reclining on top of the dining table, leashed to a hook. Its behaviour has been described as impeccable.

except among the Irish [of neighbouring districts]. It was considered a dissolute instrument."[6]

But there was also within the community the hint of an external world, provided, for example, by a first taste of exotic, aromatic coffee, thanks to the minister's wife, "a foreign woman, that is, from Nova Scotia."[7] There were also breaks in the claustrophobic solemnity provided by the tales of a Gaelic-speaking Scottish grandmother, who delighted in thunderstorms and brandy, told of witches, and refused to take life entirely seriously. Even more dramatic and sudden were the visits of a grand-uncle, Andrew Smith, a sea captain, who came to see them after every voyage, bearing wondrous gifts from abroad – silk, spice, green tea, French brandy, a white loaf of sugar – and "a breath of intelligence from the larger world" that all members of the household clearly appreciated.[8] The love of company and the generous hospitality coexisted with a faint suspicion of anyone from outside the community. Malcolm Macqueen, a distinguished Winnipeg barrister who had been born in 1878 and was a former neighbour in Orwell, gave a vivid illustration of the lack of comfort with strangers; writing to Macphail in 1933, he recalled his first meeting with the Basque portrait painter Alphonse Jongers, who had visited the Macqueen household in the company of Macphail in the late 1890s: "When he crossed the line fence I was relieved, thankful that no harm had come to us."[9] Non-Islanders were almost unknown, aside from peddlers.[10] Even Macphail's mother "was commonly described as a 'Smith woman,' that is a foreign person whose native place was some miles away."[11]

Although *The Master's Wife* is autobiographical, it is more than that. It is an almost joyous affirmation of the virtues and pleasures of Macphail's ancestral way of life, a point Université Laval classicist Maurice Lebel underscored when reviewing it in *Le Devoir*: "Ce livre renferme toute une philosophie de la vie. Il serait relativement facile d'en extraire toute une série de pensées profondes qui se lise comme des maximes. On sent que l'auteur y a condensé les résultats de son expérience du monde et des hommes."[12] The memoirist linked the world of art with the world of work in Orwell:

> To live is an art. The material at hand must be subdued to the purposes of life. The essence of art is economy, that nothing be wasted. To write as Mr. Kipling writes, to draw as *Mr. Punch* draws, to paint as Ver Meer paints, to live as we lived, is merely to practice economy, without waste, without meanness. The writer who wastes words becomes a journalist; the draughtsman who wastes lines, a fumbler searching blindly; the painter wasting colour a striver after impressions he has never felt.
>
> Art is management of words, sound, line, colour. Economy is the highest art in the management of a house. In life, as in every work of art, this note must be true and dominant over all else.[13]

At the same time that Macphail celebrated the community, he did not present an idyllic picture of a people without crime or malice. He reported the theft of the master's saddle, which was to be an unsolved crime (although his mother "always hinted that she knew the one who stole it".[14]) He told of the killing of his mother's protective Newfoundland dog: "This faithful creature was poisoned by a distant neighbour, and she [his mother] spent many years in discovering the poisoner. For the rest of her life she watched with slow delight the decadence of him and his family into distress."[15] Macphail also related another unsolved crime, the murder of Ann Beaton, a woman in the nearby district of Orwell Rear (now Lyndale), which had occurred several years before his birth. Although there was never punishment under the law, within the area there was a prime suspect, another woman. The event was so exceptional that the known details, such as the place of discovery of the body and the murder weapon itself, a heavy grubbing hoe (commonly used for clearing land by digging up roots and stumps), were discussed decade after decade.[16] Macphail recalled, "The grandmother, always courageous, was one of the first on the spot, and she could ever after secure willing service by a promise to tell what it was she saw."[17]

In *The Master's Wife*, Macphail excelled particularly at conveying the community's attitude to education. For his mother, "the school was the open door of escape."[18] Her children absorbed the message, and referring to the farmwork that had to be done, Macphail wrote, "We worked thinking only of escape."[19] When the opportunity came, at Prince of Wales College in Charlottetown, he saw that "it was well understood that the intention in coming to school was to escape from work by sitting in a professor's chair or on a judge's bench, by standing in the pulpit or before the altar, or moving at leisure in professional or political office."[20] Teaching, it is clear, was a continuation of the escape. When he gained the coveted position at Malpeque grammar school in 1883, it was as though "I was free of work forever."[21] The lesson of his mother had stayed with him: "scholastic achievement was only a means in life and not life itself." In fact he confessed, "I was never a student. I never became a scholar. Even my professional studies were perfunctory … I was spoiled by reading … I was too careful to learn no more than the academic law demanded, and I learned that little too easily."[22]

It was in the late 1920s that Macphail began work on *The Master's Wife*. Many of his closest associates died in the early years of that decade – E.W. Thomson, James Mavor, Sir William Peterson, Paul T. Lafleur, Marjorie Pickthall, and John St Loe Strachey – and the death of these old friends may have had much to do with his concern for retrospective writing in his later years. It is not certain that he originally planned for his memoir to be published. In a letter in 1927 to Tait McKenzie, one of his most intimate friends since their days together as McGill students, Macphail referred to a 200-page manuscript he was sending by registered mail: "I have no doubt of the intrinsic and personal quality. I cannot judge if it is of general or universal interest." His further comment, "It was written as a mere record for Jeffrey and Dorothy [his children]," makes it clear that he was referring to an early version of *The Master's Wife*. He explained, "No human eye has yet seen it. Now, I begin to suspect it has a general interest."[23]

Several weeks earlier he had informed McKenzie that the sculptor Henri Hébert, a fellow member of the Pen and Pencil Club, had, "at his own request," made an "excellent" bust of Macphail. "I want a bronze [made] for

Jeffrey and Dorothy,"[24] he told McKenzie. At age sixty-two, he was taking stock and thinking in terms of what he would be leaving behind for his children. Already in 1924, he had sat for a Jongers portrait, in academic robes. At the time of Jongers's death twenty-one years later, the Montreal *Gazette* praised his studies for their "strength and realism, with a superb sense of color" and indicated that the Macphail portrait was considered among the best, if not the very best of his works.[25]

The manuscript Macphail was preparing would be dedicated to the children. By 1929 he described the book as finished.[26] He then submitted it to Dorothy and Jeffrey separately for judgment. Each told him that it was too personal, and he made changes on the basis of their suggestions. Through the last decade of his life he continued to revise the manuscript, and many years later his daughter stated that he was probably working on it as late as the early part of 1938 – that is, as long as he was writing, since he was ill for several months prior to his death.[27] She also stated that he probably would have published it in 1939 had he lived to do so.[28] He appears to have taken more care with this work than with any other; but even by 1929 he had considered it to be the best book he had written. It reads with extreme ease, and as one of Macphail's maxims was "easy reading is hard writing,"[29] there can be no doubt that he worked on this book as he had worked on few writing projects. After all, in it he was saying the most important things – about himself, his parents, his social environment, his cultural heritage, and his beliefs.

Yet Macphail's position in relation to community values appears ambiguous at some points. He clearly preferred the relatively secular, worldly, and humanistic attitudes of his mother's relatives to the strict sabbatarianism and intense earnestness of his father, who seemed to epitomize the predominant outlook in Orwell. The Smiths provided, he wrote, "a pagan refuge from the problems of sin, of its punishment, and even from the complicated process of the salvation from it."[30] In an interview in 2000, a perceptive nephew referred to him as "more Smith than Macphail."[31] Moreover, he and the other children had no doubt that their place was not on the farm. Commenting on the sometimes harsh domination of life by the elemental forces of nature, Macphail wrote, "Of one thing we were all convinced from the first: we would escape from the land and the ice."[32] Thus although he eventually based his social criticism on his affection for the local way of life, especially the farming component of it, and his hostility to all that undermined it, he himself had taken the first opportunity to break loose from it. Perhaps this is an example of what he describes as "that fatal capacity to see the paradox of things, that is, both sides of a subject at the same time."[33]

It should be emphasized that in addition to the personal significance for Macphail of the way of life he portrayed in *The Master's Wife*, it was crucial for his intellectual formation. Stephen Leacock once remarked that underneath all of Macphail's half-bantering talk over drinks in Montreal about rural life, especially the rural life he had experienced as a boy, there "was a deep-seated feeling that the real virtue of a nation is bred in the country, that the city is an unnatural product."[34] He believed strongly that the largely self-sufficient farming he had known in Orwell, with its independence, dignity, approximate equality, and virtual absence of poverty, formed the ideal basis for society. He was critical of western Canadian farming, with its single-crop production, its high levels of investment in machinery, and its dependence on (and consequent vulnerability to) the international market for the single crop. It was too much like an industry transplanted into the countryside. But the "mixed" family farm, producing to meet most of the needs of its own members, meant that farmers and their families were largely independent of international markets and of the marketplace in general. People were valued as people, not as factors of production. This was the way of life that provided Macphail with the basis for his social criticism and his steadfast opposition to the industrialization and urbanization of Canada.

Finally, *The Master's Wife* is important for the originality of presentation that it displayed. It has been referred to as a novel,[35] apparently because of the novelistic technique of presentation through the mind of a child, which Macphail likens to "the mind of a dreamer by night." The characters, community, and events in *The Master's Wife* are real, yet by use of the free-associating perspective of the child and the unfettered movement through time – through decades upon decades in this case – allowed by dreams, "the whole figment," as Macphail writes, "has the force of intense reality."[36] It also draws the reader in from the start with an unusual sensation of freshness and immediacy. An ingenious approach to telling his family's story, it works exceptionally well. One critic, Janice Kulyk Keefer, has declared:

> The effect upon the reader of the first chapter of *The Master's Wife* can be likened to the effect on the viewer of the opening dream sequence in Ingmar Bergman's *Wild Strawberries*; both free us from our rigid expectations of linear narrative and the logic it builds by. Instead of a

conventional sequence of events and observations, Macphail gives us a teeming sea of perceptions, the acuity, starkness, or complexity of which derive from his refusal to categorize as good or evil any of the subjects he treats.[37]

Macphail had attempted many creative forms over the years: poetry, a novel, drama, historical writing, translation, the short story, and above all the essay. This memoir, presented through a child's eyes, is, like the creation of the *University Magazine*, one of his great successes, possibly his greatest.

A semi-autobiography, a document in Canada's social history, a statement of a social and political philosophy, beautifully written and structured in a unique way, *The Master's Wife* is a book of rare richness. The historian Daniel Cobb Harvey – also a Prince Edward Islander by birth, also a Prince of Wales alumnus, and the leading Maritime historian of his era – characterized it as Macphail's "*apologia pro vita sua*, and an impressionistic study of his native community."[38] The text is testimony to a full life and is evidence that the author never lost sight of who he was, the forces that had shaped him, and where he had come from. But beyond the content of his affirmation of a traditional way of life, *The Master's Wife* is a work of art, written by a man who was a supreme artist in words. As Pelham Edgar wrote shortly after Macphail's death, "his artistic impulse was as strong as his convictions."[39]

THE HISTORY AND RECEPTION OF *THE MASTER'S WIFE*

Macphail published fragments of the manuscript that was to become *The Master's Wife* in the form of short stories, personal reminiscences, and even brief dramas. His recollections of "The Old School" (Uigg grammar school), "The Old College" (Prince of Wales), and "The Old University" (McGill) were delivered over national radio in October and December 1937, and subsequently published in a variety of print media.[40] But he did not live to place the entire manuscript before the public in book form. It appeared in print late in the year following his death. His two children had *The Master's Wife* published through a private arrangement with a printer. The result was an aesthetic success. A handsome volume with a fine selection of photographs of leading characters, there is no doubt that Macphail would have been proud of it. Yet *The Master's Wife* was brought into the world with a double disability: it was launched shortly after the start of a world war that preoccupied public attention, and its author had died a year earlier. By the time the war was over, the book was "old news" – six years old – and Macphail had been dead seven years. In fact, there was a third problem. The method of simply working with a printer, with its lack of linkage to a system of distribution, and the circumstances of 1939 combined to bury the book in terms of public consciousness. Over the next several decades, one of the few writers to give it extended treatment was Pelham Edgar, who made it a major focus of an article he wrote on Macphail for the Queen's Quarterly in 1947.[41]

The book became a sort of hidden treasure in Canadian literature. Although born, raised, and educated in Prince Edward Island, the present author first learned of it as an undergraduate at McGill University in the honours history program during the mid-1960s. This resulted from a conversation with a senior professor, John Irwin Cooper, who had been at McGill long enough – first as a doctoral student and then as a professor – to have vivid memories of Macphail, a distinctive figure on campus with his intermittently worn eyepatch. Macphail's name had come up, probably because the professor knew the student was from Prince Edward Island and/or because the student, aware of the Macphail property in Orwell with its impressive granite pillars at the entrance to the lane, knew vaguely that Macphail had some connection with McGill – a subject about which Cooper knew a great deal. A specialist in the history of Quebec with an encyclopedic knowledge of Canadian history in general, he recommended The Master's Wife as the best memoir or book of any kind on the post-pioneering generation in the rural Canada of the nineteenth century. Intrigued, the student sought out the book that same day in the stacks of the university's Redpath Library and, having picked it up, could not put it down and read it right through. The next day he came back and read it a second time.

In 1977, after years of periodic prodding, a national publishing house, McClelland and Stewart, produced an inexpensive paperback edition of The Master's Wife for its prestigious New Canadian Library series, with a brief introduction by the present writer.[42] This provided national distribution for the book, which had long been available only through shops specializing in rare books, and in some libraries. At last it began to receive the circulation and recognition it deserved; and the second edition went through more than one printing, although without the correction of production errors and omissions made in the course of the first printing, which the publisher had promised to the author of the introduction.[43] But despite any problems of detail, the cardinal facts about this reprint are that whereas the original edition put hundreds – perhaps five hundred – copies into print, the New Canadian Library edition placed several thousand in bookstores and libraries; and the book's very inclusion in the series guaranteed a measure of scholarly and critical attention.

Ten years after the initial appearance of the second edition, Janice Kulyk Keefer published a landmark book of literary criticism concerning Maritime writing, *Under Eastern Eyes: A Critical Reading of Maritime Fiction*.[44] In this volume she focuses on the way Macphail revealed the Orwell of his youth through the mind of a child and praises "the peculiar honesty and almost total absence of nostalgia" in the book.[45] Her use of the qualifying adverb "almost" is linked to the fact that she finds the last two chapters "disappointing in tone and conception, perhaps because in them Macphail deals with his post-Orwellian adult life, and a degree of self-consciousness, sentimentality, and pompousness infects the narrative."[46] She argues that what "gives to this narrative its curious power … [is that] we have Macphail reinhabiting the mind of childhood, yet with the mobility which adult experience and understanding permit."[47] In her view, this method allows him to portray his community "with an uncanny detachment that permits us a perfectly dual vision – we see the people of Orwell as they saw themselves, and as they were there to be seen."[48]

Kulyk Keefer highlights the book's transcendence of convention, and entirely because of *The Master's Wife* she ranks Macphail with such major Maritime writers as Thomas McCulloch, T.C. Haliburton, and Joseph Howe, the giants of Nova Scotia's "golden age."[49] Yet he is unlike those earlier writers in one aspect: "What immediately strikes the reader of Macphail's text is that community – which had functioned for McCulloch and Haliburton as an observable, exigent fact, as part of the hard currency of reality – has here become more a matter of dream and, to complete the analogy, frozen asset."[50] Macphail's presentation of Orwell through, in his words, "the mind of a dreamer by night"[51] is thus understood as a product of the 1920s. That decade, as modern historians have documented, was catastrophic for the Maritime region, since the benefits negotiated through the Confederation agreement and in the succeeding generation were stripped away. Jobs disappeared, and hundreds of thousands of people left for greener pastures, most never to return except as visitors, often only decades later. Historian John G. Reid estimates that "perhaps as much as one-fifth of the entire population of the region" left during the 1920s.[52] This was when Macphail conceived the book and did most of the writing, and Kulyk Keefer links it to Frank Parker Day's conflict-ridden *Rockbound*, published late in the same decade.[53] With the book's power, its rich texture, and its complexity, it is, in Kulyk Keefer's view, "one of the finest and oddest pieces of prose to be found in Maritime, or Canadian literature as a whole."[54]

Other writers have also marvelled at the special nature of Macphail's achievement. In the first edition of *The Oxford Companion to Canadian Literature*, published in 1983, J.M. Bumsted, in his article "Historical Writing in English," characterizes *The Master's Wife* as "*sui generis*" for its blend of autobiographical memoir, history, and novelistic technique. He astutely notes that the book's defiance of neat categorization as either literature or history has been a factor contributing to its being unjustly neglected.[55] Writing in 1985, Kenneth MacKinnon, professor of English at Saint Mary's University and a specialist in Atlantic Canadian regional literature, places the author in a Gaelic context: "The traditional chronicler in Gaelic has to perform a variety of allied literary, scholarly, historical, and genealogical functions. Macphail manages these separate roles with surprising insight and great economy of expression."[56]

In an article published in 2000 as part of a volume on the literature of small islands, Brent MacLaine, a literature professor at the University of Prince Edward Island, considers Macphail's book alongside fictional works by Day and Alistair MacLeod. He finds their commonality to be the presence, at their centres, of intelligent and precocious male children maturing in economically and culturally confining circumstances in communities on islands of Atlantic Canada. The focus of much of each is the crucial initiation of the young male into the world of books while incurring the censure, hostility, or suspicion of at least some of those around him.[57] *The Master's Wife* is clearly now part of the regional literary canon. Indeed, Peter Hay, a Tasmanian geographer, poet, and essayist at the University of Tasmania, wrote in 2002, "The Master's Wife is one of the world's great literary evocations of place ... Atlantic Canada stands ... as the global capital of place-writing, and within this corpus The Master's Wife stands pre-eminent." Hay stated outright that the book is "on any standard of assessment, one of the great writings of the departing century," and he declared "its modest profile ... [to be] inexplicable."[58]

Many readers of the book have found that they need to reread it. MacKinnon refers to "re-reading *The Master's Wife* [as] an addiction" and attributes this to Macphail's use of humour: "The juxtaposition of local folk rooted in traditions of the Highland Scots with an array of contrasting provincial and cosmopolitan people permits a number of opportunities for a variety of ironic and comic explorations of incongruity ... The frequency of examples of a finely shaded range of humour is remarkable."[59] Kulyk Keefer also makes a relevant comment with regard to the urge to reread: "The thumbnail sketches of Macphail's family and neighbours ... are twined together in the complex fashion of genealogical tables, so that the whole becomes a continuum difficult to grasp or place until the entire narrative has unfolded."[60] Realization of this grows as the reading progresses, for, as MacKinnon states, "The entire work seems at first to be a sequence of well-crafted but discontinuous anecdotes."[61] In the experience of the present author, older persons of similar cultural backgrounds to that of Macphail, when first introduced to the book in the late 1960s and the 1970s, cited the following as reasons they wished to reread: what they viewed as the absolute authenticity of the character types presented; what MacKinnon refers to as "the communication of the texture of life";[62] and the quality of the prose. But Kulyk Keefer's point undoubtedly has much force: the structure of the book imposes rereading on the person who has taken to it.

The belated scholarly attention has come because the book is now accessible, for it is clear from references in the work of a number of writers that they have relied on the 1977 edition or, in the second half of the 1990s and later, a third edition. In 1994 the Institute of Island Studies at the University of Prince Edward Island published a facsimile reprint of the original edition, using the same photographs and adding, by the present author, a new, larger introduction, explanatory notes, and corrigenda. This edition also includes photographs of Macphail's mother on the front cover and Macphail himself (in 1897, at age thirty-two or thirty-three) on the back cover; a previously unpublished poem in his honour, "The Spirit," written by a fourteen-year-old grandson shortly after his death; and a preface by Harry Baglole, the director of the institute, who was strongly committed to the book.[63] The facsimile reprint meant that at last the book would have broad distribution in its original format. In 2002 the facsimile edition went through a new printing.

Original in conception, Macphail's memoir was meticulously executed, both by himself and by his children, who saw it through the production process after his death. But in the decades following its first appearance in print in 1939, for several reasons it did not achieve the distribution and the attention it merited. Since its second and third editions in 1977 and 1994, it has emerged from the shadows and has been recognized, particularly by specialists in the literature of Atlantic Canada, as a complex, sophisticated piece of work in which Macphail – brilliant stylist and arch-critic of modern life – reached the apex of his creativity and wedded originality in technique with a deeply traditional combination of roles.

MACPHAIL AND PRINCE EDWARD ISLAND: HIS HOME

Since the mid-1970s there has been a renewed appreciation of Macphail in Prince Edward Island. During the summer of 1975 the present author delivered an address, "Sir Andrew Macphail and Orwell," to a full house in the building that had housed the grammar school in Uigg that he had attended almost a century earlier. The lecture was based on a doctoral dissertation on Macphail as a social critic, completed for the University of Toronto the previous year, and it was published as the lead article in the inaugural fall – winter 1976 number of a new semi-annual periodical, the *Island Magazine*. Over the next twelve years, that issue sold more than seven thousand copies.[64] In 1976 the Caledonian Club of Prince Edward Island released a vinyl recording entitled *"Island Scotch ...": A Medley from the Scottish Tradition in Prince Edward Island*, which consisted of musical selections linked by excerpts from *The Master's Wife* read by the Reverend Donald A. Campbell, a Presbyterian clergyman with an outstanding voice. The album cover describes the book as a "classic account of early Scottish family and community life in Prince Edward Island."[65] In the wake of its republication, Island historian David Weale, an influential tastemaker in the province, declared it to be "possibly the best book written on the social history of Prince Edward Island."[66]

But as knowledge of Macphail's achievements grew, the public also became aware of a problem. Macphail's family had given his property in Orwell, encompassing approximately 140 acres, to the provincial government in 1961, expecting that it would be used as a park for the benefit of the public.[67] Unfortunately, the Prince Edward Island government did little to maintain it over the succeeding decades, despite very occasional displays of energy, optimistic announcements, promising studies, and professions of good intent.[68] "Such a lot of talk goes on & not much achieved," Dorothy Lindsay, Macphail's daughter, commented succinctly in 1979.[69] There were occasional voices raised, some persistently, but to no apparent avail.[70] By the late 1980s the park was no longer in use, and highway signs directing the public to it had been removed. The house was in an advanced state of dilapidation, and there were fears that it would not remain standing for long. Vandals broke windows and doors, and even set a fire inside the house.[71] In fact, the provincial government had all but abandoned responsibility for it.

What followed over 1988–89 can only be described as an impressive display of "people power." Interested persons from different parts of Prince Edward Island, including some summer residents, expressed publicly their

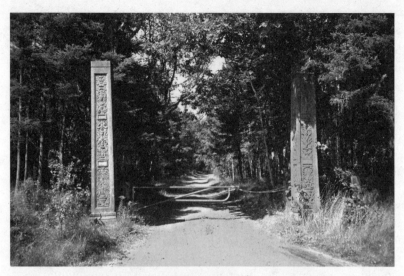

The pillars, 1987. Note the barrier between the pillars, closing the lane that was then the main entrance to the Macphail property. The highway signs directing the public to the park had also been removed by this time.

serious concern over the failure to maintain the property.[72] In the course of doing so, they highlighted the importance of Macphail in Island history, as well as the inherent beauty of the site. They organized an informal group known as Friends of Macphail to raise public awareness of him and his achievements, and to pressure the Liberal government, led by Joseph A. Ghiz, into making a commitment to save the house and to keep the property intact; the latter was a consideration, because there was an inclination on the part of some in authority to dump the house on Macphail's descendants and retain the land that had come with it in 1961. The local newspaper story reporting the formation of the Friends stated that they aimed to prevent the home from ending up "as just another old house rotting in the woods of rural P.E.I."[73] During the autumn of 1988 they mustered two work parties to repair the roof and board up windows so as to prevent further damage over the coming winter; this was volunteer labour performed with donated materials.[74] They held socials and engaged in other public activities to build support. When the present writer was invited to deliver a public lecture, "Sir Andrew Macphail and Prince Edward Island" on 10 April 1989 at the Hon. George Coles Building, Charlottetown, under the auspices of the Prince Edward Island Museum and the Institute of Island

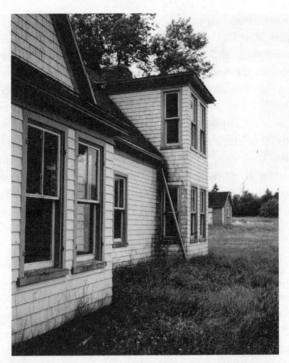

The Macphail Homestead, 1988. This photograph gives some notion of the unkempt appearance of a property that had formerly been a model of good care and attention to detail.

Studies, the Friends prepared relevant displays and provided refreshments. Approximately a hundred people, including the cabinet minister responsible, attended.

On 8 May 1989, during an election campaign, the government promised to take action.[75] Following this, the Friends established the Sir Andrew Macphail (of Orwell, P.E.I.) Foundation Inc. Incorporated in 1990, it is a non-profit charitable organization, and using money from both provincial and federal government sources and private donations, it restored the house beautifully. By 1993 the foundation had it fully open to the public; the date of the official opening was 1 August. Since then, the Macphail Homestead has operated a small conference centre and a licensed restaurant, has catered to private groups, and has held fundraising events. Occasionally there are public lectures and activities reflecting Macphail's interests. The farm property surrounding the house now features three nature trails,

a wildlife nursery, and an ecological forestry project; the on-site interpretation presents Macphail as a prophet of sustainable land use.[76] All this has
resulted from an exceptional community, or "civil society," effort that over-
came official indifference.

The sense of commitment was rooted in recognition of Macphail's significance in defining a distinctive Prince Edward Island way of life that
places value on the non-material aspects of local culture. It is now generally accepted that Macphail, particularly because of *The Master's Wife*, ranks
with Milton Acorn and Lucy Maud Montgomery at the summit among
writers drawing their inspiration from the Island.[77] Although rarely stated
explicitly, one of the reasons motivating some Friends was that Macphail and
his work represented an antidote to the somewhat contrived and too nice
view of Prince Edward Island rural life associated with the Montgomery
oeuvre. This saccharine representation of the Island past was linked particularly with the commercial exploitation of *Anne of Green Gables* that fed
the large-scale tourist industry.[78] As an example of the distortion of values
that had become evident, since the 1980s the large Cavendish Cemetery
where Montgomery is buried is entered under an arch identifying it as the
"Resting Place of L.M. Montgomery," a labelling that seems presumptuous
at best, given that the cemetery was founded in 1835. A large area around
Cavendish – the northern half of Queens County, amounting to some 15
to 20 percent of the province – is presented in government-issued promotional literature as "Anne's Land."[79]

More than half a century earlier, Macphail had expressed reservations
about tourism on the Island. They surfaced in a newspaper report. His
position was that the Island "was a place of great charm; and that charm
should be preserved not alone for profitable visitors but especially for
those who live there permanently." He argued, among other things, that if
tourists "are too much encouraged they will take away the amenities of the
country from those who like to live quietly."[80] Such sentiments were of a
piece with the new emphasis on Prince Edward Island identity and the distaste for pandering to mass tourism, which such Island writers as the historians Harry Baglole and David Weale had begun to express in the 1970s.
During 1973, the centennial year of the Island's entry into Confederation
– an anniversary that prompted much soul-searching – Baglole stated
tersely, in referring to the beauty of the rural landscape, that "tourism …
is both dependent on, and destructive of, that beauty."[81] In an eloquent
and somewhat caustic short piece, "Tourism – The Big Sell," also written
in 1973, Weale contended that hospitality, which had been practised as an

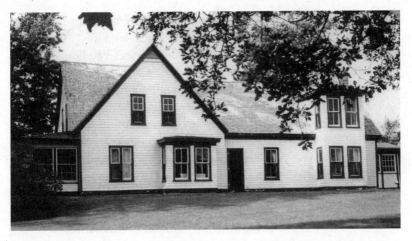

East side of the homestead, as restored. This photograph was taken in the
2003-05 period.

authentic expression of a tradition – for its own sake, simply as appropriate
behaviour – was being professionalized and commodified, thus undermin-
ing the real attractiveness of Island life.[82] The new awareness of Macphail
fitted well with that critical sensibility founded on intense local patriotism.[83] Tourists in droves were being directed to a house where a fictional
or invented character might have lived, had she ever lived, while the Island
government was letting decay the real home of a real author of stature
comparable to Montgomery, which had been presented to them in good
repair in a pristine setting, rich in interpretive potential in terms of Prince
Edward Island history.[84]

Yet the difficulties relating to the house are not over, for, since the initial
act of assisting in restoration, the provincial government has not provided
any ongoing funding. The roots lie in the decision of the Ghiz government
in 1989 to furnish "one time only" money, thus dealing with an immediate issue, and to hand over continuing responsibility to the volunteers. In
legal terms, the situation is that the property remains owned by the provincial government through the Department of Transportation and Public
Works but is leased to the non-profit group of volunteers. This arrangement, in a twist of circumstances that would probably not be anticipated
by a non-lawyer, has left the operators of the property liable to provincial
taxation which, given the lack of resources, has become a significant factor

in determining the fate of the property.[85] This state of affairs has been high-lighted by a grandniece of Macphail, Jean Macphail Weber (the grand-daughter of his elder brother Finlay), who in 1958–61 had been involved in family discussions leading to the original donation, and who has had a lengthy career in museum work in the United States. She has become intimately involved in work at the homestead in recent years, and in 2003 she pointed out in a letter to the premier, Progressive Conservative Patrick Binns, that "the current assessment of taxes immediately threatens the exist-ence of the Homestead and violates the spirit in which the family gave the property to the Government in the first place." She also noted, "The activ-ities of the Homestead fall within the realm of museum services, which are not elsewhere taxable."[86]

There is, in addition, a problem with what might be termed the "fine print" of the 1989 decision. The government proceeded in steps: first returning the property to the family in 1990,[87] then accepting it back the next year in a deal shorn of the conditions which Macphail's daughter had insisted on thirty years earlier. In 1961 conditions numbers 14 and 15 had stated explicitly that the government was not to sell or otherwise alienate any part of the property and that "if at any future time it is decided by the Government that the Park is of no value to the people of Prince Edward Island or that it cannot be maintained according to the conditions herein set forth," it was to revert to Mrs Lindsay or her heirs.[88] But since 1991 the provincial government has had the power, if it sees fit, to dispose of the property in any way it pleases, without any liability.[89]

It is not at all clear that the volunteers realized when they assumed responsibility for the Macphail Homestead that in the process of making new arrangements the provincial government had dealt itself a free hand with respect to the ultimate fate of the house and the land.[90] Events in 2004 gave some indication of the fragility of the situation. Substantial property tax arrears had accumulated, creating a financial crisis for the board of dir-ectors, who resigned. The Binns government forgave the arrears (which, if paid, would have bankrupted the site), but left its decision on the matter so late that the homestead did not open as early as usual.[91] When it did open in mid-July it was with reduced staff and activities, and only thanks to the dedication of a small number of persons, led by Weber. The dilemma facing the Macphail Foundation is as follows. If the government were to hand over ownership of the property to the volunteers, the liability for tax-ation would disappear, but so would any legal obligation, even theoretical, of the government for the care and maintenance of the property. The

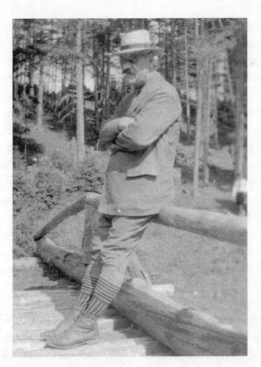

Macphail in rural setting. Clearly taken in the interwar years, probably in Orwell, this photograph caught Macphail in his characteristic arms-folded pose. Note the patch over his left eye, which is just visible here.

taxation liability has come to act, whether intentionally or not, as a lever providing an incentive for the volunteers to relieve the government of any responsibility.

Hanging over the volunteers is the real possibility of the sale of the property and destruction of the house - in other words, the thwarting of the intent of the donation of 1961. The conveyance from the family to the government in 1991 even refers explicitly to the eventuality that the property might be "sold to a private party," and it sets out how the proceeds of such a sale might be disposed of: a donation in Macphail's memory to the University of Prince Edward Island. This unhappy fact gives the board of governors of the university a vested interest in the failure of both the foundation and the homestead.[92]

The arrangements made in the early 1990s have not proved to be practicable. The existence of the foundation acts as a safeguard, yet the foundation itself does not have a secure existence. Whatever the intentions of the Ghiz government at the time, the concrete provisions have left the property with inadequate support and have specified a beneficiary for the demise of the homestead as a recognized and recognizable historic site. In 2007 the responsibility for future policy regarding the homestead passed to a new Liberal government led by Robert Ghiz, son of the former premier.

MACPHAIL AND PRINCE EDWARD ISLAND: ORAL HISTORY

The interest in Macphail prompted Katherine Dewar, one of the founders of the Friends of Macphail, to undertake an oral history project in 1990 at the suggestion of Baglole.[93] A nurse educator who had taught interviewing skills, she sought out persons who remembered Macphail and drew out of them stories of their personal connections with him, and also their perceptions of him. Because it was 1990, these people, for the most part, recalled the Macphail of the 1920s and especially the 1930s. What the interviewees from Orwell and nearby districts spoke of was a generous, kindly man who provided summer employment for young people on his property and invariably paid well above the standard local rates. This was of some consequence in the Great Depression, when any paid work was difficult to find. Furthermore, he took a real interest in them, giving them advice on their future: 'You would be suited to teaching," "You should think seriously about becoming a nurse," and so on.[94] For some of them, the money they earned on his property during the summers meant the difference between being able or not being able to pursue such ambitions. In other words, his wages and mentoring changed their life courses.

A man who worked for Macphail for ten summers, starting in his teens around 1928, remembered that he typically had about eight summer hires, perhaps three inside the house and five outside, or four in and four out. He described Macphail as "an excellent person to work for," and in all his years labouring on the property he never heard him speak harshly to any of the youngsters he employed; he was "very tactful" when correcting them. There was no fear of him, and there was no question of his authority. He was precise about what it was he wanted them to do and how they should do it; he would start them on a job and then return periodically to see how they were progressing. These tasks could include keeping the path next to the stream on his property free of debris, trimming the trees in front of his house, burning the brush, and so on; in general, their role was to keep things "very neat" around the property. Approaching the entrance to the house "the trees were trimmed so neatly you could see every sprig of grass under the trees."[95] This requirement was consistent with the apparently exceptional commitment to tidiness in his house on Peel Street, which was a matter of occasional amusement to friends like Leacock.[96] A granddaughter reported that he disliked "mess."[97]

Macphail was as clear, possibly even clearer, about what he wanted his summer employees not to do. For example, he made it known to them that they were not to harm any creatures, saying to one who took up an axe with the intent of killing an errant snake, "No, no, no, no – that's my pet snake!"[98] He was actually reputed to have had a pet snake for several years, with a name apparently something like "Susie," which would follow him up the lane to his house and was eventually killed by an unknown person[99]; but he used that expression so often that the deeper message was conveyed. If he thought the boys were working too hard, he would say, "Sit down on this nice clean stump" – an expression he used so frequently that they sometimes mimicked him, saying it among themselves when away from the property, for example, at a dance. The person who provided this anecdote eventually became Macphail's chauffeur on trips to Charlottetown (using his father's automobile), and during the entire time they were together Macphail would quiz him on matters of grammar, proper English usage, and so on. For example, he would ask, "What would you say: 'between the fence and I' or 'between the fence and me' – and *why* would you say that?" He recalled that Macphail would not let him away with simply guessing at the right answer. As someone who later spent some years as a teacher in rural schools, he stated with emphasis that Macphail, with his instruction on grammar and proper expression, was "a great teacher." He thought that he probably learned more from him than from his formal schooling.[100]

Another summer employee recalled working for Macphail as a teenager. On one occasion he fixed the fireplace under his supervision, with Macphail giving very precise, step-by-step directions.[101] He appears to have to liked to instruct, whether on correct English usage or on how to set the table – in the former case, "every chance he had."[102] A granddaughter reported that the local workers "thought he was terrific, but it had to be done his way."[103] Several informants stated that he did not overwork them. At the same time, it was understood that the tasks had to be performed to his standard, or a worker would not be asked back the next year; but there were no scoldings or dramatic firings.[104]

In addition to hiring locally, Macphail patronized many general stores in the area, a fact that was noticed and much appreciated by merchants,

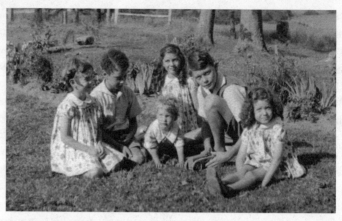

Sir Andrew Macphail's grandchildren at Orwell, summer 1934. These are the
children of Lionel M. Lindsay and Dorothy Macphail. (*Left to right*): Elspeth,
Jeffrey, Alan, Meg, Robin, Eleanor. The Orwell River is in the background,
suggesting that the photo was taken at the home occupied during the summers
by James Alexander Macphail, Andrew's brother.

since Macphail's custom was significant, with his family, guests, and parties.[105] In the 1930s, for example, a group coming from Montreal might
consist of twenty members of all ages.[106] A relative then on Prince Edward
Island recalled, "They would charter a Pullman car which would take them
from Montreal to Charlottetown without intervention."[107] A woman inter-
viewed by the present author in 1970 recalled Macphail's response when a
younger member of his family sent a considerable store of canned goods in
advance from Montreal, on grounds of lesser cost. Macphail was already on
the Island when the purchases arrived and, unwilling to tolerate this devia-
tion from his usual practice, gave all the goods away. In the face of protests
once the family member arrived, he underscored his rationale by referring
to a fable that made the point of how important a bit of extra business
was to rural storekeepers, compared with the unimportance for people in
his family's situation of spending a few more dollars than they would in
Montreal for the equivalent.[108]

Stories of Macphail's generosity came through in more than one of the
interviews conducted in 1990. An informant whose father did occasional
work on the property as a carpenter related that Macphail knew that his
father liked to hunt and asked whether he had a gun. The carpenter replied
that he did but it was not in good repair. Macphail pointed to a shotgun

on the wall and told him to take it home with him, keep it there, and not bring it back until he told him to; he never asked for it back.[109] In the community at large, there was another reason for appreciation of his presence: if anyone had a fire or other disaster, Macphail was there the next day with the offer of either materials or financial assistance. "He hated to see anyone suffering," his young chauffeur recalled.[110] His generosity was also felt within his family. In 2000 a nephew of Macphail, a man who went on to become professor of physics at McGill University, revealed in an interview with the present author that his uncle discreetly paid off the debts on his parents' farm in rural Prince Edward Island during the 1930s.[111] One of Macphail's longtime colleagues in the Faculty of Medicine at McGill commented after his death, "He hid his generous deeds as most men hide their sins."[112] There appears to have been considerable truth in this statement, for circumstantial evidence and various scraps of information point to other instances of rendering significant assistance and having a policy of doing so quietly.[113]

One man who had been a Church of Scotland student minister when he first encountered Macphail in 1931 "marvelled at" how attentive Macphail had been to every word he spoke when he was in the pulpit. He wondered what he, a young person, a student, could say that would be interesting or new to someone of Macphail's eminence and experience. He found Macphail's attitude encouraging and speculated that it may have been his way of expressing his support. Macphail's demeanour led the minister to describe him as "extremely humble," and he related that through the years during pastoral visits he found him "very easy to talk to ... [He] made me feel comfortable." They discussed spiritual matters, world events, people, and other subjects. He observed that Macphail was alert and understanding with regard to other people's feelings, put everyone at ease, and embarrassed no one. A member of the minister's church who had been employed by Macphail as a housekeeper in Montreal for many years told him that Macphail was kind and considerate to work for, although "very firm on protocol" when entertaining. Before Macphail left Orwell for the last time, in the summer of 1938, he gave a mutual connection a personal cheque for $100 (a considerable sum in the 1930s) to convey to the young minister as a gift. The minister believed this was an indication that Macphail knew that his illness was terminal – "I think he realized that this was it" - and that he would not be returning. In spite of the cordial relationship and Macphail's rigorous church attendance when at Orwell, the minister wondered, given Macphail's relentless emphasis on "following the old ways" (such as using a bucket to get water from his well, when most people had switched to a pump by the 1930s), whether "tradition" was his real religion.[114]

In a follow-up interview in 2003, the minister, who by then was ninety-four, stressed that Macphail "didn't parade his intelligence to me" and that in mixing with the fellow worshippers at the little church in Kinross he attended when on the Island, "he didn't raise a barrier with anyone regardless of status. Anyone could approach him." He remembered vividly Macphail on his left as he looked down from the pulpit, listening as though rapt; and he recalled how Macphail would take his Bible and Church of Scotland hymn book and psalm book out of his pocket, and untie a string and bow that bound them, probably following a ritual of his father. When he had visited Macphail during his illness in the summer of 1938 he had not realized that this would be the last time. It was only after he received the $100 cheque and heard that, in Charlottetown, Macphail had been taken onto the Montreal train on a stretcher, that he realized the gravity of his condition.[115]

The interviewees in Prince Edward Island also remembered a man who on occasion entertained lavishly at his rustic summer home.[116] The son of Murdoch MacKinnon, who served as lieutenant governor from 1919 to 1924, related that Macphail had made it known to his father that whenever he had special guests to entertain, he would be willing to provide hospitality at Orwell.[117] There was always plenty of alcohol even though this was during Prohibition in the province. Macphail would explain to his guests that the Island government had allowed him to import his summer's supply on condition that it was for his personal use only; he was not at liberty to give any of it to others. But he would also tell his guests that although he could not *give* them alcohol, there was alcohol on the premises in several locations, and if they *found* any, they were welcome to make use of it.[118]

Among the interviewees was a woman who, as an eighteen year old, had been the cook in Macphail's house during the summer of 1938, when he was in the final months of his life. She estimated that her monthly payment was twenty dollars, and that this was approximately double the norm for such work at that time in that area; it provided her with her board at Prince of Wales College for the autumn term. She recalled that Macphail did not go out much that summer. Yet although not as mobile as previously, he was not entirely bedridden and in fact got up every day. He continued to have a bracing shower in the stream below his house, where a waterfall had been created by building a dam; sometimes he went there and splashed around in the cold water before breakfast, and sometimes he did so before his evening meal. That summer he was occasionally driven to his stream. He generally had his standard breakfast of oatmeal porridge late, perhaps at 9 or 10 AM and in the company of his brothers if they were in Orwell.[119] The late breakfasts were not really a break with routine, for he was a famously late riser, after working far into the night - "sometimes most of the night," according to his daughter.[120] It was also part of his routine when in Orwell to have a whisky and water brought to him in his bedroom at 11 AM, announcing to anyone in earshot that "good whisky and good water will never hurt you."[121] The imbibing continued in 1938, as the cook remembered: he and his family members "had their drinks all the time." Yet that summer there was nothing comparable to his usual round of entertaining. When his former cook was asked whether he had been at all irritable in the face of his diminished capacity for physical activity, she replied with an emphatic "no." Until that moment in the interview she had been somewhat subdued in tone.[122]

The testimony in these interviews is remarkably consistent. Macphail made an enormously positive impression on the local young people through his generosity, his obvious interest in them as individuals, his concern for their welfare and their prospects, his good humour, and the respect with which he treated them. Each year they awaited his arrival with real anticipation.[123] The older generation in his native district cherished his presence also; an employee of his daughter recalled in an interview in 1970 that during his final illness "some of the old Scotsmen of Orwell-Uigg used to parade outside his window playing the bag-pipes – which he greatly appreciated."[124]

Clearly, Macphail was deeply attached to his native province, to members of his family, and to the people of his district. He expressed this attachment in many different ways, from the loving care he took in maintaining his family home and its environs in the state he had known it in his youth to the advocacy of a rural way of life and the composition of *The Master's Wife*. Prince Edward Island was, in his mind, inseparable from agriculture. After he was gone, there was a period when his name went into eclipse on the Island. Since the mid-1970s this has changed, and he has achieved new recognition as a spokesman for the traditional Prince Edward Island version of farming as representing a distinct way of life. The overdue attention to *The Master's Wife* has also meant new recognition of Macphail as a significant literary figure, beyond his previously well-accepted reputation as an essayist. Recognition comes in different forms; in Macphail's case, one is the way in which popular written guides for visitors to Prince Edward Island direct one towards his family home, now restored – one of a kind as an authentic rural residence from the nineteenth century surviving in public hands.[125] His standing as an important part of Prince Edward Island's history and culture has been secured.

Placing Andrew Macphail

CANADIAN MAN OF LETTERS

Andrew Macphail was a unique figure in English Canadian intellectual and cultural history, and there are several major aspects of his distinctiveness. He has long been a recognized master of the essay as a genre, having published specimens in Britain and the United States as well as Canada. His reputation in this respect has endured and has been repeatedly reconfirmed. In 1997 an article on him was included in a major international project on the essay that resulted in a book of more than a thousand pages, published in London.[1] The author of the more general entry on the Canadian essay in English that appears in that tome brackets the works of Macphail, Archibald MacMechan, and Bliss Carman as indicating the coming of age of the essay as a literary form in English-speaking Canada.[2]

Among Macphail's writings that are not essays, one remarkable work stands out in a category by itself: *The Master's Wife*. Although highly original in conception and execution, because of the circumstances of its posthumous publication and probably also because of its non-adherence to conventional forms, approximately two generations elapsed before it received serious recognition and critical attention. Led by Kenneth MacKinnon, literary scholars have belatedly placed the book within the contexts of the Gaelic chronicling tradition, Maritime literature, the literature of small islands, and generally the literature of "place-writing."[3]

At a popular level on Prince Edward Island, the subject matter and quality of *The Master's Wife* have made Macphail into an iconic figure. In turn, this has led to a re-examination of his world view and the remarkable breadth of his interests and achievements, encompassing his writing, his agricultural experiments, his founding of the *Canadian Medical Association*

Journal, and his frontline service in the First World War at an age when it would be unthinkable for most. He has now been recognized as a person exemplifying commitment, both verbal and practical, to a rural way of life, particularly the type of agriculture traditionally pursued on the Island, and as a forerunner to advocacy of sustainable development. In fact, the book has made his reputation on the Island imperishable, because of the excellence of the writing, the documentation of a vanished past, the manifest authenticity of the portraiture of people and community, and the compellingly imaginative use of the perspective of a child – all of which have provoked curiosity about Macphail himself.

One exceptional contribution Macphail made to Canadian cultural development in the first two decades of the twentieth century was his role as editor and ultimate financial backer of the *University Magazine.* The periodical marked a notable advance in the development of Canadian letters. Not only did it provide one of the few outlets for certain types of writing, such as the essay,[4] but it set a new standard of excellence and reached the widest audience of any quality Canadian quarterly at any time. The creative vigour of Macphail was largely responsible for this success. In 1907 Canada may have been ready for such a journal, but many at the time thought the venture a leap in the dark. Macphail himself contributed more than faith: he was adamant that all contributors must be paid, and he virtually excluded footnotes and other scholarly paraphernalia that might intimidate the non-academic readers he hoped to attract. Although he did not close the periodical to dissenting views,[5] he placed his imprint on it as surely as Goldwin Smith did on his various publications. Despite an absence of four years because of the First World War, Macphail was the journal's most frequent contributor, more than equalling the combined output of the two next most frequent contributors.[6]

The *University Magazine,* an unparalleled phenomenon in prewar Canada by virtue of both its quality and its circulation, was Macphail's, and its achievements were his. This was acknowledged by his contemporaries,[7] and he rapidly attained a prestige that is easily underestimated in an era when no comparable periodical exists. His journal played a role similar to those of Smith and Henri Bourassa – as a non-partisan institution designed to influence public opinion in a particular direction. As its editor and leading contributor, he came virtually to embody the magazine in the public mind.

Macphail's own writing was as non-specialized as his journal, concerning which one modern critic, Paul Matthew St Pierre, has made the following observation: that it provided Macphail and his contributors "with a forum for ideas, most significantly ideas outside their own professional spheres."[8] Indeed, Macphail emerges as the most notable native Canadian example of what a British writer, John Gross, has described as the "man of letters." By the late nineteenth century, this expression

> was very definitely coming to suggest a writer of the second rank, a critic, someone who aimed higher than journalism but made no pretence of being primarily an artist. Up until the First World War men of letters in this sense were a familiar part of the [British] literary landscape; then the term fell into disrepute.
>
> It was a useful term, and nothing has really taken its place ... But if the phrase is obsolete, it is largely because the concept it describes is obsolete too ... Instead of men of letters, there are academic experts, mass media pundits, cultural functionaries.[9]

Like his British counterparts, Macphail covered the ground of all these specialists. He also fitted the mould in that his period of greatest prominence was prior to the First World War. After the war it was evident that the secure bourgeois world of the nineteenth century was splintering on many levels. Among the indicators were the decline of the holistically minded generalist, writing with a confident air of omnicompetence, and the complementary rise of the specialist, careful not to step outside his accredited terrain.

Another symptom, specific to Canada, was the failure to establish a successor to the conservative, national, and broadly focused *University Magazine*. Within a year of its demise, three important new journals were founded: the progressive *Canadian Forum*, the regional *Dalhousie Review*, and the specialist *Canadian Historical Review*.[10] Macphail's choice of British periodicals in which to publish his essays further symbolized his own predominantly nineteenth-century style. Although the *Spectator* was the only financially profitable weekly of the Edwardian age, Gross states that "during the long editorship of J. St Loe Strachey it increasingly lost its hold on younger readers, and among the *avant-garde* it became a by-word for stuffy gentility."[11] In fact, Macphail's "American Woman" article, with its reactionary message, appears to have been one of the most controversial pieces to appear in Strachey's *Spectator*. By the twentieth century, the *Quarterly Review* was also in the process of a long decline, until its discontinuation in 1968.[12]

Macphail stood squarely in another British literary tradition: the romantic, anti-industrial sensibility of such men as John Ruskin and William Morris. He shared their belief that modern industry, with its division of labour, was creating a fragmented man who found no pleasure in his work. Craftsmanship, art, and the capacity to appreciate beauty were all being undermined. Macphail read these authors, used their imagery, and adopted many of their polarities: the "organic" was commendable and natural; the "mechanical" was reprehensible and artificial.[13] "The essence of art," he wrote in 1933, in words he could as easily have written for the Montreal *Gazette* in the late 1880s, "is selection, selecting from nature what is beautiful";[14] he was making a contrast with the undiscriminating eye of the camera. Nonetheless, verbal similarities with Ruskin and Morris are not sufficient reason to infer that this tradition was the source of his world view.

MISINTERPRETING MACPHAIL

The historian and physician Samuel E.D. Shortt has devoted a chapter of a book, *The Search for an Ideal*, published in 1976, to Macphail (the chapter is entitled "Andrew Macphail: The Ideal in Nature") and has also produced two brief articles or essays on him, which appeared subsequently. In summary, his thesis is that "Macphail's social thought was a unified whole, growing naturally out of his idealistic, evolutionary metaphysics."[15] Shortt commenced his book with a quotation drawn from an article by Arnold Haultain, entitled "A Search for an Ideal" and published in 1904, stating that at the end of the nineteenth century men found themselves at an intellectual precipice – their old convictions challenged, they were unsure of where to turn and were searching for a new synthesis.[16] Among the fundamental problems with this argument as it applies to Macphail are that Shortt fails to appreciate the significance of Prince Edward Island and its history for the main body of Macphail's writings; and that, having decided that Macphail had found his "ideal" in "nature," the notion becomes a Procrustean bed - anything in Macphail's varied writings that can be enlisted to support this thesis is used, whether in context or not. In fact, Macphail's reading in metaphysical matters was extremely eclectic and his pronouncements were ad hoc. Reviewers have drawn attention to the conceptual fuzziness of Shortt's argument and have questioned his grasp of the terminology he employs, for example, treating empiricism and positivism as equivalents.[17]

Compounding these difficulties are a disturbing number of basic factual errors, easily avoidable, in Shortt's account of Macphail's life and family background.[18] The lack of careful reading of sources is evident time and again, and extends well beyond matters of biographical detail. On the first page of his chapter on Macphail, Shortt asserts that he wrote sonnets that amounted to "stormy jeremiads" on the issues confronting society.[19] If so, this is not evident from surviving material, and when examining the list of Macphail's writings that Shortt includes in his bibliography it is apparent that he is referring to sonnets which Andrew's brother Alexander published in the *University Magazine*, and which are clearly identified as Alexander's, not Andrew's.[20] The evidence that does survive makes it clear that when Andrew did write sonnets or other poems, they tended to be on such themes as romance, love, and sorrow.[21]

It may be asserted that in themselves some of the criticisms about factual errors and the misattribution of writings are inconsequential for Shortt's interpretation. But there are additional difficulties with the quality of the research that must raise questions about the soundness of the argument. For example, in commenting on Macphail and the doctrine of laissez-faire, Shortt writes that he "confided that the work of John Maynard Keynes 'instils doubt.'"[22] Yet there is no evidence that Macphail ever read *The General Theory of Employment, Interest and Money* (1936) or other related publications by Keynes or, if he did, that they influenced him in any way. The book Macphail was referring to when he wrote in a published article – not "confided" – that Keynes's work "instils doubt" was *The Economic Consequences of the Peace* (1919), his classic criticism of the Treaty of Versailles; the article was published in 1920.[23] The carelessness of the research and documentation that went into Shortt's discussion of Macphail and his writings, when wedded with imprecise use of concepts and an unsettling tendency to quote him entirely out of context, has the effect of making any case constructed on such foundations deeply flawed.[24] Indeed, Shortt's interpretation cannot be considered a serious contribution to understanding Macphail.[25]

RURAL LIFE

Macphail's system of thought and his peculiar affinities evolved out of the clash in values he perceived between the rural Scottish Canadian hinterland of his early years and the metropolis where he worked and lived as an adult. This contradiction in value systems can be traced to the radically different ways of life in which they were rooted. But it is not enough to apply the amorphous terms "ruralist" and "agrarian" to Macphail.[26] These concepts are sufficiently inclusive to embrace anything ranging from plantation slavery to "independent" farming to corporate agriculture. In each system of production the locale is the countryside rather than an urban area, and the basic resource is the land itself. Neither "ruralism" nor

"agrarianism" conveys any further precision. They are not specific enough
to explain Macphail's isolation from and lack of enthusiasm for the western Canadian farmers' movement. After all, he was sinking into despair
at a time when three provinces were electing farmers' governments and
when the farmers' presence in Ottawa was at its peak, its smashing electoral successes having bent, if not broken, the traditional two-party political system of Canada. Some spokesmen for the farmers' movement welcomed Macphail's writings; *The Grain Growers' Guide* and E.A. Partridge
reprinted sections of his denunciatory essays.[27] But the attraction was not
mutual. Macphail did not believe that his aspirations and theirs were identical. His failure to respond to their movement was not solely because of its
militant reformism, for his objections went deeper. The mixed farming he
advocated was meant to operate in an environment fundamentally different from that of the western grain growers.

The rural Prince Edward Island of Macphail's youth had been a society
in which people lived little affected by forces beyond their own communities.[28] There is, of course, no denying that the Island in the late nineteenth
century was part of a larger commercial whole; yet the districts with which
Macphail was familiar came particularly close to the ideal of self-sufficiency.
Farming was mixed, and the farmers were men of wide talents. They were
not commercial, "one-crop" farmers, and the market was of only periph-
eral significance to their lives. These farmers produced primarily for use,
not for exchange and the accumulation of treasure. The predominance of
this mode of production was the essential characteristic of the social ideal
Macphail enunciated in the *University Magazine* and elsewhere: the mixed
farm operated by the labour of a family, with minimal use of machinery,
which could be obtained only by taking surplus products of the farm to
the marketplace, with its entanglements.[29]

Western farmers had erred with their single crops and expensive
machines, for their well-being had come to depend on their position in a
much larger whole, the international market. By the very nature of their
farming they were compelled, if they wished to be successful, to adopt the
value system of the entrepreneur: single-minded dedication to efficiency
in the production of one commodity.[30] Such a way of life left little room
for the love of one's fields and animals, as distinguished from their produc-
tivity. Its skills and surprises would resemble those of the marketplace, and
the focus of the farmer's attention would have to be as much there as in
his community. Producing a single commodity, the prairie farmer was, as a
result, fully integrated into the industrial system; he was not independent,

regardless of any illusions he might have in times of prosperity. His ultimate goal would be to secure a fair deal in the marketplace.[31] To use a
favourite metaphor of Macphail, the two types of farmer belonged to different worlds. For one, the problem was the abuses or maladjustments in
the system; for the other, it was the system itself. Hence it is not surprising
that Macphail, a self-declared spokesman for the eastern Canadian brand
of mixed farming, should choose to remain aloof from the farm organizations of the day, based as they were on business farming.[32]

Macphail's precision in stating the essentials of his social vision has a
dual explanation. His insistence that each farmer own his land arose in
part from the peculiarities of Prince Edward Island's social and economic
history. In the eighteenth century the colony had been divided into townships of approximately 20,000 acres, which were distributed among persons who had claims on the British government, leaving almost no Crown
land for working settlers to acquire. The proprietors, and especially their
agents, did not surrender their holdings without a struggle, and the land
question dominated Island politics for most of the nineteenth century.[33]
Indeed, the system of leasehold tenure was finally liquidated only after the
Island's entry into Confederation.[34] The land on which Macphail had been
born and on which he had spent his early years had been rented land. In
The Master's Wife, he wrote, "A man who lives on his own land and owes no
man anything develops all the dignity inherent in his nature."[35]

This consciousness of the need for each man to own the means of his
subsistence – a "freeholder ideology"[36] – was reinforced among Scottish
(and Irish) Islanders by bitter memories of the dangers of anything less
than clear legal title to the land. Macphail's affirmation that the family, not
the individual, was the true unit of civilized society can also be traced to his
Highland cultural inheritance. Money as the social bond was entirely foreign to traditional Highland society. Thus, in the crucial matter of family
solidarity as well as the nature of his "agrarianism," Macphail was a thor-
ough product of his ancestors in both the new and the old worlds. The
writings of a Ruskin may have provided him with a vocabulary, but the
basic perceptions came from his own experience and that of his kin.

An important part of Macphail's uniqueness lies in the fullness with
which he expressed what the political theorist C.B. Macpherson characterized as the simple market concept of society. The defining characteristic of
such a society is that each individual (or head of a family) has the land or
other resources with which to obtain a living by exercising of his labour
power. Since one cannot control the labour power of others, there is little

scope for accumulation. The resulting ethic is: "All individuals seek ration-
ally to maximize their utilities, that is, to get the most satisfaction they
can for a given expenditure of energy or goods, or to get a given satisfaction for the least possible expenditure of energy or goods."[37] This matched
exactly what Macphail described as the ethic of farmers: "Their theory of
life is to take what they can get, be it much or little. The more they get the
less they work. They do not love work for its own sake."[38] As the situation
became more desperate, if not hopeless, he became more explicit, both in
denouncing the dominant social trends and stating the losing alternative.
Certainly, no other contemporary Canadian commentator set forth such a
complete world view, and Macphail's medical training probably accounts
in considerable part for this, because its emphasis on seeing the patient as
an interrelated whole would reinforce any tendency to conceptualize society in holistic terms, rather than as the sum of discrete phenomena.[39]

MACPHAIL IN PERSPECTIVE

Among Macphail's contemporaries, Bourassa's Nationalist League and
such "red tories" as Stephen Leacock belonged, like the western farmers,
to the "other world."[40] They looked forward as well as backward and tried
to introduce shock absorbers into the process of industrialization. There
is no doubt that Macphail, Bourassa, and Leacock shared many insights.
But what differentiated Macphail was his refusal to accept the new industrial order; in this sense his dissent was more profound. Perhaps his greater
tenacity than Leacock in adhering to the old is partially explained by
the fact that he returned each summer to Orwell rather than to Orillia.
There was little qualitative change in rural Prince Edward Island for several generations.[41] Macphail related in *The Master's Wife*, when referring
to the farm implements on his property at Orwell, "The cart was made by
an elder of the church. Fifty-four years afterwards, as appeared from the
Master's books, I sent for this same man to survey the cart, as I suspected
it required some repairs. He admitted that the vehicle had not lasted as
long as it should, and he feared he 'must have put bad stuff in it.' He was
willing to make the replacements free of charge, as he wished to maintain
his reputation for sound work."[42] Orillia, on the other hand, was being
overwhelmed by metropolitan influences and penetrated by urban, industrial values.[43] As the critic F.W. Watt has remarked, the sins of Mariposans
are forgivable only by virtue of their small scale; the vices are the same as
those of the city.[44] In such a situation, Leacock's perception of the gap in

values between the old and the new could not be as clear-cut as that of Macphail, whose neighbours were scarcely likely to be dabbling in Cuban real estate. Leacock's comment in his obituary article on Macphail – "I am certain that he never quite knew what he believed and what he didn't"[45] – applied more to himself than to the deceased. Both were caught up in a tremendous social upheaval; Macphail knew exactly where he stood on the matter. All who accepted the basic change in balance between town and country, with its attendant specialization in human functions, were of the "other world."

Although Macphail may be one of a kind in English Canadian intellectual history, his tone in decrying the advance of modernism in the 1920s is not so uncommon in the perspective of world history. The sociologist and historian Barrington Moore Jr has advanced the concept of "Catonism" to describe a more general phenomenon:

> Where commercial relationships have begun to undermine a peasant economy, the conservative elements in society are likely to generate a rhetoric of extolling the peasant as the backbone of society … The key elements in the rhetoric … appear in the West as early as Cato the Elder (234–149 B.C.) who operated his own *latifundium* with slave labour. It is fitting, therefore, to label this complex of ideas with his name … Catonism … denies the need for further social changes, especially revolutionary ones … An aura of moral earnestness suffuses Catonist arguments. This morality is not instrumental; that is, policies are not advocated in order to make humanity happier … and certainly not in order to make people richer. They are important because they are supposed to contribute to a way of life that has somehow proved its validity in the past …
>
> This way of life is supposed to be an organic whole and, of course, being connected with the soil is essential to making it organic. Indeed, "organic" and "whole" are favourite cloudy terms in Catonism. The organic life of the countryside is supposedly superior to the atomised and disintegrating world of modern urban civilization … Art must be "healthy," traditional, and above all easily comprehensible. Catonist artistic notions center on folk and provincial art.[46]

If the word "farmer" is substituted for "peasant," Macphail emerges as the closest there is to an English Canadian Catonist. In his translation of *Maria*

Chapdelaine and in *The Master's Wife* the positive side is visible: his celebration of the values of the simple folk. And in his 1920s criticism of the
alleged decline of Western civilization the denunciatory aspect is evident.

Macphail must also be placed within the context of imperialism in
Canada. An outspoken advocate, he shared many of the characteristic
imperialist attitudes,[47] and the main distinguishing emphases are best
explained in terms of his social assumptions. He believed firmly in the
monarchy, the British connection, and the parliamentary system, with its
organic link between executive and legislature. Hand in hand with these
articles of faith went an oft-repeated traditionalist critique of the American
system of government. In these respects, Macphail was entirely orthodox.

Yet as an ardent free-trader and admirer of French Canada, Macphail
was in a minority within the imperialist movement. His support for free
trade and opposition to protection, which led him to write more than any
other imperialist on the negative effects of the tariff, had very specific historical roots, and these did not lie in a doctrinaire commitment to free markets.[48] In his view, the early years of Britain's free trade era had coincided
with demographic and economic growth in the Maritimes; protection had
brought stagnation and depopulation to his native region. Seen in these
terms, free trade became almost a state of nature from which the nation
had fallen. Over his adult years he had watched protection decisively alter
the balance between town and country, thus changing the very character of
Canada. Furthermore, the equation of protection and imperialism implied
the identity of pecuniary and familial values – a point of view he, as a conservative, found completely repugnant.

Macphail did not oppose protectionism in all cases. In "The Freedom
of England," published in 1930, he advocated that the mother country, now
liberated from its imperial responsibilities, adopt a high tariff on agricultural goods, even against the dominions. At first sight this would appear to
be a considerable reversal. In Macphail's heyday as a current commentator,
he had been a steadfast free-trader and generally an antistatist. "All that the
farmer required was to be left alone,"[49] he had said in 1920. Yet ten years later
he was recommending protection to Great Britain although it, "of all political systems, is the most prone to evil."[50] Nonetheless, the problem of consistency lessens when it is noted that the appeal was couched in the same
"agrarian" sentiments as his earlier arguments in favour of reciprocity: "A
duty on agricultural products would mean the restoration of the English
country, and result in cheaper and better food … Rural England lies like a
land under an interdict, with the population dead; or rather like some fair

creature bound by an enchantment, and preserving her bondage by muttering the old bewitchment – Free food, Free trade."[51] It is clear that trading relationships between states were less important in Macphail's worldview than the rural-urban question. Such international arrangements were simply instruments to be used for the maintenance or furtherance of the rural proportion of the population.

With regard to French Canada, what Macphail beheld seemed to be a realization of his conservatism: a traditional society in which the cleric was honoured, families were large, the woman was in the house, only the gifted children were in school, and divorce was unknown. Unlike most of his fellow imperialists, he did not desire that the influence of French Canada be contained or in any way marginalized; his deep commitment to the ideal of an orderly, conservative society compelled admiration, not grudging tolerance. Thus the explanation for each of his major deviations from the mainstream of imperialist thought lies in the nature of his social vision. Free trade and French Canada seemed to him to have been vital supports of the way of life he valued and hence deserved his advocacy.

In summation, Andrew Macphail was one of the central figures in the English Canadian intelligentsia for a generation. His period of greatest recognition and influence was 1907 to 1914, when he forged the *University Magazine* into a national quarterly of exceptional quality and readability, with a remarkably large circulation. Aside from his editorial work, he distinguished himself by his power and versatility as a writer and by his translation of the British literary tradition of romantic anti-industrialism into Canadian terms. Yet Macphail cannot be reduced to a formula of "a Canadian Ruskin." On all matters, including his imperialism, he displayed an extraordinarily consistent conservatism that was firmly rooted in the soil of Prince Edward Island, and even of his ancestral home, the Scottish Highlands. In 1905 he wrote, "The first fact to establish in estimating a personality is the environment of the man; his class, and hence the habitual bent of his mind; his family and friends; in short, his outlook upon the world."[52]

Macphail's social and political criticism emerged out of the encounter between his conservative value system and the capitalistic mores of urban, industrial society. The resultant body of writing was unmatched in the clarity of its statement of the basic postulates of simple market society. This lucidity of thought, made possible by his own specific background, led him to grapple with fundamental problems in the changing social

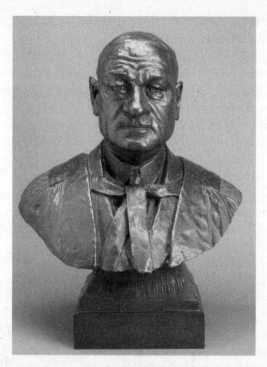

Bust of Macphail, made in 1927 by sculptor Henri Hébert, a fellow member of the Pen and Pencil Club. It is part of the permanent collection of the Confederation Centre Art Gallery in Charlottetown.

relationships of early-twentieth-century Canada. No doubt it was this capacity to penetrate to the core of a situation that accounted, at least in part, for his wide appeal in the years prior to the First World War, when the changes Canada was going through had not yet taken on an air of finality. He must have voiced the feelings of many Canadians who had been born in the countryside but had moved to the city.[53] In this respect Andrew Macphail, despite his conscious attempt at popularization, is part of a tradition that has always been in a distinct minority in Canadian intellectual history – that of dealing in a philosophical manner with fundamental social questions of one's own time and place.[54] Many years after his death his posthumous publication, *The Master's Wife*, in which he recreated the society of his youth, brought him new recognition for literary creativity. It is now understood, particularly in Prince Edward Island and by literary scholars, to be his *chef d'oeuvre*.

Notes

ABBREVIATIONS

BL Beaverbrook Library, London, UK
BUA Bishop's University Archives, Lennoxville, PQ
DCB *Dictionary of Canadian Biography*
DUA Dalhousie University Archives, Halifax
KCL University of King's College Library, Halifax
LAC Library and Archives Canada, Ottawa
MMCH McCord Museum of Canadian History, Montreal
MRB McGill University Rare Book Room, McLennan Library
MUA McGill University Archives
MUA(AFM) McGill University Archives, Archives of the Faculty of Medicine
OL Osler Library of the History of Medicine, McGill University
PARO Public Archives and Records Office, Charlottetown
QUL Queen's University Library
UD University of Durham Department of Palaeography and Diplomatic, UK
UPA University of Pennsylvania Archives and Records Center, Philadelphia, USA
UTA University of Toronto Archives
UTRB University of Toronto Rare Book Room
VUA Victoria University Archives, Toronto

INTRODUCTION

1 Macphail, "John McCrae: An Essay in Character," in McCrae, *In Flanders Fields and Other Poems*, 128

2 Rudyard Kipling to Andrew Macphail, 20–30 Nov. 1908, Kipling-Macphail volume, Sir Andrew Macphail Papers (in private possession when used). All references henceforth to the "Macphail Papers" will denote this collection. The papers of Macphail's brothers, father, and grandfather will be identified by using the given names of each.

3 Fourth Earl Grey to John St Loe Strachey, 14 Oct. 1907 (private), John St Loe Strachey Papers, BL

4 See Lawrence J. Burpee, "Co-operation in Historical Research," *University Magazine* 7 (Oct. 1908): 360–70.

5 See Lawrence J. Burpee, "A Plea for a National Library," *University Magazine* 10 (Feb. 1911): 152–63.

6 See John Edward Hoare, "A Plea for a Canadian Theatre," *University Magazine* 10 (April 1911): 239–53.

7 Stephen Leacock, "Greater Canada: An Appeal," *University Magazine* 6 (April 1907): 132

8 See Robertson, "Andrew Macphail," in Chevalier, ed., *Encyclopedia of the Essay*, 512–13.

9 In fact, Macphail himself saw his Island as representing an alternative to the developing industrial civilization of Canada; see Macphail, "Prince Edward Island," press cutting from a PEI newspaper, n.d. [Oct. 1912], Burland-Macphail Scrapbook, Macphail Papers.

10 See Weale and Baglole, *The Island and Confederation*; Robertson, "Sir Andrew Macphail and Orwell," *Island Magazine* 1 (Fall–Winter 1976): 4–8.

11 A recent scholar has stated, "For the greater part of the 20th century V.S. Pritchett almost singlehandedly preserved the tradition of the English man of letters." Rogers, "V.S. Pritchett," 676.

CHAPTER ONE

1 Macphail, "John McCrae: An Essay in Character," in McCrae, *In Flanders Fields and Other Poems*, 112

2 Although William Macphail Sr (1802–52) and his son William Macphail (1830–1905) spelled their last names "McPhail," for the sake of consistency of usage they will be referred to as "Macphail" throughout this book, since Andrew Macphail spelled his name "Macphail" for most of his adult life. He maintained the traditional family spelling until about 1893 (age 29).

3 See Macphail, *The Master's Wife*, 31–3, in which the dates of emigration and removal to PEI are given as 1832 and 1838, respectively. I have accepted instead the dates given in 1865 by William Macphail in his notes for the preparation of a "Family Record," as reproduced in Lindsay-Macphail

Scrapbooks 1, Macphail Papers. The collection, when used, consisted of seventeen bound volumes and several thousand items, including some 3,273 letters, not in bound form. In the notes, any references to material in bound form in the Macphail Papers will be identified as such; all other sources from the Macphail Papers may be assumed to be unbound material. *The Master's Wife* is generally an accurate source, in spite of the two factual errors already cited. Originally published posthumously by his children one year after Macphail's death, it has gone through two additional publications, in 1977 and 1994, each with an introduction by Ian Ross Robertson. The third edition is a facsimile of the original text and reproduces the original illustrations; it includes a list of "Incorrect Dates and Ages" (255).

4 Statement signed by John Henderson, 29 Aug. 1844, William Macphail Sr Papers (in private possession)

5 See Macphail, *The Master's Wife*, 26, 28; William Macphail to Andrew Macphail, 14 Aug. 1885, William Macphail Papers (in private possession). Hereafter, all references in the notes to "Macphail" will mean Andrew Macphail.

6 Hobsbawm, *Industry and Empire*, 301–3. Also see Richards, *A History of the Highland Clearances*, vol. 1, ch. 8, and vol. 2, ch. 17.

7 Hugh Macphail to William and Mary Macphail, 12–14 Sept. 1836, William Macphail Sr Papers. Also see table 2 in Mellor, "Population," 42; Macphail, *The Master's Wife*, 30.

8 See Macphail, *The Master's Wife*, 245.

9 J.A. Sims (?) to William Macphail Sr, 4 Sept. 1840 [original emphasis], William Macphail Family Papers, PARO. Professor Rusty Bittermann of St Thomas University brought this collection to my attention.

10 I have adopted Macphail's spelling, although Rayburn, *Geographical Names of Prince Edward Island*, 92, renders it "Newtown."

11 Lake, *Topographical Map of Prince Edward Island in the Gulf of St. Lawrence*

12 See document dated 15 May 1843; and Malcolm [Macqueen] to Catherine Macphail Jackson, 28 March 1950, William Macphail Family Papers, PARO.

13 Statement signed by John M. Stark, 2 Oct. 1854, William Macphail Papers. Also see Macphail, *The Master's Wife*, 33-5; teaching license of William Macphail, dated 28 Oct. 1847; press cutting of PEI origin, 18 Jan. 1904, Lindsay-Macphail Scrapbooks 1, Macphail Papers; interview with Mrs John Campbell, 18 Aug. 1971; Robertson, "William McPhail," DCB 13: 671–2. The locations of the adjacent districts of Upper and Lower Newton are indicated in *Illustrated Historical Atlas of the Province of Prince Edward Island*, 119-20. Unless otherwise indicated, all interviews cited were conducted by the present author.

14 For an account of the troubles that Stark encountered and that led to his return to Scotland in 1857, see Robertson, "Religion, Politics, and Education in Prince Edward Island, from 1856 to 1877," 1–15.

15 William Macphail's wife will be referred to in the notes as "Catherine
    Macphail." Her daughters will be identified by their maiden names as long
    as they are single; after marriage they will be identified as, for example,
    "Maggie Macphail Jenkins."

16 See Macphail, *The Master's Wife*, 16-17. Macphail had less definite informa-
    tion about the maternal side of his mother's family; see 8.

17 Macphail, *The Master's Wife*, 6

18 "Family Record," Lindsay-Macphail Scrapbooks 1, Macphail Papers. The
    Family Record has the following information: "Legitimate children
    though born only eight months after marriage which was satisfactorily
    accounted for by the Doctors in the fact that it was the first confinement
    of a young woman by the children. The lives of both Mother and children
    were despaired of for a time."

19 His full name was John Andrew Macphail, but as he ceased to use the
    name John outside his family after about 1893, he will be referred to as
    "Andrew" throughout this book. The other Macphail children who sur-
    vived birth were William John James, b. 2 April 1859; Margaret Ann, b.
    3 February 1861, Finlay Smith, b. 2 September 1862; Mary Isabella, b. 24
    March 1866; Janetta Clark, b. 14 April 1868; James Alexander, b. 25 January
    1870; William Matheson, b. 18 March 1872; Catherine Elizabeth, b. 20 April
    1874; John Goodwill, b. 18 December 1877.

20 See William Macphail to James Alexander Macphail (his brother), 26 Sept.
    1859, 3 Jan., 20 Feb. 1860, 4 Jan., 6 June 1861, William Macphail Papers;
    Macphail, *The Master's Wife*, 37, 165; Assignment of Lease of 100 acres on
    Lot 50 from Caroline Fletcher, administratrix, to William Macphail, 7 May
    1864, Land Title Documents, Leases and Related Documents, Lease No. 109
    [a file containing several documents], Lot 50, PARO; Orwell W.I. [Women's
    Institute], *Orwell: Good Days in Orwell, History of Orwell, PEI*. The location
    of the farm can be seen in *Illustrated Historical Atlas of the Province of Prince
    Edward Island*, 104; *Atlas of Province of Prince Edward Island, Canada, and
    the World*, 71. Regarding the terms of leasehold tenure in colonial Prince
    Edward Island, see Robertson, *The Tenant League of Prince Edward Island*,
    8, 19–24; on 280 the author mistakenly refers to Macphail as having been
    born on the Selkirk Estate.

21 William Macphail to James Alexander Macphail, 26 Sept. 1861; William
    Macphail to Donald Lamont, 2 April 1852 (draft letter marked "confi-
    dential"), Dec. 1852 (draft letter in verse), 13 Jan. 1853 (in verse); William
    Macphail to James Alexander Macphail, 21-24 June 1859, 20 Feb. 1860,
    William Macphail Papers; entry for 20 Sept. 1856, manuscript copy of diary
    kept by William Macphail during a two-month cruise, Lindsay-Macphail
    Scrapbooks 1, Macphail Papers.

22 The "McDonaldites" claimed to be the true representatives of the Church
    of Scotland in PEI and were named after their founder, the Rev. Donald
    McDonald (1783–1867); see Macphail, *The Master's Wife*, 33, 126, 136.
    Regarding McDonald and his movement, see the following publications

by David Weale: "Donald McDonald," *DCB* 9: 480–1; "'The Minister': The Reverend Donald McDonald," 1–6; "The Time Is Come! Millenarianism in Colonial Prince Edward Island," 35–48.

23   Macphail, *The Master's Wife*, 58. Also see 52–62, 68–9, 197–8; William Macphail to Macphail, 31 Oct. 1889, Macphail Papers. On "earnestness," see Houghton, *The Victorian Frame of Mind*, ch. 10.

24   Interview with Mrs Dorothy Lindsay, 21 Sept. 1970

25   See S.N. Robertson, "The Public School System," 380a, 383a–7a; I.R. Robertson, "Religion, Politics, and Education in Prince Edward Island, from 1856 to 1877," 254–322, especially 261; William Macphail to Catherine Macphail, 30 Nov., 21 Dec. 1868; William Macphail to James C. Pope, 28 Oct. 1871; William Macphail to W.D. Stewart, 12 Jan. 1874; undated petition of the School Trustees of Hazel Grove [*ca.* 1877]; William Macphail to Edward Manning, 7 and 13 Dec. (two dates on this draft), 13 Dec. (a second draft) 1878, William Macphail Papers; Macphail, *The Master's Wife*, 57.

26   See Robertson, "William McPhail," *DCB* 13:671-2. The institution had a prior history of scandal, which had led to construction of a new building in 1880. See Rogers, "John Mackieson," *DCB* 11:566; Shephard, "An Island Doctor: The Life and Times of Dr. John Mackieson, 1795–1885," and *Island Doctor*, 90–2, 112–16; Rider, "'A Blot Upon the Fair Fame of Our Island': The Scandal at the Charlottetown Lunatic Asylum, 1874," 3–9; MacBeath, "Sir William Wilfred Sullivan," *DCB* 14:981–3.

27   Macphail, *The Master's Wife*, 25; also see 14, 70–2, 75, 145, 148–9.

28   Ibid., 10; also see 68–9.

29   Ibid., 66–7. See especially ch. 2, entitled "The Spar-Maker," and ch. 3, "Her People."

30   Macphail, *The Master's Wife*, 115, 117

31   Ibid., 114

32   Ibid., 4

33   Ibid., 80

34   Ibid., 79; also see 77–8.

35   See Hobsbawm, *Industry and Empire*, 305–6; Clark, *Three Centuries and the Island*, 91, 102–14, and figs. 43, 44 on 90; Malcolm Campbell, William Macphail, and Murdoch Lamont to the Synod of [?], 17 Aug. 1869 (marked "not sent"), William Macphail Papers.

36   William Macphail to Wellington Dixon, 4 June 1878, William Macphail Papers. Also see Macphail, *The Master's Wife*, 174–88.

37   Macphail, "The Old School," Charlottetown *Patriot*, 28 Dec. 1937. Also see Macphail, *The Master's Wife*, 173; Macphail, "The Education of the People," *Saturday Night*, 12 Aug. 1911.

38   Macphail, *The Master's Wife*, 177. Also see 174–6.

39   Ibid., 93, 145

40   See Bruce, *A Century of Excellence*, in which she provides a compelling portrait of Anderson. Also see her "Alexander Anderson," *DCB* 15:24–6.

41   Macphail, *The Master's Wife*, 177, 179. Also see "Alexander Anderson," in
      MacKinnon and Warburton, eds., *Past and Present of Prince Edward Island*,
      330–2; Robertson, "Religion, Politics, and Education in Prince Edward
      Island, from 1856 to 1877," 262–4; Alexander Anderson to Macphail, 19 Nov.
      1908, Macphail Papers. Anderson, for his part, came to admire greatly the
      scholarly accomplishments of the Macphail family and Uiggers in general;
      see Anderson to Macphail, 17 Sept. 1895, Macphail Papers

42   McGill's reasons for honouring Anderson are embodied in "Extracts from
      the Minutes of Corporation of McGill University – Meeting held October
      26th, 1887," Macphail Papers, and they bear out Macphail's description
      of him.

43   See William Macphail to Macphail, 26 April 1881; Margaret (or "Maggie")
      Macphail (his elder sister) to Macphail, 6 April 1881; George W. Sutherland
      to Macphail, Dec. 1885, Macphail Papers; Macphail, "The Old College,"
      Charlottetown *Patriot*, 3 Jan. 1938; Macphail, "The Old University," *McGill
      News* 19 (Spring 1938): 28; Macphail, *The Master's Wife*, 178–80.

44   See William Macphail to Macphail, 10 Nov. 1881; Donald McLeod to
      Macphail, 7 Nov. 1881; Donald McLeod to "My dear old chum" [James
      H. Good], 25 Nov. 1881; anon. [Miss Bertie Fowler] to "Dear Friend"
      [Macphail], Oct. 1881; "Jack" [Fowler] to "Dear friend" [Macphail], 22 April
      1882; Maggie Macphail to Macphail, 6 Sept. 1881, 10 April 1882, Macphail
      Papers; Macphail, "The Old College," Charlottetown *Patriot*, 3 Jan. 1938;
      interview with Mrs Dora Campbell and Mrs Helen Chauvin, 30 Sept. 1970.

45   See Gillis et al., *Leap over Time*, Table of Contents and 81. Rayburn,
      Geographical Names of Prince Edward Island, 21, has Belfast comprising fewer
      districts, but the generalization arises from Gillis et al., and they are refer-
      ring to the larger area. The location of the school can be seen in *Illustrated
      Historical Atlas of the Province of Prince Edward Island*, 127. Regarding the his-
      tory of the school in Melville, see Gillis et al., *Leap over Time*, 81–8; for a list
      of the teachers who taught in Melville, see 88. The district was also known
      as Raasa, the name of a small Hebridean island off the Isle of Skye, and in
      some Prince Edward Island circles Raasa and the nearby Rona (named for
      another small Hebridean island and later known as Mount Vernon) were
      mocked as being typical of a certain sort of Island-Scottish Protestantism.

46   Although by 2007 there was little sign of habitation or of a former com-
      munity, at one time Melville had had a store, a post office, a mill, and a rail-
      way station, as well as a school; see Hornby, ed., *Belfast People*, 25, 31. I thank
      Marian Bruce for providing me with references regarding Melville.

47   Macphail to William Macphail, 11 Sept. 1882 [original emphasis]. Also see
      William Macphail to Macphail, 18 Sept. 1882, Macphail Papers; Macphail,
      The Master's Wife, 181.

48   See William Macphail to Macphail, 14 Aug. 1882; Macphail to William
      Macphail, 11 Sept. 1882; A.D. Fraser to Catherine Macphail, 14 Dec. 1882;
      Fraser to Macphail, 22 Dec. 1882, Macphail Papers.

49 For a detailed map of the community of Malpeque (although not naming it as such, but rather using the archaic place name of Princetown Royalty), with individual landholdings identified in 1880, and showing the location of Fanning Grammar School, see *Illustrated Historical Atlas of the Province of Prince Edward Island*, 77; also see 85. The school building, which ceased being used as a school in 1969, still stands but was moved 2.5 km to Cabot Beach Provincial Park in 1993 and has been restored. The intent of the move was to save the building, which had greatly deteriorated, from demolition; both the move and the restoration have been the result of a determined effort by a committee of volunteers.

50 Macphail, *The Master's Wife*, 182; also see 184; Clark, *Three Centuries and the Island*, 57, 70; Macphail to Thomas MacNutt, n.d. [1935]; James M. McGougan to Macphail, 21 Oct. 1885; William [?] Hodgson to Macphail, 1 Nov. 1885, Macphail Papers. See Malpeque Historical Society, *Malpeque and Its People 1700-1982*.

51 Macphail to MacNutt, n.d. [1935], Macphail Papers; this letter, written "precisely" fifty years after Macphail's departure from Malpeque, summarizes his experiences in the community. The letter to MacNutt was published in the Charlottetown *Guardian* of 29 Jan. 1935.

52 Charles R. Rogers to Macphail, 24 Jan. 1883, Macphail Papers

53 Macphail, *The Master's Wife*, 184. Also see Thomas Le Page to Macphail, 11 Feb., 2 April 1883; William Macphail to Macphail, 6, 18 Sept. 1882, 1 Feb. 1883, Macphail Papers. From the start of his teaching career, Andrew had shown a decided indifference to the teaching of Sabbath schools; see Macphail to William Macphail, 11 Sept. 1882, Macphail Papers.

54 Information courtesy of Dr John A. Johnston, curator of the National Presbyterian Museum, telephone interview, 28 Oct. 2007. Also see press cuttings from [presumed] Charlottetown *Patriot*, mid-April 1885; Charlottetown *Herald*, 26 Aug. 1885; Sutherland to Macphail, Dec. 1885, Macphail Papers; Buggey, "John Keir," *DCB* 8:451–3. There is a Keir Memorial Museum in Malpeque.

55 Moir, *Enduring Witness: A History of the Presbyterian Church in Canada*, 117.

56 See Fabrius Cassius Funny Fellow, *An Address to Prince Edward Island, by a Native*; Malpeque Historical Society, *Malpeque and Its People 1700–1982*, 287–9. The point of view on the land question which Keir took in his poem was that only the imperial government could make the Island *"Forever free from Rent"* [original emphasis] (11), and that colonial politicians were wasting their time. Regarding the royal commission, see Robertson, ed., *The Prince Edward Island Land Commission of 1860*, "Introduction."

57 See Macphail, *The Master's Wife*, 184–5; William Macphail to Macphail, 6, 18 Sept. 1882, 1 Oct. 1884; Good to Macphail, 20 April, 30 May, 24 Aug., 28 Sept. 1884, 2 June 1885; William J.J. Macphail to Macphail, 1 Oct., 19 Dec. 1883, 12 April 1885; W. Drysdale & Co. to Macphail, 19 April 1883; John

Dougall & Son to Macphail, 31 March 1884, Macphail Papers; Macphail
to Catherine Macphail, 24-26 Nov. 1885, Lindsay-Macphail Scrapbooks 1,
Macphail Papers; Mahoney, "William Hazlitt," 378–81. Eliot had also been
a prolific essayist, but that work largely preceded her career as a novelist, and it was her novels in which Macphail appears to have been most
intensely interested. Yet he did order, through his brother, *The Impressions
of Theophrastus Such* (1879), published one year before her death, which
has been described as "a relatively experimental ... series of fictional/essay-
istic sketches" (Hesse, "British Essay," 109); see William J.J. Macphail to
Macphail, 19 Dec. 1883, 12 April 1885, Macphail Papers; McDonagh, "George
Eliot," 247–9.

58 See Macphail to Catherine Macphail, 2 June, 29 Sept. 1884, 2 Oct. 1885,
Lindsay-Macphail Scrapbooks 1, Macphail Papers; William Macphail to
Macphail, 18–19 March 1885; Good to Macphail, 24 March, 24, 30 July, 30
Sept., 7 Oct. 1884, 8 April 1885; press cuttings from Charlottetown *Examiner*,
9 Oct. 1884; [presumed] Charlottetown *Herald*, 17 Oct. 1884; *Canadian
School Journal*, Nov. 1884 [with correction pencilled in by Macphail];
McGougan to Macphail, 20 Jan. 1886; Sutherland to Macphail, 3 Feb. 1886;
William J.J. Macphail to Macphail, 1 Oct., 19 Dec. 1883; Macphail, "In
Retrospect: Armistice Day," an address delivered at Saint John, NB, 11 Nov.
1936, 4, Macphail Papers; Macphail, *The Master's Wife*, 191–2. When he left
Malpeque for McGill University, Macphail was besieged with requests for
photographs of himself in his new setting; see, for example, William [?]
Hodgson to Macphail, 1 Nov. 1885; McGougan to Macphail, 20 Jan. 1886,
Macphail Papers.

59 Good to Macphail, 24 March 1884 [original emphasis], Macphail Papers. It
seems that both Good and Macphail retained a nominal connection with
a temperance club or institution.

60 Macphail, *The Master's Wife*, 182. Also see 69–70, 151; Good to Macphail, 9,
20 April, 28 Sept. 1884; Macphail to MacNutt, n.d. [1935], Macphail Papers.

61 Macphail to MacNutt, n.d. [1935], Macphail Papers.

62 Good to Macphail, 16 Feb. 1885, Macphail Papers. Also see Good to
Macphail, 15 Dec. 1884; William Macphail to Macphail, 1 Feb. 1883; Dixon
to Macphail, 23 Sept. 1884, Macphail Papers.

63 Good to Macphail, 16 Feb. 1885, Macphail Papers. Also see Neil McLeod
to Macphail, 23 Jan. [1885]; Macphail to MacNutt, n.d. [1935]; William
Macphail to Macphail, 9 April 1891, Macphail Papers. On Carlyle's conception of the role of work and fulfilment of duty in one's life, see Houghton,
The Victorian Frame of Mind, 243–4, 249. In contemplating his future,
Macphail considered practising medicine in India; see W.W. [?] Warburton
to Macphail, 23 Feb. 1885, Macphail Papers.

64 See the Rev. George Hodgson to Macphail, 21 July 1884; William J.J.
Macphail to Macphail, 4 Feb., 1 March 1885; Gawaliel Gillis to Macphail, 22
April 1885; Sir William Dawson to Macphail, 30 May 1885, Macphail Papers.

65 Macphail, *The Master's Wife*, 182–3. Also see 181, 188; Macphail to Lord
    Beaverbrook, 20 Nov. 1934, Lord Beaverbrook Papers, BL; William Macphail
    to Macphail, 22 June, 14 Aug. 1885, Macphail Papers.
66 Macphail to MacNutt, n.d. [1935], Macphail Papers
67 Ibid.
68 Leacock, "Andrew Macphail," *Queen's Quarterly* 45 (Winter 1938): 451. This
    evocative piece has recently been reprinted in Bowker, ed., *On the Front
    Line of Life*, 107–12.
69 Macphail, *The Master's Wife*, 184

CHAPTER TWO

1 Macphail to Catherine Macphail, 8 Jan. 1894, Burland-Macphail Scrapbook,
   Macphail Papers
2 William J.J. Macphail to James Alexander Macphail, 1 March 1892,
   Macphail Papers
3 Macphail to Catherine Macphail, 2 Oct. 1885, Lindsay-Macphail
   Scrapbooks 1, Macphail Papers. Also see Wellington Dixon to Macphail, 8
   Aug. 1885; William J.J. Macphail to Macphail, 11 Oct. 1885, Macphail Papers;
   Lavigne and Rodrigue, *Les rues de Montréal*, 71. Cf. Cooper, *Montreal*, 85, 91.
4 Macphail, *The Master's Wife*, 184. Also see Macphail to Catherine Macphail,
   2 Oct. 1885, Lindsay-Macphail Scrapbooks 1, Macphail Papers; Macphail,
   "The Old University," *McGill News* 19 (Spring 1938): 28. Lucy Maud
   Montgomery made a similar observation when she enrolled in Dalhousie
   College and studied Latin: "We are at Virgil now and are in Book v of
   the Aeneid – we studied the VI at P.W.C." Entry for 20 Jan. 1896, Rubio and
   Waterson, eds., *The Selected Journals of L.M. Montgomery*, 1:155.
5 For illustrations of McGill in 1875 and 1882, see Frost, *McGill University*,
   vol. 1 (hereafter cited as Frost, *McGill 1*), 236, 294; the 1875 illustration gives
   a better notion of the physical setting.
6 Macphail, "Personal Tribute" [to John Redpath Dougall], *Montreal
   Witness*, [18 Sept.] 1935. Also see Macphail, "The Old University," *McGill
   News* 19 (Spring 1938): 28–9; Macphail, *The Master's Wife*, 95; Macphail,
   "John McCrae: An Essay in Character," in McCrae, *In Flanders Fields and
   Other Poems*, 120–1; Cooper, *Montreal*, 59–61. On Dawson and Darwin,
   see O'Brien, *Sir William Dawson*, ch. 5; Berger, *Science, God, and Nature in
   Victorian Canada*, 39–40, 45–6, 56–64; Eakins and Eakins, "Sir John William
   Dawson," *DCB* 12:230–7, especially 234. The other "righteous man" was
   John Dougall of the *Montreal Witness*, who was strongly committed to
   sabbatarianism and temperance; see Snell, "John Dougall," *DCB* 11:270–1.
   For Andrew's estimate of Dawson twenty years later, see "Sir William
   Dawson," *McGill University Magazine* 5 (Dec. 1905): 12–29, especially 24–8;
   for a detailed scholarly account of the Dawson years at McGill, see Frost,
   McGill 1, chs. 8–11.

7   See Lady Margaret Dawson to Macphail, 12 Dec. [1885], Macphail Papers;
    Macphail, "The Old University," *McGill News* 19 (Spring 1938): 28–9;
    Macphail, *Essays in Fallacy*, 131–2; Macphail, *The Master's Wife*, 185. Regarding
    Johnson, see Frost, *McGill 1*, 186, 201, 207n35, 270, 273.

8   Macphail to Catherine Macphail, 24–26 Nov. 1885, Lindsay-Macphail
    Scrapbooks 1, Macphail Papers

9   William J.J. Macphail to Macphail, 11 Oct. 1885, 10 Dec. 1888; William
    Macphail to Macphail, 26 Oct. 1885, 12 April 1886; John Alden, Publisher,
    to Macphail, 26 Feb. 1886; Mary J. Macphail (aunt) to Macphail, 24 Feb., 14
    May 1886; Janet Macphail (aunt) to Macphail, 25 Feb., 14 May 1886; Donald
    Montgomery to Macphail, 5 March 1886; H.H. Curtis to Macphail, 14, 23 May
    1886, Macphail Papers; press cutting from Charlottetown *Examiner*, 2 June
    1903 (on William Macphail's retirement), Lindsay-Macphail Scrapbooks 1,
    Macphail Papers; Macphail, "The Old University," *McGill News* 19 (Spring
    1938): 28; Macphail, *The Master's Wife*, 187–8; Harte, "Canadian Journalists
    and Journalism," *New England Magazine*, new series, 5 (Dec. 1891): 436. The
    article by Harte contains the most comprehensive and probably the most
    accurate account of Macphail's journalistic career through 1891, as the infor-
    mation was solicited from Macphail himself; see Harte to Macphail, 3 March
    1891, Macphail Papers.

10 Montreal *Gazette*, 21 Nov. 1890; also see Charles W. Curtis to Macphail, 3
    Feb. 1886; program of Arts Undergraduate Dinner, 27 Jan. 1886; program
    of "Faculty of Arts Undergraduate Conversazions," 6 Feb. 1888, Macphail
    Papers; Macphail, *The Master's Wife*, 68–9; interview with Mrs Dorothy
    Lindsay, 10 Sept. 1970.

11 *McGill Fortnightly*, 27 Oct. 1892, 1, MRB; this publication introduced itself as
    the successor of the *University Gazette*. See Frost, *McGill 1*, 287–8.

12 See *McGill Fortnightly*, 27 Oct. 1892, 1, MRB; *University Gazette*, 10 May 1889,
    139–40, 2 June 1890, 220, 1 Dec. 1888, 44, and 5 Dec. 1889, 24, MRB.

13 See Perceval-Maxwell, "The History of History at McGill," 8–10. I thank
    Professor Perceval-Maxwell for access to his paper. The Faculty of Arts
    Minute Book, III, 218–19, MUA, does not name the petitioners. McGill did
    not appoint a specialist in Canadian history until the 1930s; Frost, *McGill
    University*, vol. 2 (hereafter cited as Frost, *McGill 2*), 146, 183n13.

14 See *University Gazette*, 10 Feb. 1890, 105; letter by Macphail, n.d., in *University
    Gazette*, 24 March 1890, 186, MRB. The masthead of the former number
    announced that the *University Gazette* was becoming a weekly.

15 See Harte, "Canadian Journalists and Journalism," 436; William Macphail
    to Macphail, 14 Aug. 1885, 12 Sept. 1890; certificate signed by E.S. Blanchard,
    24 Feb. 1891, Macphail Papers; Macphail to Catherine Macphail, 24–26 Nov.
    1885, 27 Sept. 1887, 15 April 1888; Macphail to William Macphail, 7 May 1888;
    press cutting from Charlottetown *Examiner*, 2 June 1903, Lindsay-Macphail
    Scrapbooks 1, Macphail Papers; interview with Mrs Dorothy Lindsay, 21
    July 1970; Macphail, *The Master's Wife*, 208.

16 Macphail to Catherine Macphail, 15 April 1888, Lindsay-Macphail
   Scrapbooks 1, Macphail Papers; also see William Macphail to Macphail,
   26 March 1886, Macphail Papers; Macphail, *The Master's Wife*, 187–8.
   Scholarships for medical students were rare; see Dixon to Macphail,
   23 Sept. 1884; Macphail to Alexander Macphail (brother), 12 Nov. 1889,
   Macphail Papers.

17 Macphail to William Macphail, 7 May 1888, Lindsay-Macphail
   Scrapbooks 1, Macphail Papers

18 Macphail to William Macphail, 21 May 1888, Lindsay-Macphail Scrapbooks
   1, Macphail Papers

19 See Harte, "Canadian Journalists and Journalism," 436; press cutting from
   Charlottetown *Examiner*, 1 May 1888; Macphail to Catherine Macphail,
   4 Dec. 1888, Lindsay-Macphail Scrapbooks 1, Macphail Papers. "Olla
   Podrida" is a Spanish expression meaning a hearty mixed stew of meat
   and vegetables.

20 See undated press cuttings, "Music and the Drama" Scrapbook, Macphail
   Papers. This scrapbook was compiled by Macphail himself. There are some
   42 sides filled with pasted-in reports, reviews, and commentaries, as well as
   a number of loose clippings. These pieces were unsigned, and, except for
   the "Olla Podrida" columns, would be impossible to identify as Macphail's
   without the scrapbook. None of the cuttings are dated, and many are
   untitled save for the location of the performance. Given the nature of the
   material, precise dates are not important.

21 "Music and the Drama" Scrapbook, Macphail Papers

22 Ibid.

23 Ibid.

24 Ibid.

25 See Harte, "Canadian Journalists and Journalism," 436; R.F. Easson to
   Macphail, 31 July 1889, 7 May (telegram), 22 May 1890, n.d. [early 1890]
   (telegram); William Henry Smith, "To Whom It May Concern," 18 April
   1891; William Macphail to Macphail, 31 Oct. 1889, Macphail Papers;
   Macphail to Catherine Macphail, 21 May, 4 Dec. 1888, Lindsay-Macphail
   Scrapbooks 1, Macphail Papers; Macphail, *The Master's Wife*, 181, 185.

26 Although his full name was James Alexander Macphail, he will be referred
   to as Alexander Macphail throughout the text of this study, since he eventually followed Andrew's example in discarding his first name.

27 See William Macphail to Macphail, 31 Oct. 1889, 1 Oct. 1884; Nettie
   Macphail to Macphail, 8 Sept. 1884, 27 March 1890; Belle Macphail to
   Macphail, 18 March 1886; William J.J. Macphail to Macphail, 10 Dec. 1888,
   2 Jan. 1889, 27 March 1890, 29 March 1891; Macphail to Alexander
   Macphail, 12 Nov. 1889; Alexander Macphail to Macphail, 9 May 1891,
   Macphail Papers.

28 Macphail, *The Master's Wife*, 188; also see Macphail to William J.J. Macphail,
   31 March 1891, Lindsay-Macphail Scrapbooks 1, Macphail Papers

29 See Macphail, *The Master's Wife*, 186; press cutting from Charlottetown *Examiner*, 1 May 1888, Lindsay-Macphail Scrapbooks 1, Macphail Papers. He did not specify which examination he had failed.

30 Andrew Macphail, "On Vivisection," reprint from *Montreal Medical Journal*, June 1891, 16 (revised version of "Vivisection," published in Angell, comp., *Vivisection*, 27–43; a copy of the original version is in Lindsay-Macphail Scrapbooks 1, Macphail Papers); American Humane Education Society advertisement, n.d. [closing date for entries: 1 Jan. 1891]; George T. Angell to Macphail, 19 March 1891, Macphail Papers. Macphail, *The Master's Wife*, 185, is incorrect in giving the amount of each prize as $500.

31 Macphail, "The Vivisection Controversy," n.d. [1896] (a draft essay/address); also see Macphail, "On Vivisection," *Montreal Medical Journal*, June 1891; Mrs Caroline Earle White to Macphail, 8 Jan. 1893, Macphail Papers.

32 White to Macphail, 8 Jan. 1893; also see Macphail, "The Vivisection Controversy," Macphail Papers. I have been unable to locate Macphail's checkrein pamphlet.

33 Press cutting from Charlottetown *Examiner*, 8 July 1891 (story by "M. Phail"), Lindsay-Macphail Scrapbooks 1, Macphail Papers. Also see Macphail to William J.J. Macphail, 4 April 1891; press cutting from a Charlottetown newspaper, n.d. [22, 23, or 25 May 1891], Lindsay-Macphail Scrapbooks 1, Macphail Papers; Macphail, *The Master's Wife*, 188; William Macphail to Macphail, 7, 22 April 1891, Macphail Papers; Macphail, "Johnson's Life of Boswell," Quarterly Review 253 (July 1929): 61–2.

34 Press cutting from Charlottetown *Examiner*, 8 July 1891, Lindsay-Macphail Scrapbooks 1, Macphail Papers

35 See his "Athletics in Japan," an article he published in *Outing*, copy in Macphail Papers.

36 Macphail, untitled draft manuscript, n.d. [1891 or 1892] (89 loose and unnumbered pages), Macphail Papers. Also see press cutting from a Charlottetown newspaper, n.d. [22, 23, or 25 May 1891], Lindsay-Macphail Scrapbooks 1, Macphail Papers.

37 Keating, "Jeffrey Hale Burland," DCB 14:158

38 Lewis, *Manufacturing Montreal*, 68, map 3.3. For some of the background on Burland's rise to prominence in this industry, see Galarneau, "George-Édouard Desbarats," DCB 12:247–8.

39 Press cutting from *La Presse*, Feb. 1905, Burland-Macphail Scrapbook, Macphail Papers. Also see Morgan, ed., *The Canadian Men and Women of the Time*, 132.

40 See Copp, *The Anatomy of Poverty*, 100–2; Keating, "Jeffrey Hale Burland," DCB 14:158–9.

41 Macphail to Archibald MacMechan, 20 Oct. 1914, Archibald MacMechan Papers, DUA

42 See R.S. Lea to Macphail, 9 July, 22 Sept. 1890, Macphail Papers.

43 Press cutting from unknown newspaper, 21 Oct. 1891, Burland-Macphail Scrapbook, Macphail Papers

44 When the Macphail Papers were used by the present author, they
    contained only three letters written by Georgie: two to Andrew's mother
    and one to his father – and none to Andrew. But it is clear from Andrew's
    letters to Georgie that she did write to him when they were separated for
    any period of time. It is possible that Macphail destroyed her letters to him
    or ordered them destroyed.

45 See William Macphail to Macphail, 8 Oct. 1891; Lea to Macphail, 26 June
    1891, Macphail Papers; Macphail to William J.J. Macphail, 31 March, 4
    April 1891; Macphail to William Macphail, 2 Nov. 1893, Lindsay-Macphail
    Scrapbooks 1, Macphail Papers.

46 Press cutting from a Montreal newspaper, 20 Dec. 1893; press cutting of
    unknown origin, 25 May 1894; Macphail to William Macphail, 7 March
    1894, Burland-Macphail Scrapbook, Macphail Papers.

47 Ross, "The French and English Social Élites of Montreal: A Comparison
    of La Ligue de la Jeunesse Féminine with the Junior League," 47. Also
    see interview with Mrs Dorothy Lindsay, 10 July 1970; William Macphail
    Martin to the author, electronic mail, 10, 14 Nov., 28 Dec. 2004; Julia
    Gersovitz to the author, electronic mail, 14 March 2005.

48 Kerr and Holdsworth, eds., *Historical Atlas of Canada*, vol. 3, plate 30

49 MacLeod, "Salubrious Settings and Fortunate Families: The Making of
    Montreal's Golden Square Mile, 1840-1895," 232. The term "Golden Square
    Mile" was not, according to MacLeod, used until the twentieth century;
    see 1.

50 See ibid., 1, and maps 1 and 2 (on unnumbered pages). Different authors
    give slight variations in the boundaries. Rémillard and Merrett (*Demeures
    bourgeoises de Montréal*, 17) define the western and eastern limits as Atwater
    Avenue on the west (several streets west of Cote des Neiges) and Park
    Avenue and Bleury Street (the same street, differently named: Park to
    the north of Sherbrooke Street, Bleury to the south) on the east. Westley
    (*Remembrance of Grandeur*, 25) places the western boundary at Cote des
    Neiges (she gives the name it takes south of Sherbrooke: Guy Street), the
    southern at Dorchester Boulevard (slightly north of the CPR tracks), the
    northern at Pine Avenue, and the eastern as "near Bleury." MacKay (*The
    Square Mile*, 8) states that the southern fringe moved northward over time
    as Dorchester deteriorated with the coming of "tourist hotels and bawdy
    houses" by the 1930s. Dorchester Boulevard was renamed René Lévesque
    Boulevard in 1987; see Lavigne and Rodrigue, *Les rues de Montréal: réper-
    toire historique*, 401.

51 MacLeod, "Salubrious Settings and Fortunate Families: The Making of
    Montreal's Golden Square Mile, 1840–1895," ii

52 Gersovitz, "The Square Mile, Montreal 1860–1914," 2. She cites Pine and
    Cedar Avenues to the north, University to the east, Guy and Cote des
    Neiges to the west, and Dorchester to the south, as the boundaries, and
    refers to this as "in reality a Half-Square Mile." The author wishes to

acknowledge the exceptional efforts of Elizabeth Seres, Resource Sharing Coordinator, the Bladen Library, University of Toronto at Scarborough, in gaining access for him to this thesis.

53 Cochrane was the maiden name of Georgie's mother, who had died in 1890.

54 Georgina Burland Macphail to Catherine Macphail, 26 Sept. 1896, Burland-Macphail Scrapbook, Macphail Papers

55 Press cutting from a Prince Edward Island newspaper, n.d., reprinted from *Montreal Star*, 22 April 1902, Burland-Macphail Scrapbook, Macphail Papers

56 Maggie Macphail Jenkins to Macphail, 7 Aug. 1896 [original emphasis], Macphail Papers. Also see William Macphail to Georgina Burland, 7 Nov. 1893; William Macphail to Macphail, 1 Aug. 1896, Macphail Papers; William Macphail to Macphail, 8 Nov. 1893, Lindsay-Macphail Scrapbooks 1, Macphail Papers. Nettie was the first Prince Edward Island woman to graduate from McGill; see press cutting from the Charlottetown *Examiner*, 11 May 1896, Lindsay-Macphail Scrapbooks 1, Macphail Papers.

57 Maggie Macphail Jenkins to Macphail, 7 Aug. 1896, Macphail Papers

58 Macphail to Georgina Burland Macphail, n.d. [Aug. 1896], Macphail Papers

59 Marguerite ("Meg") Stanley, granddaughter of Macphail, at the Sir Andrew Macphail Heritage Days, at the Macphail Homestead, Orwell, 29 July 2000

60 Interview with Mrs Dorothy Lindsay, 15 and 16 June 1969

61 See Macphail to Georgina Burland, 8 Aug. 1893, Macphail Papers; also see Macphail to Georgina Burland, 5 July 1893, Macphail Papers.

62 Press cutting from a Prince Edward Island newspaper, n.d., reprinted from *Montreal Star*, 22 April 1902, Burland-Macphail Scrapbook, Macphail Papers

63 Macphail to William Macphail, 5 May 1902, Macphail Papers

64 Interview with Mrs Dorothy Lindsay, 1 Oct. 1970

65 See Macphail to Georgina Burland, 15 Aug. 1893, Macphail Papers; Macphail to Catherine Macphail, 25 Aug. 1893; Macphail to William Macphail, 2 Nov. 1893, Lindsay-Macphail Scrapbooks 1, Macphail Papers; interviews with Mrs Dorothy Lindsay, 30 May, 5 Dec. 1968, 29 July 1970.

66 Leacock, "Andrew Macphail," *Queen's Quarterly* 45 (Winter 1938): 452

67 Interview with Mrs Dorothy Lindsay, 13 March 1970

68 MacMechan to Macphail, 12 Oct. 1914, Macphail Papers

69 Macphail to MacMechan, 20 Oct. 1914, MacMechan Papers, DUA

70 For accounts of the events surrounding her death and funeral, see the letters sent to William Matheson Macphail (in Winnipeg) by three of his siblings: by Andrew, 20 May 1920; by Catherine Macphail Martin "Saturday" [22 May 1920?]; by John Goodwill Macphail, 21 May, 29 June 1920, William Macphail Family Papers, PARO. Many years earlier Macphail's elder brother Finlay had moved to Southport, a rural district close to Charlottetown.

71 Macphail to William J.J. Macphail, 1 Dec. 1891, Lindsay-Macphail Scrapbooks 1, Macphail Papers

72 Macphail, *The Master's Wife*, 187; Macphail to William J.J. Macphail, 1 Aug. 1892, Lindsay-Macphail Scrapbooks 1, Macphail Papers; Alexander Macphail to William Macphail, 10 Nov. 1892; W. Abbot to Macphail, 20 April 1892, Macphail Papers

73 Macphail to William Macphail, 2 Nov. 1893, Lindsay-Macphail Scrapbooks 1, Macphail Papers; Macphail to Georgina Burland, 23 March, 30 June, 23 July, 1, 31 Aug. 1893; certificate of the United States Life Insurance Company in the City of New York, 1 Dec. 1892; certificate of the Mutual Life Insurance Company of New York, 7 Jan. 1893; certificate of the Union Life Insurance Company of Maine, 19 Jan. 1893; G.T. Ross to Macphail, 1 June 1893, Macphail Papers; entries for 31 May 1893, 19 May 1894, Minutes of the Faculty of Medicine, University of Bishop's College, vol. 2, 164, 180, BUA. Concerning the Bishop's medical faculty, see Milner, *Bishop's Medical Faculty*, and "Francis Wayland Campbell," DCB 13:153–4; Nicholl, *Bishop's University*, app. 3, 317–47.

74 See Grenier, "Thomas Joseph Workman Burgess," DCB 15:165.

75 Macphail, "The After-History of Applicants Rejected for Life Insurance," *British Medical Journal*, 15 Dec. 1900, 1697–1701; Maggie Macphail Jenkins to Macphail, 18 Dec. 1894; James Brown to Macphail, 16 Oct. 1895; A. Lapthorn-Smith to Macphail, 8 Feb. 1896; William Macphail to Georgina Burland Macphail, 11 Dec. 1898, Macphail Papers; entry for 15 Nov. 1898, Minutes of the Faculty of Medicine, University of Bishop's College, vol. 2, 321, BUA; interviews with Mrs Dorothy Lindsay, 30 May 1968, 29 July 1970.

76 Wells, *The Fishery of Prince Edward Island*, 29, 131–5, 140–3 provides the relevant background.

77 Macphail to Georgina Burland Macphail, 25 May 1896. Also see Macphail to Georgina Burland Macphail, 15, 21 May, 8 June 1896, Macphail Papers; press cutting from a Charlottetown newspaper, n.d. [mid-May 1896], Lindsay-Macphail Scrapbooks 1, Macphail Papers; press cutting from a Montreal newspaper, n.d. [1896], Burland-Macphail Scrapbook, Macphail Papers. Owing to his preoccupation with the lobster investigation, Macphail's medical practice declined temporarily; see William Macphail to Macphail, 13 March 1897, Macphail Papers.

78 See Macphail to Georgina Burland Macphail, 8 June 1896, Macphail Papers; press cutting from Charlottetown *Examiner*, n.d. [mid-June 1897]; press cutting of unknown origin, n.d. [late Aug. 1896]; press cutting from *Montreal Witness*, n.d. [late Oct. 1897], Burland-Macphail Scrapbook, Macphail Papers; press cutting of unknown origin, n.d. [1897], Lindsay-Macphail Scrapbooks 1, Macphail Papers; Macphail, *Discoloration in Canned Lobsters: Report of an Inquiry into the Causes Leading to a Deterioration in the Quality of Canned Lobsters* (33 pp.). As Bruère retired from the project before its completion, only Macphail signed the report.

79 See Gorveatt, "'Polluted with Factories': Lobster Canning on Prince Edward Island," 16–17. Also see Wells, *The Fishery of Prince Edward Island*, 144 (which misdates the field research as having been done in 1897).

80 See press cutting from a Charlottetown newspaper, 28 May 1896, Lindsay-
    Macphail Scrapbooks 1, Macphail Papers; Alexander Anderson to
    Macphail, 15, 17 Sept., 8, 22 Dec. 1895, 15 Feb. 1897; Macphail to Anderson,
    3 May 1897; Dawson to Macphail, 8 June 1892, Macphail Papers

81 See MacDermot, "Sir Andrew Macphail," *McGill News* 20 (Winter 1938):
    16; Stevenson, "Sir Andrew Macphail," *Canadian Defence Quarterly* 16 (Jan.
    1939): 210; interview with Mrs Dorothy Lindsay, 29 July 1970.

82 Macphail, untitled manuscript on the prospects of Bishop's College
    Medical Faculty, n.d. [1904]; address by Macphail at the Canadian Society
    of Authors annual dinner, Toronto, 26 Jan. 1907, Macphail Papers.

83 Minutes of the Faculty of Medicine, University of Bishop's College, 3 vols.
    (1871–82, 1882–1900, 1900–05), *passim*, BUA.

84 See entries for 13 Dec. 1904, 28 Jan., 4 Feb. 1905, Minutes of the Faculty of
    Medicine, University of Bishop's College, vol. 3, 96-102, BUA; Milner, *Bishop's
    Medical Faculty*, 293–4.

85 "To the Medical Faculty of Bishop's College" (an unsigned report on a 27
    Feb. 1905 Bishop's-McGill meeting), n.d. [1905; apparently a committee
    report prepared by Macphail; there are two versions, one a typescript, and
    one in Macphail's hand]; untitled typescript statement concerning the
    negotiations between McGill and Bishop's, n.d. [1905; apparently a state-
    ment on behalf on the Bishop's negotiating committee meant for McGill
    eyes], Macphail Papers; entries for 1, 2 March 1905, Minutes of the Faculty
    of Medicine, University of Bishop's College, vol. 3, 104–7, BUA; Masters,
    Bishop's University: The First Hundred Years, 110-12; Bensley, "Bishop's Medical
    College," 463–5; Frost, *McGill* 2, 44–5.

86 See Masters, *Bishop's University*, 111; "To the Medical Faculty of Bishop's
    College" (a report), n.d. [1905]; Macphail, untitled manuscript on the
    prospects of Bishop's College Medical Faculty, n.d. [1904], Macphail
    Papers; Class 38/3/5, Faculty of Medicine Minute Book, 437, minutes of
    meeting held 1 April 1905, MUA(AFM); Class 38/3/6, Faculty of Medicine
    Minute Book, 62, 208, 215-16, 218, minutes of meetings held 6 May 1905, 4
    May, 13 June 1907, MUA(AFM); William Peterson to Macphail, 20 Feb. 1905,
    Sir William Peterson Letterbooks, vol. 6, 365, MUA; Peterson to Macphail,
    17 May 1905, Peterson Letterbooks, vol. 7, 142, MUA; interview with E.H.
    Bensley, 23 June 1971; Bensley, "Bishop's Medical College," 463–5; accession
    681/7, McGill Board of Governors Minute Book, 429, minutes of meeting
    held 21 June 1907, MUA. The ten members of the McGill medical faculty
    present on 13 June 1907 had all attended the May 1905 meeting. On the
    matter of Macphail's connection with Bishop's, Milner (*Bishop's Medical
    Faculty*, 338) states that he resigned at a faculty meeting on 5 April 1904, but
    that his resignation was not accepted. The minutes of the faculty do not
    support this interpretation. A letter by Macphail which seemed to indicate
    an intention to resign several months hence was read at a faculty meeting
    on 5 April, yet he attended the next meeting, on 20 May, and no mention

of the matter appears in the minutes of that meeting or subsequently; see
entry for 5 April 1904, Minutes of the Faculty of Medicine, University of
Bishop's College, vol. 3, 88–9, BUA.

87 Nicholl, *Bishop's University*, 347. For a list of long-standing faculty members, many of whom were serving at the time of amalgamation in 1905, see
Milner, *Bishop's Medical Faculty*, app. C, 492.

88 Macphail, "Medicine," in Wallace, ed., *Encyclopedia of Canada*, 4:264

89 "To the Medical Faculty of Bishop's College" (a report), n.d. [1905],
Macphail Papers. For the joint report of the two negotiating commit-
tees, dated 7 March 1905, which contained the cautionary proviso that the
making of appointments "would necessarily be a work of time," see Milner,
Bishop's Medical Faculty, 295–8; also see letter of J.B. McConnell to F.W.
Frith, 4 April 1905, in Milner, *Bishop's Medical Faculty*, app. L, 515.

90 Cited in Milner, *Bishop's Medical Faculty*, 485–6; the person for whom
Macphail prepared the memorandum is unknown. During a visit to
Bishop's University Archives on 22 June 1999 there was a photocopy of this
document in the Elizabeth Hearn Milner Papers, BUA, but no indication
of the whereabouts of the original; in her book, Milner does not provide
this information and indeed gives the location of her source as "Bishop's
Medical Faculty File."

91 McGill University Calendar for 1908–09, 295, MUA

92 Class 38/3/6, Faculty of Medicine Minute Book, 216, minutes of meeting
held 13 June 1907, MUA(AFM). Macphail had put himself on record several
years earlier as opposing compulsory attendance at lectures; see "The
Attainment of Consideration," *British Medical Journal*, 15 Nov. 1902, 1612–14.

93 Interview with H.E. MacDermot, 22 June 1971

94 Ibid.; also see MacDermot, "Sir Andrew Macphail," *McGill News* 20 (Winter
1938): 16.

95 Macphail, "John McCrae: An Essay in Character," in McCrae, *In Flanders
Fields and Other Poems*, 123

96 MacDermot, "Sir Andrew Macphail," *McGill News* 20 (Winter 1938): 17; also
interview with H.E. MacDermot, 22 June 1971

97 Interview with H.E. MacDermot, 22 June 1971; MacDermot, "Sir Andrew
Macphail," *McGill News* 20 (Winter 1938): 16–17; Francis, "Sir Andrew
Macphail," *Bulletin of the History of Medicine* 7 (July 1939): 799; interview
with Mrs Dorothy Lindsay, 30 May 1968.

98 Martin, in *Canadian Medical Association Journal* 39 (1938): 509

99 Paul Potter, Hannah Professor of the History of Medicine, University of
Western Ontario, personal communication, 19 Sept. 2003. For a brief summary of the contrasting approaches to medical education in Canada, see
Waugh, "Medical Education," 1456; also see Roland, "Medical Schools," 396.
I thank Dr Raymond Wenn, DDS, for initially drawing to my attention,
on 27 Aug. 2003, the extent to which Macphail's views with respect to the
medical curriculum were ahead of his time.

100   Press cutting of unknown origin, n.d. [1909], Macphail Papers.
101   See [Macphail], "Style in Medical Writing," *Canadian Medical Association Journal* 1 (Jan. 1911): 70–3, and 15 June 1992, 2197–8; Squires, "Remembering Our First Editor," *Canadian Medical Association Journal*, 15 June 1992, 2127.
102   MacDermot, *One Hundred Years of Medicine in Canada*, 164; also interviews with H.E. MacDermot, 22 June 1971, and E.H. Bensley, 23 June 1971; Francis, "Sir Andrew Macphail," 799
103   See entries for 12, 13 Sept. 1907 (pp. 10, 42, 45–6), Canadian Medical Association Minute Book General Meetings, 1907–1925, LAC; entries for 10 June 1908 (memorandum in Macphail's handwriting, pasted into pp. 3–4), 31 May 1910 (p. 36), Canadian Medical Association Minutes Executive Council 1908 to 1927, LAC; *Montreal Medical Journal* 39 (Dec. 1910): 818; "H.E.M." [MacDermot], "Sir Andrew Macphail," *Canadian Medical Association Journal* 39 (Nov. 1938): 482; MacDermot, "Sir Andrew Macphail," *McGill News* 20 (Winter 1938): 16; Shortt, "Sir Andrew Macphail: Physician, Philosopher, Founding Editor of *CMAJ*," 324, 326; Shortt, "Essayist, Editor, and Physician: The Career of Sir Andrew Macphail, 1864–1938," 53–4; Robertson, "Andrew Macphail: A Holistic Approach," 179–80.
104   See entries for 1 Sept. 1899 (pp. 70–1), 14 Sept. 1900 (93–4), 17 Sept. 1902 (137), 25 Aug. 1903 (162), 24 Aug. 1905 (239), 20 Aug. 1906 (251–2), stapled-in material, n.d. [probably 1906], and 26 Feb. 1907 (265), Canadian Medical Association Minute Book Annual Meetings, 1896–1907, LAC; entries for 11 Sept. 1907 (1-2), 12 Sept. 1907 (9-10), 13 Sept. 1907 (42, 45–6), 9 June 1908 (49), 11 June 1908 (p. 54), 25 Aug. 1909 (72–4), Canadian Medical Association Minute Book General Meetings, 1907-1925, LAC; entry for 8 July 1914 (113–16), Canadian Medical Association Minutes Executive Council, 1908–1927, LAC.
105   [Macphail], "Style in Medical Writing," *Canadian Medical Association Journal* 1 (Jan. 1911): 70, 72. As editor of the *Canadian Medical Association Journal*, Macphail did not sign his editorials; when others wrote editorials they included their names (interview with H.E. MacDermot, 22 June 1971). Also see Macphail to Pelham Edgar, 14 Nov. 1910, James Mavor Papers, UTRB; Macphail to MacMechan, 12 July 1910, MacMechan Papers, DUA; Macphail to the fourth Earl Grey, 8 Jan. 1911, the fourth Earl Grey Papers, UD; entry for 7 June 1911 (p. 56–7), Canadian Medical Association Minutes Executive Council, 1908–1927, LAC.
106   "H.E.M." [MacDermot], "Sir Andrew Macphail," *Canadian Medical Association Journal* 39 (Nov. 1938): 482–3; also Macphail to F.J. Shepherd, 25 Sept. 1908, Macphail Papers; interviews with H.E. MacDermot, 22 June 1971, and E.H. Bensley, 23 June 1971. Macphail's name was not formally removed as editor of the *Canadian Medical Association Journal* until 1919; see entry for 27 June 1919 (pp. 145–6), Canadian Medical Association Minute Book General Meetings, 1907–1925, LAC.

107   It has proved impossible (despite the assistance of *Dictionnaire biographique
      du Canada* researchers based in Quebec City) to find the will of George
      Bull Burland, and consequently it has not been possible to determine,
      even approximately, how much money accrued to Macphail with the
      death of his father-in-law in May 1907. Burland's willingness to share with
      Macphail is not in doubt. In addition to everything cited in the present
      chapter, in 1898 he provided money for the Protestant Hospital for the
      Insane to build a pathology laboratory which Macphail, who had been
      appointed to the hospital in 1895, would direct; see Grenier, "Thomas
      Joseph Workman Burgess," DCB 15:165. Two business historians have
      determined that Macphail, in concert with his younger brother William
      Matheson who was an engineer in western Canada, pursued the possibil-
      ity of being a significant investor in a waterpower development in 1911.
      They speculate that when he apparently lost interest later in the year, it
      may have been, in some measure, because of a debilitating domestic acci-
      dent that cost him part of his eyesight permanently and meant a lengthy
      convalescence. See Armstrong and Nelles, "Competition vs. Convenience:
      Federal Administration of Bow River Waterpowers, 1906–13," 163, 170–3, 175,
      179, 217–18n39.
108   Macphail to William Matheson Macphail, 23 Feb. 1891, William Macphail
      Family Papers, PARO.
109   See Macphail to William Macphail, 24 Sept. 1899; William Macphail
      to Macphail, 28 Jan. 1896, 20, 28 Sept. 1899, 5 April, 2 Aug. 1901,
      Macphail Papers.
110   See Macphail to Georgina Burland Macphail, 29 Dec. 1896,
      Macphail Papers.

CHAPTER THREE

1   Montreal *Gazette*, 8 Aug. 1894; also see W.F. Torrance to Macphail,
    30 Dec. 1891, Macphail Papers.
2   See Macphail to Georgina Burland Macphail, 22 Aug. 1895,
    Macphail Papers.
3   Entries for 19 March, 16 April, 26 Nov. 1898, 24 Feb. 1900, Pen and Pencil
    Club Minutes vol. 1, 117, 119, 121, 141, MMCH
4   Entry for 4 Jan. 1902, Pen and Pencil Club Minutes, vol. 1, 153, MMCH
5   Entry for 20 Feb. 1897, Pen and Pencil Club Minutes, vol. 1, 103, MMCH.
6   See Gersovitz, "The Square Mile, Montreal 1860–1914," 45
7   See Cox, *Fifty Years of Brush and Pen*; Williamson, *Robert Harris*, 144, 149, 150.
    The Cox pamphlet concludes with a list of members elected, 1890–1937, in
    the sequence of their election (8–10). The exclusion of women from the
    club was one reason given in 1894 for the founding of the Women's Art
    Association of Canada, Montreal Branch; see McLeod, *In Good Hands*, 91.
8   Moritz and Moritz, *Stephen Leacock*, 114

9   Macphail, "John McCrae: An Essay in Character," in McCrae, *In Flanders Fields and Other Poems*, 84. Also see Leacock, "Andrew Macphail," 446–8; entry for 18 Feb. 1905, Pen and Pencil Club Minutes, MMCH.

10   Macphail, "John McCrae: An Essay in Character," 127–8

11   Photograph of Macphail with "Miss Dorothy" and "Mr. Percy Taylor," n.d. [*ca.* 1907], Burland-Macphail Scrapbook, Macphail Papers

12   See entries for 22 Jan. – 28 April 1898, Pen and Pencil Club Minutes, vol. 1, 115–19, MMCH.

13   Macphail, "John McCrae: An Essay in Character," 128

14   See entry for 29 Feb. 1908, Pen and Pencil Club Minutes, vol. 2 [pages in this volume are unnumbered], MMCH. Harris's text is reproduced in Williamson, *Robert Harris*, app. 1, 202–7.

15   Try-Davies, *A Semi-Detached House and Other Stories*, dedication; the cover states "by J. Try-Davies illustrated by Robert Harris." Also see entry for 27 Oct. 1900, Pen and Pencil Club Minutes, vol. 1, 145, MMCH. In 2007 the Confederation Centre Art Gallery in Charlottetown had a mini-exhibition on the collaboration of Harris and Try-Davies. There is a copy of the book, which is rare, in the Harris Collection at the Gallery.

16   See entry for 18 April 1914, Pen and Pencil Club Minutes, vol. 3, 12–15, MMCH.

17   Entry for 5 Dec. 1908, Pen and Pencil Club Minutes, vol. 2

18   See Wagg, *Percy Erskine Nobbs*, 67–74; "P.E.N. [Percy E. Nobbs]," "Praise of Fence," *McGill University Magazine* 4 (May 1905): 233–41; Macphail, "Design," *Queen's Quarterly* 44 (Spring 1937): 29. Some of Nobbs's bold proposals for buildings on the McGill campus that were never built continue to provoke hostile commentary; see Reynolds, "The Campus That Never Was," 29.

19   Entry for 15 March 1902, Pen and Pencil Club Minutes, vol. 1, unnumbered page between 154 and 155, MMCH.

20   Entry for on 1 Feb. 1902, Pen and Pencil Club Minutes, vol. 1, 154, MMCH.

21   For more on Leacock's contributions to the Club, see Moritz and Moritz, *Stephen Leacock*, 115.

22   See entry for 30 March 1901, Pen and Pencil Club Minutes, vol. 1, 150, MMCH. For a self-portrait by Dyonnet, dated 1940, see Sisler, *Passionate Spirits*, 195.

23   Entry for 29 Nov. 1919, Pen and Pencil Club Minutes, vol. 3, 169, MMCH

24   Entry for 19 Jan. 1901, Pen and Pencil Club Minutes, vol. 1, 148, MMCH

25   Entry for 3 April 1897, Pen and Pencil Club Minutes, vol. 1, 105, MMCH

26   Entry for 23 March 1907, Pen and Pencil Club Minutes, vol. 2 [unnumbered pages]; also see entries for 21 Dec. 1907, vol. 2 [unnumbered pages]; 1 May 1920, vol. 3, 189, MMCH

27   Entry for 11 Nov. 1922, Pen and Pencil Club Minutes, vol. 3, 225, MMCH

28   Entry for 24 Jan. 1920, Pen and Pencil Club Minutes, vol. 3, 173, MMCH

29   Leacock, *Montreal*, 312

30 Entry for 6 April 1912, Pen and Pencil Club Minutes, vol. 2 [unnumbered pages], MMCH; also see entry for 27 Jan. 1912, Pen and Pencil Club Minutes, vol. 2 [unnumbered pages], MMCH.

31 Macphail, *Essays in Puritanism*, "Note" (on an unnumbered page). Also see Macphail Notebooks, vols. 1,2, and 3 *(ca.* 1900–05); War Diaries, vol. 2, 10 Jan. 1916, Macphail Papers; Macphail, ed., *The Book of Sorrow*, Preface; interviews with Mrs Dorothy Lindsay, 30 May 1968, 13 March 1970. Papers on Fuller, Edwards, Wesley (in two parts), Winthrop (also in two parts) are indicated in the entries for 10, 24 Jan., 3 Oct., 7 Nov., 26 Dec. 1903, 20 Feb. 1904, Pen and Pencil Club Minutes, vol. 1, 159, 163–4, vol. 2, unnumbered pages, MMCH. It is not clear when he delivered his paper on Whitman; the minutes vary considerably in the amount of information included.

32 Macphail, *Essays in Puritanism*, 79; all page references to this book will be to the American edition, whose pagination differs from that of the British edition.

33 William Macphail to Macphail, 12 Jan. 1905, Macphail Papers; also see Macphail, untitled manuscript on "Best Work and Why," n.d. [1929], Macphail Papers. The San Francisco *Chronicle* even described Macphail as Voltairian in his approach to theology, and a Presbyterian journal launched an attack on the book for its "superficiality," "ridicule," "would-be smartness," and "flippancy"; see reviews in *Chronicle*, 9 July 1905, and [Toronto ?] *Westminster*, 1 July 1905, Macphail Papers.

34 Macphail, *Essays in Puritanism*, 3–30; also see review in Montreal *Gazette*, 22 April 1905, Macphail Papers.

35 Review in *New York Times*, 29 April 1905, Macphail Papers. Macphail's friend E.W. Thomson attributed these faults to the origins of the papers and insufficient revision before publication; see review by "E.W.T" in *Winnipeg Free Press*, 25 March 1905, Macphail Papers.

36 Review in *Baltimore News*, 29 April 1905; also see review in London (England) *Spectator*, 25 Feb. 1905; review in *British Medical Journal*, 30 June 1906, all in Macphail Papers.

37 Review by W. Wilfred Campbell in Ottawa *Evening Journal*, 20 May 1905, Macphail Papers. Also see, for example, reviews in *New York Times*, 29 April 1905, and *Providence Journal*, 5 April 1905, Macphail Papers.

38 See review in Boston *Zion-Herald*, 11 July 1906, Macphail Papers. The book was published in New York in 1906.

39 See entry for 30 Oct. 1897, Pen and Pencil Club Minutes, vol. 1, 110, MMCH. Also see entries for 27 Nov. 1897, 19 Feb. 1898, Pen and Pencil Club Minutes, vol. 1, 112, 116, MMCH.

40 Macphail Papers

41 Review in Philadelphia *Westminster*, 8 Sept. 1906, Macphail Papers. Also see Waite, "The Canadian Historical Novel," 4, 8–9.

42 Macphail, untitled manuscript on "Best Work and Why," n.d. [1929], Macphail Papers. Also see reviews in Charleston, SC, *News*, 8 July 1906, and Philadelphia *Church Standard*, 21 July 1906, Macphail Papers.

43 Review in London (England) *Tribune*, 8 Aug. 1906, Macphail Papers. Also see Roper, "New Forces: New Fiction 1880–1920," 281.

44 Thomson to Macphail, n.d. [1905 or 1906], Macphail Papers

45 Review in *Chicago Evening Post*, 30 June 1906, Macphail Papers

46 Review in *Cleveland Plain Dealer*, 12 Aug. 1906, Macphail Papers

47 See review in *Cleveland Plain Dealer*, 12 Aug. 1906; review in *Chicago Evening Post*, 30 June 1906, Macphail Papers.

48 In addition to *Essays in Puritanism*, see "Sir William Dawson," *The McGill University Magazine* 5 (Dec. 1905): 12–29; "The Attainment of Consideration," *British Medical Journal*, 15 Nov. 1902, 1612–14; "Vivisection," in Angell, comp., *Vivisection*, 27–43. One relatively recent critic, Ronald W. McBrine, has denied that Macphail was an essayist, on the following grounds: "The five selections in *Essays in Puritanism* ... are long treatises on Puritanism as exemplified by ... [the five subjects]. Macphail intended his remarks in each instance to be objective and analytical ... His essay is not a test or an attempt. It is a treatise in which he examines material seeking to arrive at conclusions" (McBrine, "The Development of the Familiar Essay in English Canadian Literature from 1900 to 1920," 44–5). The point is well taken, but as McBrine fails to provide a better alternative word than "treatise," I shall continue to use Macphail's own term, "essay." On the distinction between the familiar essay and the treatise, see Buechler, "Treatise," in Chevalier, ed., *Encyclopedia of the Essay*, 853–4. Also see Conron, "Essays 1880-1920," in Klinck et al., eds., *Literary History of Canada*, 342–4. Conron complains that "Macphail's concept of the essay tended towards straight discursive writing" (343). But he and McBrine see "discursiveness" as one of the fundamental characteristics of the essay; see Conron, "Essays 1880–1920," 340, and McBrine, "The Development of the Familiar Essay," ii, 4.

49 For an illustration of the changing proportions of English and French Canadians within Montreal between 1881 and 1931, see Dickinson and Young, *A History of Quebec*, 202, fig. 6.4; for a more detailed breakdown, see Frost, *McGill* 2, 126.

50 Sutcliffe, "Montreal Metropolis," 22

51 Entry for 3 Aug. 1894, Minutes of the Faculty of Medicine, University of Bishop's College, vol. 2, 192-3, BUA

52 Unfortunately, Macphail's surviving letters from his student years give no hint about his views – or even awareness – of the furor over the hanging of Louis Riel, or the associated French-English tensions in Montreal. The explanation may lie in the fact that most of his correspondents were family members and others who were in contact with family members. Thus, his reticence about the dramatic conflicts playing out in the city where he was studying could be understandable as a desire not to cause anxiety for them.

53 See entries for 17 Nov., 1 Dec. 1906, Pen and Pencil Club Minutes, vol. 2 [unnumbered pages], MMCH.

54 The only reference to the South African War in Macphail's surviving correspondence was as follows: "I can at least write you a letter wishing you all a Merry Christmas if I cannot send much in the way of presents. The unhappy war has so disturbed things here that everyone is just trying to hold on till the turn of the year"; Macphail to Catherine Macphail, 20 Dec. 1899, Burland-Macphail Scrapbook, Macphail Papers.

55 Jean Ménard, preface to Dyonnet, *Mémoires d'un artiste canadien*, 10–11. Although Dyonnet and Lafleur were the most active French-speaking members, it should not be inferred that they were the only francophones; distinguished persons such as the architect Ernest Cormier and the sculptor Henri Hébert also joined. In 1924 the francophone Basque portraitist Alphonse Jongers was identified in the minutes as "the oldest active member of the Club excepting Dyonnet." See entry for 19 Jan. 1924, Pen and Pencil Club Minutes, vol. 3, 244, MMCH.

56 See Keating, "Jeffrey Hale Burland," *DCB* 14:158–9; Rémillard and Merrett, *Demeures bourgeoises de Montréal*, 90–1. In the latter, on page 90, there is a photograph of the front of the house, and on 91 there is a photograph of a portion of what must have been a large garden (since 1973, partially filled in by townhouses).

57 MacKay, *The Square Mile*, 192. Also see 192, 217; and Rémillard and Merrett, *Demeures bourgeoises de Montréal*, 216–17, which includes two photographs of the house.

58 Macphail to Georgina Burland, 5 July 1893, Macphail Papers

59 Gentilcore and Matthews, eds., *Historical Atlas of Canada*, vol. 2, plate 49

60 Westley, *Remembrance of Grandeur*, 24; also see 37.

61 MacKay, *The Square Mile*, 192

62 *The Concise Oxford Dictionary*, 8th edn (1990), 496. See Gournay "Gigantism in Downtown Montreal," 154–5, 201–2n4.

63 Ibid. The hotel building was converted into "Les Cours Mont-Royal" in 1988.

64 Frost, *McGill* 2, 51

65 See Noonan, "William Henry Drummond," in Benson and Toye, eds., *The Oxford Companion to Canadian Literature*, 2nd edn, 333; Edwards, "William Henry Drummond," *DCB* 13:286.

66 Macphail to James Mavor, 25 April 1907, Mavor Papers, UTRB

67 See Robertson, "The Historical Leacock," 46.

68 See entry for 8 Jan. 1921, Pen and Pencil Club Minutes, vol. 3, 197, MMCH.

69 Rémillard and Merrett, *Demeures bourgeoises de Montréal*, 19: "It attained a degree of refinement unequalled in Canada, with its numerous very exclusive clubs, sporting teams, magnificent receptions, the celebrated art collections of some of its members, and the homes in city and country with their trained staff."

70 Ibid. Also see Gersovitz, "The Square Mile, Montreal 1860–1914," 33.

CHAPTER FOUR

1 *McGill University Magazine* 1 (Dec. 1901): 13. Also see Peterson to Moyse, 22 May 1906, Peterson Letterbooks, vol. 9, 169, MUA.

2 See McNally, "*The McGill University Magazine*, 1901–1906: An Evaluation and a Bio-bibliographical Analysis," 6, table 1, which classifies the articles "by broad subject."

3 See speech of E.B. Greenshields in proposing a toast to the health of Macphail at the University Club, Montreal, 10 March 1909, 15, Macphail Papers; accession 681/7, McGill Board of Governors Minute Book, 362, minutes of meeting held 25 May 1906, MUA; Peterson to Greenshields, 20 June 1906, Peterson Letterbooks, vol. 9, 292, MUA; Macphail to Edgar, 14 Nov. 1910, Mavor Papers, UTRB.

4 McNally, "*The McGill University Magazine*, 1901–1906," 1. Also see McNally, "Canadian Periodicals and Intellectual History: The Case of the *McGill University Magazine/University Magazine*, 1901–1920," 69–78. Heggie and McGaughey have compiled and published *The University Magazine, 1901–1920: An Annotated Index*, which includes brief summaries of prose contributions, except in instances where the title makes the content self-evident (e.g., "Greek Heroines"). As the dates in the title suggest, their index includes the *McGill University Magazine*, but their list of references, published in 1997, does not include the two works by McNally cited here (1976 and 1980).

5 See McNally, "*The McGill University Magazine*, 1901–1906," 74. Also see 10, 12, 14.

6 Shortt, *The Search for an Ideal*, 16. See McNally, "Canadian Periodicals and Intellectual History," 72.

7 McNally, "*The McGill University Magazine*, 1901–1906," 3; also see 4.

8 Ibid., 11; also see 6, table 1.

9 Ibid., 97

10 Ibid., 6, table 1

11 Ibid., 51

12 Ibid., 68

13 Peterson to Moyse, 22 May 1906, Peterson Letterbooks, vol. 9, 169, MUA; Peterson to Macphail, 19 June 1906, Peterson Letterbooks, vol. 9, 287, MUA; Peterson to Greenshields, 20 June 1906, Peterson Letterbooks, vol. 9, 292, MUA; Peterson to John W. Cunliffe, 20 June 1906, Peterson Letterbooks, vol. 9, 291, MUA; Peterson to Charles W. Colby, 20 June 1906, Peterson Letterbooks, vol. 9, 297, MUA; speech by Macphail at the Canadian Society of Authors annual dinner, Toronto, 26 Jan. 1907; Shepherd to Macphail, 24 Sept. 1908; Macphail to Shepherd, 25 Sept. 1908, Macphail Papers; Macphail, "John McCrae: An Essay in Character," in McCrae, *In Flanders Fields and Other Poems*, 51; Macphail to Byron Edmund Walker, 1 June 1907, Sir Edmund Walker Papers, UTRB; interview with H.E. MacDermot, 22 June 1971; Collard, "Sir William Peterson's Principalship, 1895–1919," 79, 81.

Not everyone was sanguine about the prospects for reorganization; see McGill Corporation Minute Book no. 6, 334, minutes of meeting held 8 June 1906, MUA.

14 Leacock, "Andrew Macphail," 449–50. No comprehensive files on the editing of the *University Magazine* have survived. In the present author's first letter to Mrs Dorothy Lindsay, Macphail's daughter, 4 Feb. 1968, he inquired about surviving files of the *University Magazine*; Mrs Lindsay responded, "My father kept his records for 15 years or so after the Magazine closed up and then I suspect destroyed them. Also I think a good part of the records would have been accounts and a great deal else done by personal talks" (Mrs Dorothy Lindsay to the author, 11 Feb. 1968).

15 Peterson to Colquhoun, 6 Nov. 1906, Peterson Letterbooks, vol. 9, 373, MUA. Also see Peterson to W.P. Ker, 13 Nov. 1906, Peterson Letterbooks, vol. 9, 395, MUA; Peterson to Smith, 6 Nov. 1906, Peterson Letterbooks, vol. 9, 374–5, MUA;

16 *University Magazine* 6 (Feb. 1907). The word "main" was deleted after the first number.

17 Macphail to MacMechan, 11 Dec. 1907, MacMechan Papers, DUA. Macphail maintained this emphasis over the years; see Macphail to MacMechan, 3 Oct. 1913, MacMechan Papers, DUA; Macphail to Mavor, 23 Sept. 1919, Mavor Papers, UTRB.

18 McNally, "*The McGill University Magazine*, 1901–1906," 12

19 Macphail, *Essays in Politics*, 73. "What Can Canada Do," the essay from which the citation comes, was first published in the *University Magazine* 6 (Dec. 1907): 397–411. Also see Peterson to Macphail, 17 Dec. 1906, Peterson Letterbooks, vol. 9, 492, MUA. The five articles appeared in the Oct. 1907, Dec. 1907, Oct. 1908, Dec. 1908, and April 1909 numbers. For the *Review of Historical Publications Relating to Canada*'s notice of this series, see the *Review* 12 (1908): 73; 13 (1909): 55–6; and especially 14 (1910): 7–9.

20 Clark, *Three Centuries and the Island*, 121, table 5.

21 These calculations are based on ibid., 125, table 6.

22 Macphail to MacMechan, 11 Dec. 1907, MacMechan Papers, DUA

23 Macphail to MacMechan, 2 April 1907, MacMechan Papers, DUA. Also see Macphail to Mavor, 23 Oct. 1907, Mavor Papers (in private possession).

24 See speech by Greenshields, a member of the McGill Board of Governors, in proposing a toast to the health of Macphail at the University Club, Montreal, 10 March 1909, 16, Macphail Papers. The occasion was a dinner in his honour, as editor of the magazine; about fifteen people were present. See entry for 10 March 1909, E.B. Greenshields Diaries 2, MMCH; also see entry for 3 Oct. 1908, Greenshields Diaries 2, MMCH.

25 Edgar, "Sir Andrew Macphail: An Appraisal," *Canadian Author*, 16 (Autumn 1938): 7. For a modern assessment of Pickthall's work, see MacGillivray, "Marjorie Pickthall," in Benson and Toye, eds., *The Oxford Companion to Canadian Literature*, 918–20

26 See Macphail to Walker, 25 April 1908, Walker Papers, UTRB; MacMechan to Macphail, 4, 9 Nov. 1908, Macphail Papers; Robert Falconer to Macphail, 31 Jan., 1 May 1911, Sir Robert A. Falconer Papers, UTA.

27 See Copp, *The Anatomy of Poverty*, 32.

28 MacMechan, *Head-waters of Canadian Literature*, 202–3. Also see 201.

29 See "The University Magazine; A Statement submitted to the Board of Governors of the University of Toronto," n.d. [Feb. or March 1907], Falconer Papers, UTA; Walker to Sir William M. Clark, 7, 10 Jan. 1907; Walker to Edgar, 10 Jan. 1907; Edgar to Walker, 21 Jan. 1907; Walker to C.A. Chant, 18 Jan. 1907, Walker Papers, UTRB; Peterson to Arthur E. Childs, 24 Jan. 1907, Peterson Letterbooks, vol. 10, 100, MUA. Leacock was to have accompanied Macphail and Peterson but was unable to make the trip.

30 Speech by Macphail at the Canadian Society of Authors annual dinner, 26 Jan. 1907, Macphail Papers. .

31 See Macphail to Edgar, 14 Nov. 1910, Mavor Papers, UTRB; Macphail to Edgar, 27 Feb. 1907; "The University Magazine; A Statement submitted to the Board of Governors of the University of Toronto," n.d. [Feb. or March 1907], Falconer Papers, UTA; Macphail to Walker, 25 April 1908, Walker Papers, UTRB.

32 MacMechan, *Head-waters of Canadian Literature*, 202; *University Magazine* 6 (April 1907), inside cover

33 Walker to Clark, 10 Jan. 1907, Walker Papers, UTRB; Macphail to Edgar, 1 Feb. 1907, Falconer Papers, UTA; Macphail to Edgar, 14 Nov. 1910, Mavor Papers, UTRB; Macphail to Grey, 8 Jan. 1911, Grey Papers, UD

34 See Wallace, ed., *The Macmillan Dictionary of Canadian Biography*, 593; press cutting from *Montreal Herald*, 17 July 1907, McGill University Scrapbooks 2, 228, MUA; Frost, *McGill* 2, 4, 5, 7, 43, 95–6, 108–9; entry for 16 Dec. 1899, Pen and Pencil Club Minutes, vol. 1, 138, MMCH; entry for 18 Dec. 1909, Pen and Pencil Club Minutes, vol. 2, MMCH.

35 See Thompson, *William Morris*, 355–6, 366.

36 See Wallace, ed., *The Macmillan Dictionary of Canadian Biography*, 505; Story, *The Oxford Companion to Canadian History and Literature*, 520; Ferns and Ostry, *The Age of Mackenzie King*, 18-19; interview with E.H. Bensley, 23 June 1971; Bowker, "Truly Useful Men," ch. 4; Shortt, *The Search for an Ideal*, 119–35; Sperdakos, *Dora Mavor Moore*, 17–32; Panayotidis, "James Mavor," DCB 15:723–5. Bowker and Sperdakos, in her book on Mavor's daughter, convey the personality of this unusual Torontonian effectively.

37 Bowker, "Truly Useful Men," 126

38 Peterson to Mavor, 5 April 1916, Peterson Letterbooks, vol. 27, 27, MUA; see Bowker, "Truly Useful Men," 148–9. Regarding relations with Leacock and Wrong, see Edgar, "Stephen Leacock," 178–9; Bowker, "Truly Useful Men," 85.

39 Sperdakos, *Dora Mavor Moore*, 21. Sperdakos has informed the author that the phrase comes from Mavor's grandson, the famed producer, playwright,

and actor James Mavor Moore; Sperdakos to the author, electronic mail, 25 Feb. 2003.

40 See Bowker, "Truly Useful Men," especially ch. 4, on his role within the university. Regarding Mavor and the arts, see 145–6; regarding Macphail and the *Economic History of Russia*, see 138–9. Also see Shortt, *The Search for an Ideal*, 123.

41 Murray, *Working in English*, 39

42 Ibid., 19. Also see Wallace and Woodhouse, "In Memoriam: William John Alexander," 1–33; MacLure, "Literary Scholarship," 230–1; Harris, *English Studies at Toronto*, 200.

43 See Murray, *Working in English*, ch. 2.

44 Griffiths, *The Splendid Vision*, 85

45 See Stevens, "Sir James David Edgar," *DCB* 12: 291–4; Breault, "Matilda Ridout (Edgar, Lady Edgar)," *DCB* 13: 869–71; Griffiths, *The Splendid Vision*, 84–5.

46 See Wallace, ed., *The Macmillan Dictionary of Canadian Biography*, 213–14; Story, *The Oxford Companion to Canadian History and Literature*, 239–40; MacLure, "Literary Scholarship," 224–5; Pacey, "Literary Criticism in Canada," 114; Friedland, *The University of Toronto*, 119; Harris, *English Studies at Toronto*, 52.

47 Waite, *The Lives of Dalhousie University*, 1: 295

48 See Wallace, ed., *The Macmillan Dictionary of Canadian Biography*, 480; Story, *The Oxford Companion to Canadian History and Literature*, 499-500; Pacey, "Literary Criticism in Canada," 114; MacLure, "Literary Scholarship," 230–1; Shortt, *The Search for an Ideal*, 41–57; Waite, *The Lives of Dalhousie University*, 1: 158–62, and 2: 15; Baker, "Archibald MacMechan," 511–12.

49 Baker, *Archibald MacMechan*, back cover

50 See ibid., 94–102.

51 Macphail to MacMechan, 11 Dec. 1907, MacMechan Papers, DUA. On at least one occasion Macphail suggested that the Toronto members of the board put together a number; see Macphail to Mavor, n.d. [2 Feb. 1908], Mavor Papers (in private possession). The figure of fifty includes an anonymous piece by MacMechan and excludes numerous short editorial pieces by Peterson in the 1915–19 period. It should also be borne in mind that after 1914 Walton was in Egypt, and that after 1916 Alexander and Mavor had no formal connection with the magazine, although in 1919 the latter did contribute an article.

52 See Peterson to Alexander, 13 April 1916, Peterson Letterbooks, vol. 27, 67, MUA.

53 Grey to John St Loe Strachey, 14 Oct. 1907 (private), John St Loe Strachey Papers, BL. Also see Peterson to Macphail, 9 April 1907, Peterson Letterbooks, vol. 10, 362, MUA.

54 Macphail, *Essays in Politics*, 10–11. The articles on the Ashburton Treaty, which appeared anonymously, were written by James White, chief

geographer for the Canadian Department of the Interior; see Macphail, *Essays in Politics*, 275–6; White to Macphail, 30 Oct. 1908, Macphail Papers. In many of Macphail's essays he used "England/English" interchangeably with "Britain/British," and often he used the former when the latter would seem to have been more appropriate – uncharacteristic lapses in accepted usages.

55 Macphail, *Essays in Politics*, 18–19; also see 5–6. Strachey took very favourable notice of this article; see press cutting from *Spectator*, 2 Nov. 1907, 656–7, Macphail Papers.

56 Cited in Macphail, *Essays in Politics*, 251–2.

57 Grey to Lord Elgin, 14 Oct. 1907, Grey Papers, LAC; also see Grey to Elgin, 9 April 1907, Grey Papers, LAC. For the appreciation of this series by the colonial editor of the *Times* of London, see L.S. Amery to Macphail, 29 April 1909, Macphail Papers.

58 See Grey to Strachey, 14 Oct. 1907 (private), Strachey Papers, BL; Grey to Bryce, 14 Oct. 1907; Grey to Elgin, 14 Oct. 1907; Grey to Lord Knollys, 14 Oct. 1907, Grey Papers, LAC; Kipling-Macphail volume, Introduction by Macphail, n.d. [mid-1920s?], Macphail Papers. After they met, Kipling allowed Macphail to publish in the *University Magazine* an address he had delivered at McGill.

59 Grey to the Earl of Crewe, 18 Feb. 1909, Grey Papers, LAC; also see Grey to Strachey, 17 Feb. 1909, Strachey Papers, BL. Regarding these negotiations, and Grey's role in bringing them about, see Noel, *Politics in Newfoundland*, 41–51, 58, 62–4; Miller, "Albert Henry George Grey, 4th Earl Grey," *DCB* 14: 440.

60 Press cutting from Montreal *Gazette*, 11 Dec. 1907, McGill University Scrapbooks 2, 241, MUA

61 *Review of Historical Publications Relating to Canada*, 12 (1908): 72–3. This favourable notice does not seem to have been simply the courtesy owing to beginners, for it was regularly repeated in the ensuing years; see, for example, *Review* 16 (1912): 52–3.

62 Macphail to MacMechan, 11 Dec. 1907, MacMechan Papers, DUA

63 See press cutting from Toronto *Globe*, 17 Dec. 1908, Macphail Papers.

64 Press cutting from Montreal *Daily Herald*, 18 Dec. 1908, Macphail Papers

65 See press cutting from Toronto *Daily Star*, 23 Dec. 1908.

66 Milner, "The Higher National Life," 429. Also see Marquis, "English-Canadian Literature," 523.

67 Robertson, "Sir Andrew Macphail as a Social Critic," 360–6, appendix: "*The University Magazine* Coterie."

68 Macphail to Walker, 1 Feb. 1907, Walker Papers, UTRB. Of the twelve leading contributors to the *University Magazine*, three were non-academics (Pickthall, Thomson, and Hamilton). No article by Walker ever appeared in the *University Magazine*.

69 See MacMechan to Macphail, 4 Jan., 11 Oct. 1912, Macphail Papers.

70   McNally, "*The McGill University Magazine*, 1901–1906," 73; also see 85–6.

71   For indexes and summaries of the contents of the *University Magazine*,
     see Jones, "A Content Guide and Index to *The University Magazine*,
     Vols. IX–XIX, 1910–1920"; Heggie and McGaughey, comp., *The University
     Magazine, 1901–1920*. Jones does not give a reason for commencing the
     study in 1910 rather than 1907; Heggie and McGaughey (1997) do not
     appear to have been aware of the Jones thesis (1954), for they state without
     qualification, "*The University Magazine* ... has never been indexed" (8).

72   See Macphail to Mavor, 17 Sept. 1913, Macphail Papers. There can be little
     doubt that the circulation exceeded 4,500, the number which Macphail,
     in the Dec. 1919 number of the *University Magazine,* implied had been
     its peak. See Macphail to Grey, 9 Dec. 1911, Grey Papers, UD; Macphail to
     MacMechan, 2 Jan. 1912, MacMechan Papers, DUA; Macphail to Walker, 6
     Feb. 1912, Walker Papers, UTRB; "To Readers," *University Magazine* 18 (Dec.
     1919), inside cover.

73   See Peterson to Macphail, 9 April 1907, Peterson Letterbooks, vol. 10,
     362, MUA; Macphail to Walker, 25 April, 1 June 1908, Walker Papers, UTRB;
     Greenshields to Sir William Van Horne, 9 Dec. 1909, Sir William Van
     Horne Papers, MUA.

74   Walker to D.B. Dewar, 6 May 1908; Macphail to Walker, 25 April 1908;
     Walker to Macphail, 29 April 1908, Walker Papers, UTRB; Van Horne to
     Greenshields, 27 Dec. 1909, Van Horne Papers, MUA; Macphail to Edgar, 14
     Nov. 1910; Macphail to Mavor, 2 June 1913, Mavor Papers, UTRB; Macphail
     to Mavor, 17 Sept. 1913, Macphail Papers; *University Magazine* 9 (Dec. 1910),
     inside cover. In February 1909 the price of a single issue had been raised
     from 25 to 35 cents.

75   Walker to Edgar, 3 June 1908, Walker Papers, UTRB. As well as president of
     the Bank of Commerce, Walker was a member of the University of Toronto
     Board of Governors.

76   Macphail to Thomson, 30 Oct. 1913. Also see Mavor to Macphail, 16 Sept.
     1913; Macphail to Mavor, 17 Sept. 1913, Macphail Papers; Macphail to Mavor,
     2 June 1913, Mavor Papers, UTRB; Macphail to MacMechan, 3 Oct. 1913,
     MacMechan Papers, DUA; Macphail to Mavor, 9 Oct. 1913, Mavor Papers
     (in private possession). In the two last-cited letters, Macphail mentioned
     having been faced by Morang with a $3,800 deficit, which he paid; this was
     prior to the final settlement.

77   See Peterson to Grey, 6 March 1915, Peterson Letterbooks, vol. 24, 381, MUA;
     Walker to Macphail, 4 June 1908; Edgar to Walker, 4 Nov. 1910; Walker to
     Edgar, 8 Nov. 1910; Walker to Falconer, 8 Nov. 1910, Walker Papers, UTRB;
     Greenshields to Van Horne, 8, 29 Dec. 1909, Van Horne Papers, MUA;
     Falconer to Macphail, 22 Feb. 1909, Falconer Papers, UTA; Macphail to
     Edgar, 14 Nov. 1910, Mavor Papers, UTRB.

78   See Greenshields to Van Horne, 8, 29 Dec. 1909; Van Horne to Greenshields,
     2 Jan. 1910, Van Horne Papers, MUA; Macphail to Greenshields, 19 June

1908, 10 Jan. 1910; Greenshields to Macphail, 6 Jan., 26 Oct. 1910, E.B.
Greenshields Scrapbook, MMCH; Macphail to Walker, 25 April, 1 June 1908,
Walker Papers, UTRB; Macphail to Edgar, 14 Nov. 1910, Mavor Papers, UTRB;
Peterson to Maurice Hutton, 12 March 1909, Peterson Letterbooks, vol.
13, 2, MUA; Peterson to Macphail, 28 Feb. 1918, Peterson Letterbooks, vol.
30, 213, MUA; draft appeal for funds for the *University Magazine*, 20 Oct.
1911 (unsigned); "General Statement; University Magazine," 31 Dec. 1917,
Falconer Papers, UTA; Macphail to MacMechan, 28 March 1914, MacMechan
Papers, DUA. Regarding Greenshields, see Gordon Burr, "Edward Black
Greenshields," *DCB 14:* 437–8.

79 Address by Macphail at the Canadian Society of Authors annual dinner,
Toronto, 26 Jan. 1907, Macphail Papers

80 Shortt, *The Search for an Ideal*, 17, refers to the "poor circulation figures" of
the magazine, but despite the array of numbers he cites it is not clear what
number he would consider to have been an indicator of success; nor does
he present comparative numbers for such other periodicals as the *Queen's
Quarterly* or the later *Dalhousie Review* and *University of Toronto Quarterly*,
which might place the *University Magazine* figures in perspective.

81 See Macphail to MacMechan, 3 Aug. 1913, MacMechan Papers, DUA;
Macphail to Mavor, 18 Jan. 1913, 23 Jan. 1914, Mavor Papers, UTRB; Macphail,
"John McCrae: An Essay in Character," 52–3. It would appear that members
of the editorial board paid for their own subscriptions; see Peterson to
Morang & Co., 15 April 1911, Peterson Letterbooks, vol. 16, 333, MUA.

82 The following did appear: André Siegfried, "Les partis politiques en
France," *University Magazine*, 7 (Feb. 1908): 153–68; Henri Lebeau, "Eugene
Le Roy," *University Magazine* 8 (Dec. 1909): 634–48; Louis Perdriau, "Le
modernisme catholique," *University Magazine* 13 (April 1914): 327–41; René
du Roure, "Le traité de paix," *University Magazine* 18 (Dec. 1919): 482–5
(prose); and Charles E. Saunders, "À Jeanne d'Arc," *University Magazine*
19 (April 1920): 170–1 (poetry). Max Ingres, "Aux champs de Flandre,"
University Magazine 19 (Feb. 1920): 118, is a translation of John McCrae's
poem *In Flanders Fields*. Several items, despite French titles, were in fact
written in English; an example is a sonnet by E.B. Greenshields, "La dou-
leur qui veille," *University Magazine* 8 (Oct. 1909): 421.

83 N.A. Belcourt, "French in Ontario," *University Magazine* 11 (Dec. 1912): 551–61

84 Macphail, Postscript to Belcourt, "French in Ontario," *University Magazine*
11 (Dec. 1912): 561

85 For more on this injury, see pp. 148–9, below.

86 See Sir Robert Borden to Macphail, 28 Sept. 1914 (telegram), Sir Robert
Borden Papers, LAC; interview with Mrs Dorothy Lindsay, 30 May 1968;
Macphail to Peterson, 13, 30 Jan. 1915, Sir William Peterson Papers, MUA;
Peterson to Grey, 6 March 1915, Peterson Letterbooks, vol. 14, 381–2, MUA;
entry for 15 April 1915, War Diaries, vol. 1, Macphail Papers.

87 MacMechan to Macphail, 23 March 1912, Macphail Papers

88 This was a reference to the fact that the "Doctor Macphail" nameplate never came down during Macphail's lifetime. See p. 43, above.

89 Edgar, "Sir Andrew Macphail," *Queen's Quarterly* 54 (Spring 1947): 9–10.

90 Leacock, "Andrew Macphail," 446

CHAPTER FIVE

1   Macphail, "John Knox in the Church of England," *University Magazine* 6 (Feb. 1907): 15–23

2   Macphail, *Essays in Politics*, 122–31. For all articles appearing in *Essays in Politics* as well as the *University Magazine*, citations will be to the page numbers in the book. Angus McFadyen was the name of an early acquaintance of Macphail; the significance, if any, of this coincidence is not clear. See William J.J. Macphail to Macphail, 13 Feb. 1877, Macphail Papers.

3   Macphail, *Essays in Politics*, 29–31

4   Ibid., 23. Macphail's visits had occurred in 1892, 1893, 1896–97, and 1902; he was also to be in Britain in June 1907.

5   Macphail, *Essays in Politics*, 26

6   Ibid., 27; also see 25.

7   Ibid., 29; also see 27–8.

8   Ibid., 31

9   Macphail is referring to the proposal that Britain, then a "free trade" country, institute a preference for Canadian imports.

10 Macphail, *Essays in Politics*, 32–3; also see 34.

11 Ibid., 35

12 Ibid., 31. Also see 35; Leacock, "Greater Canada: An Appeal," *University Magazine* 6 (April 1907): 134–6; Berger, *The Sense of Power*, 260-1.

13 Macphail, *Essays in Politics*, 36

14 See Grey to Elgin, 14 Oct. 1907, Grey Papers, LAC; Grey to Strachey, 14 Oct. 1907 (private), Strachey Papers, BL; Hodgins, *British and American Diplomacy Affecting Canada* and *The Alaska Boundary Dispute*; Munro, "English-Canadianism and the Demand for Canadian Autonomy: Ontario's Response to the Alaska Boundary Decision, 1903," 189–203.

15 Munro, "English-Canadianism and the Demand for Canadian Autonomy," 199

16 See "x.x.x." [James White], "The Ashburton Treaty: A Diplomatic Victory or Defeat," *University Magazine* 6 (Oct. 1907): 291–8; D.A. MacArthur, "The Alaska Boundary Award," *University Magazine* 6 (Dec. 1907): 412–26; James White, "Oregon and San Juan Boundaries," *University Magazine* 7 (Oct. 1908), 398–414; "***" [James White], "The Ashburton Treaty: An Afterword," *University Magazine*, 7 (Dec. 1908), 560–3.

17 Macphail, *Essays in Politics*, 4

18 Ibid., 10; also see 5, 11-15.

19 Ibid., 7

20 Ibid., 6, 15–17.
21 Ibid., 247. For this article Macphail adopted the title of the series, "British Diplomacy and Canada."
22 Ibid., 248–50.
23 Ibid., 254–90.
24 Ibid., 279–80; also see MacArthur, "The Alaska Boundary Award," *University Magazine* 6 (Dec. 1907): 426. For Macphail's more extravagant assertions on behalf of the British diplomatic record, see his *Essays in Politics*, 253, 265, 299.
25 "A Canadian" [James White], "The Long Sault Dam," *University Magazine* 9 (April 1910): 263. See White to Macphail, 23 March 1910, Macphail Papers
26 See Macphail to Laurier, 22 March 1910, Sir Wilfrid Laurier Papers, LAC; Macphail to MacMechan, 14 Feb. 1910, MacMechan Papers, DUA; Grey to Laurier, 1 March 1909, 12 Feb. 1910, Grey Papers, LAC.
27 See Bryce to Grey, 25 Oct. 1907; Crewe to Grey, 5 May 1909 (private and confidential), Grey Papers, LAC; Northcliffe to Grey, 19 April 1909; Amery to Macphail, 29 April 1909, Macphail Papers; Strachey to Grey, 26 Oct. 1907; Grey to Strachey, 2 Jan. 1908 (private), Strachey Papers, BL.
28 Strachey to Grey, 15 Jan. 1908, Strachey Papers, BL. Also see press cutting from *Spectator*, 2 Nov. 1907, 656–7, Macphail Papers; Hodgins to Strachey, 30 Dec. 1907; Strachey to Hodgins, 13 Jan. 1908, Grey Papers, UD.
29 See Macphail to Mavor, 23 Oct., 22 Nov., 4, 30 Dec. 1907, n.d. [*ca.* 2 Jan. 1908], n.d. [*ca.* 12 Jan. 1908], n.d. [*ca.* 19 Jan. 1908], n.d. [2 Feb. 1908], 17 Feb., 9 March 1908; Macphail to Hodgins, 30 Dec. 1907, n.d. [*ca.* 19 Jan. 1908], 2, 6 Feb. 1908; Mavor to Hodgins, 10 Feb. 1908; Hodgins to Mavor, 11, 17 Feb. 1908, Mavor Papers (in private possession).
30 See *Review of Historical Publications Relating to Canada*, 13 (1909): 55–6, and 14 (1910): 7–9.
31 See Macphail, *Essays in Politics*, 11, 248.
32 Amery to Macphail, 29 April 1909, Macphail Papers. Also see Grey to Strachey, 14 Oct. 1907 (private), Strachey Papers, BL; Grey to Elgin, 14 Oct. 1907, Grey Papers, LAC.
33 Grey to Crewe, 8 April 1909, Grey Papers, LAC
34 See Macphail to Grey, 29 March 1909, Grey Papers, UD; press cutting from Montreal *Gazette*, 13 April 1909, Macphail Papers; Macphail, *Essays in Politics*, 247.
35 Macphail, *Essays in Politics*, 64, 67; also see 65–6.
36 See ibid., 77–81.
37 Ibid., 72–3
38 Ibid., 80–1, 73–7
39 Ibid., 81–3. At the census of 1900–01 the population of the United Kingdom exclusive of Ireland was reckoned at 37 million, and thus Macphail was characterizing approximately one-third of the population as being unprofitably employed. See Ensor, *England 1870–1914*, 269.

40 Macphail, *Essays in Politics*, 83–4
41 Ibid., 89; also see 82–5.
42 See press cutting from a Montreal newspaper, n.d. [Jan. 1908], Macphail Papers, for substantial excerpts; also see press cutting from an Ottawa newspaper, n.d. [Jan. 1908], Macphail Papers. The excerpts match verbatim certain paragraphs of the article that appeared in the *University Magazine* of Feb. 1908.
43 See Macphail Papers for a typescript copy.
44 Macphail, *Essays in Politics*, 38–9. Cf. Rudyard Kipling, "Ad Universitatem," *University Magazine* 6 (Dec. 1907): 450–1.
45 Macphail, *Essays in Politics*, 40; also see 38–9.
46 Ibid., 40; also see 41.
47 Ibid., 44; also see 43
48 Cited in ibid., 41
49 See Macphail, *Essays in Politics*, 41–3.
50 Ibid., 40
51 Ibid., 41
52 Ibid., 44–5
53 Ibid., 46; also see 60, 45, 49.
54 Ibid., 61; also see 62.
55 Ibid., 59
56 Ibid., 60
57 Ibid., 85; also see 60.
58 Ibid., 45 (sequence of Macphail's words altered)
59 Macphail, "The Whole Duty of the Canadian Man," address delivered to the Canadian Club of Saint John, NB, 26 March 1908, 7–8, Macphail Papers; also see 6. A lengthy summary of the address was published in the Saint John *Sun*, 27 March 1908; see press cutting in Macphail Papers. It would appear that Macphail deviated slightly from his prepared text.
60 Macphail, "The Whole Duty of the Canadian Man," 9, Macphail Papers; also see 8.
61 Ibid., 8
62 Ibid., 18
63 Ibid., 17
64 Ibid., 18
65 Macphail utilized sections from "Loyalty – To What," "The Patience of England," "What Can Canada Do," and "The Dominion and the Spirit." Parts of the address later appeared in "The 'American Woman,'" "Protection and Politics," "The Psychology of Canada," and "Why the Conservatives Failed."
66 Macphail, "The Whole Duty of the Canadian Man," 4, Macphail Papers; also see 3.
67 Ibid., 4–6
68 Ibid., 6; also see 4.

69 Strachey to Macphail, 13 May 1908, Macphail Papers. From a random sample of the *Spectator* of this period, it would appear that considerably less than half of the weekly numbers carried such signed "Letters." As the articles, even reduced in size, were thrice the normal length, Strachey paid Macphail £9, the fee for three contributions. See Strachey to Macphail, 20 July (confidential), 20 Jan. 1908, Macphail Papers; Grey to Strachey, 2 Jan. 1908 (private); Strachey to Grey, 15 Jan. 1908, 4 Feb. 1909 (confidential), Strachey Papers, BL; Strachey to Grey, 16 Jan. 1904, 30 May 1906 (private), Grey Papers, UD.

70 Thomas, *The Story of the Spectator, 1828–1928*, 92; also see 87–91; Fulton, "*The Spectator*," 807–8. Strachey attained his most widespread influence in the struggle against Chamberlain's Tariff Reform movement. See Thomas, *The Story of the Spectator, 1828–1928*, 91, 102; interview with W.J. Igoe, 7 July 1971.

71 See Macphail to Grey, 20 Feb. 1909, Grey Papers, UD.

72 Macphail, "The 'American Woman' - I," *Spectator*, 3 Oct. 1908, 497

73 See ibid., Macphail, "The 'American Woman' – II," *Spectator*, 10 Oct. 1908, 537. But see especially the expanded version published in Macphail, *Essays in Fallacy*, 25–8, 30–1. For an attempt at an historical explanation of the flourishing of the type on American soil, based on a physiological analogy, see Macphail, "The 'American Woman' – I," 497.

74 Macphail, "The 'American Woman' – I," 497; also see Macphail, "The 'American Woman' – II," 537.

75 Macphail, "The 'American Woman' – II," 538. The sentence sequence is altered and there are minor changes in content in Macphail, *Essays in Fallacy*, 54. Also see Macphail, "The 'American Woman' – I," 498.

76 Macphail, *Essays in Fallacy*, 39; also see Macphail, "The 'American Woman' – I," 497–8.

77 Substantial portions of "The Whole Duty of the Canadian Man," including much of the citation on pp. 97–8, above, were integrated into "The 'American Woman'" verbatim. Macphail also published parts of "The 'American Woman'" in an Ottawa ladies' magazine centred on Government House; see Macphail, "The Authority of the Woman," *May Court Club Magazine* 1 (Oct. 1908): 14–18.

78 *Spectator*, 3 Oct. 1908, 498

79 *Spectator*, 10 Oct. 1908, 539

80 Strachey to Macphail, 27 Nov. 1908 (confidential), Macphail Papers. Also see Strachey to Macphail, 20 July 1908 (confidential), Macphail Papers. For the letters published by Strachey, see *Spectator*, 10–31 Oct. 1908, 539, 584–5, 626–7, 671.

81 Macphail to Strachey, n.d. [Oct. or Nov. 1908] (draft letter), Macphail Papers. Also see Frank B. Tracy to Macphail, 19, 30 Oct. 1908, Macphail Papers; Kipling to Macphail, 20-30 Nov. 1908, Kipling-Macphail

volume, Macphail Papers. Tracy was editor of the prestigious *Boston Evening Transcript*.

82 Strachey to Grey, 4 Feb. 1909 (confidential), Strachey Papers, BL. For a similar criticism of Macphail's *Essays in Puritanism*, see review in Boston *Christian Register*, 18 May 1905, Macphail Papers. Also see the speech by E.B. Greenshields in proposing a toast to the health of Macphail at the University Club, Montreal, 10 March 1909, 13–15; Strachey to William Osler, 1 Dec. 1909, Macphail Papers.

83 See Grey to Strachey, 17 Feb. 1909, Strachey Papers, BL; Macphail to Grey, 20 Feb. 1909, Grey Papers, UD. A typed, undated copy of the relevant sections of Strachey's 4 Feb. 1909 letter to Grey, with no provenance indicated, survives in the Macphail Papers.

84 R. Tait McKenzie to Macphail, 5 Oct. 1908, Macphail Papers. McKenzie had contributed to the second issue of Macphail's quarterly: "The University and Physical Efficiency," *University Magazine* 6 (April 1907): 168–78. Also see the speech by Greenshields in proposing a toast to the health of Macphail at the University Club, Montreal, 10 March 1909, 14, Macphail Papers; Macphail to Grey, 20 Feb. 1909, Grey Papers, UD.

85 See Strachey to Macphail, 21 Jan. 1909 (confidential), Macphail Papers. On at least one occasion Strachey used his good offices with other British editors on Macphail's behalf, but apparently to no avail; see Strachey to Macphail, 27 Nov. 1908 (confidential), Macphail Papers.

86 Macphail, *Essays in Politics*, 159–60. On the question of when a tariff becomes protective, see 149–50. The article "Protection and Politics" appeared in the April 1908 number of the *University Magazine*, 7: 529-45.

87 See Macphail, *Essays in Politics*, 141–7; also see 132–3.

88 Ibid., 155

89 Ibid., 134; also see 153, 137–8.

90 Ibid., 155; also see 150, 152–3.

91 Ibid., 158–9

92 Ibid., 156, 158.

93 See p. 78, above.

94 Macphail, *Essays in Politics*, 177, 179. Also see 167 ff.

95 Ibid., 179; also see 177–83. Borden had suggested that Laurier use the preference to extract concessions from the British.

96 Macphail, *Essays in Politics*, 181; also see 180.

97 Ibid., 182

98 Ibid., 190–1. For Macphail's comments on the illiberalism of the Liberals, see 179, 183–4, 189–90. His analysis of the Conservative role in the 1905 crisis caused some heated public discussion among Conservative supporters; see press cuttings from Montreal *Gazette*, 1, 2, 4, 5 Jan. 1909, letters from "Conservative" and "Old Conservative," Macphail Papers. For an interpretation disputing Macphail's emphasis on Conservative shortcomings and

instead attributing the result to the strength of the Liberal position, see
press cutting from Charlottetown *Guardian*, 22 Dec. 1908, Macphail Papers.

99   Macphail, *Essays in Politics*, 192

100 Macphail, "How Canada Looks at American Tariff-Making," *American
     Review of Reviews* 39 (Jan. 1909): 85; also see 86–7.

101 Strachey to Macphail, 21 Jan. 1909 (confidential), Macphail Papers. Also see
     Macphail to Strachey 6 Jan. 1909 (draft letter), Macphail Papers.

102 Macphail, "A Canadian View of Reciprocity and Imperialism," *Spectator*,
     6 March 1909, 372; also see 373. This "Letter" incorporated sections of the
     American Review of Reviews article.

103 Strachey to Grey, 4 March 1909 (confidential), Strachey Papers, BL. Grey
     sent the letter on to Macphail; see Grey to Macphail, 16 March 1909,
     Macphail Papers. Also see Strachey to Macphail, 24 Feb. 1909 (confiden-
     tial); Macphail to Strachey, 10 March 1909, Macphail Papers.

104 Macphail, "A Canadian View of Reciprocity and Imperialism," *Spectator*, 6
     March 1909, 372

105 Macphail, *Essays in Politics*, 114; also see 90–5, 100.

106 Ibid., 114

107 Ibid., 101; also see 116.

108 Ibid., 114–15

109 Ibid., 103–11.

110 Ibid., 118

111 Ibid., 108–9, 93, 113. He did concede that an autonomous Canada would
     not have to face a racial issue comparable to that of the United States: "We
     have not impending over us the fearful Nemesis of the negro" (106).

112 Macphail, *Essays in Politics*, 117. The Montreal *Gazette* approvingly repub-
     lished much of the article under the heading "A Contrast and a Warning";
     see press cutting dated 15 Feb. 1909, Macphail Papers.

113 Strachey to Grey, 4 March 1909 (confidential), Strachey Papers, BL. Also see
     Grey to Strachey, 17 Feb. 1909, Strachey Papers, BL; Amery to Macphail, 2
     March 1909, Macphail Papers; Kipling to Macphail, 20–30 Nov. 1908, 13–28
     Dec. 1908, Kipling–Macphail volume, Macphail Papers; Kipling had been
     shown an advance copy.

114 Strachey to Macphail, 24 Feb. 1909 (confidential), Macphail Papers.

115 Peterson to Macphail, 6 Nov. 1908, Peterson Letterbooks, vol. 12, 664, MUA

116 Macphail, *Essays in Politics*, 195. The essay, which was chapter 9 in the
     book, incorporated sections of "The Whole Duty of the Canadian Man,"
     "How Canada Looks at American Tariff-Making," and "A Canadian View
     of Reciprocity and Imperialism." Macphail had at one point considered
     using the title of the new essay for that of the book; he may have taken the
     expression from a letter written by Kipling, in which the latter urged him
     to tell Viscount Milner, then on a visit to Canada, "about the *psychology* of
     Canada – the growing mental pains and confusions of a new country etc.
     etc." [original emphasis]. See Macphail to Strachey, 6 Jan. 1909 (draft letter),

Macphail Papers; Kipling to Macphail, 26 Sept. 1908, Kipling-Macphail volume, Macphail Papers. The nine reprinted papers in *Essays in Politics* appeared in the following order: "The Patience of England," "Loyalty – To What," "The Dominion and the Spirit," "What Can Canada Do," "New Lamps for Old," "A Patent Anomaly," "Protection and Politics," "Why the Conservatives Failed," and "British Diplomacy and Canada."

117   Macphail, *Essays in Politics*, 202. Also see 196–200.

118   Ibid., 203–8

119   Ibid., 224–5; also see 214. In private, Macphail had made his views known at least to Grey some time before this. See Macphail to Grey, 31 Oct. 1908, Grey Papers, LAC; Grey to Macphail, 2 Nov. 1908 (private and confidential), Macphail Papers; Grey to Strachey, 17 Feb. 1909, Strachey Papers, BL. For a dismissive response to Macphail's point of view, see Sir Richard J. Cartwright to Grey, 4 Nov. 1908 (private), Grey Papers, LAC.

120   Macphail, *Essays in Politics*, 226

121   See ibid., 235.

122   Ibid., 223; also see Macphail to Strachey, 10 March 1909, Macphail Papers.

123   Macphail, *Essays in Politics*, 213; also see 214–15.

124   Ibid., 240; also see 217-18, 243.

125   Ibid., 239; also see 209–10.

126   Ibid., 239

127   Ibid., 244; also see 239–40, 243.

128   Bertrand Russell, preface to Horowitz, ed., *Containment and Revolution*, 5. Also see Macphail to Mavor, 6 Nov. 1908, Mavor Papers (in private possession); Amery to Macphail, 2 March 1909; review in London *Morning Post*, 26 Aug. 1909, by "E.B.O.," Macphail Papers.

129   *Review of Historical Publications Relating to Canada*, 14 (1910): 1

130   Ibid., 4

131   Ibid., 2

132   Ibid., 3. An Oxford professor of imperial history perceived in the origins of the book a source of strength: "The essays were ... written at different times, and they often repeat the same note, but the effect is the more impressive, the passionate conviction expressed resembling the recurring motive music of a Wagnerian opera." Review in *United Empire*, June 1910, 421, by Hugh E. Egerton, Macphail Papers.

133   *Review of Historical Publications Relating to Canada*, 14 (1910): 4

134   Press cutting from a Charlottetown newspaper, n.d., citing the *Contemporary Review*, August 1909, Macphail Papers; also see review in Toronto *Globe*, 16 Oct. 1909, Macphail Papers.

135   Review in London *Morning Post*, 26 Aug. 1909, by "E.B.O.," Macphail Papers

136   Review in *Baltimore News*, 8 Oct. 1909, Macphail Papers; also see review in *Indianapolis News*, 26 Nov. [?] 1909, Macphail Papers.

137   See Strachey to Macphail, 27 Sept. (confidential), 8 Nov. (confidential) 1909; Athenaeum dinner list for 13 Dec. 1909; Osler to Macphail, 1 Nov.,

6 Dec. 1909; Strachey to Osler, 1 Dec. 1909; Charles L. Graves to Macphail, 11 Dec. 1909, 11 March 1910, Macphail Papers; Kipling to Macphail, 17 July, 2 Dec. 1909, Kipling-Macphail volume, Macphail Papers; press cutting from Charlottetown *Guardian*, n.d. [Dec. 1909], Burland-Macphail Scrapbook, Macphail Papers; *Spectator*, 18 Sept. 1909, 419; Macphail to Laurier, 23 Nov. 1909, Laurier Papers, LAC; Macphail to Strachey, 27 Oct. 1909, Strachey Papers, BL.

138 Kipling to Macphail, 20–30 Nov. 1908, Kipling-Macphail volume, Macphail Papers. Also see *Review of Historical Publications Relating to Canada* 14 (1910): 1.

139 Kipling to Macphail, 17 July 1909, Kipling-Macphail volume, Macphail Papers

140 Review in Toronto *Globe*, 16 Oct. 1909, Macphail Papers

141 Laurier to Macphail, 24 Oct. 1909, Macphail Papers. Also see Macphail to Laurier, 6 Oct. 1909, Laurier Papers, LAC.

142 Thomson to Macphail, 31 Oct. 1909, Macphail Papers. Also see Macphail to Mavor, 20 Nov. 1909, Mavor Papers (in private possession).

143 Review in *United Empire*, June 1910, 421, by Egerton, Macphail Papers. On the requisite qualities for an imperialist, and particularly an imperialist statesman, see Macphail to Strachey, 27 Oct. 1909, Strachey Papers, BL.

CHAPTER SIX

1 Macphail, untitled manuscript on "Best Work and Why," n.d. [1929], Macphail Papers

2 Macphail, *Essays in Fallacy*, vi. This may have been the longer version which John St. Loe Strachey had him cut down for publication in the *Spectator*; see pp. 99–100, above.

3 Macphail, *Essays in Fallacy*, 42. This sentence does not appear in the earlier version.

4 This paper ("The Psychology of the Suffragette") was read to the Empire Club of Canada (Toronto) on 20 Jan. 1910, and is to be found in *Empire Club Speeches*, 102–27. Several minor additions were made, and one paragraph, from *Essays in Fallacy*, 87–8, was deleted. Page references will be to the fuller version. In February he spoke to the University of Toronto faculty members on "The American Woman"; these addresses caused some reverberations in Toronto. See Macphail to Mavor, 2 Jan., 8 Feb. 1910, Mavor Papers, UTRB; Frank Wise to Macphail, 12 April 1910, Macphail Papers.

5 Macphail, "The Psychology of the Suffragette," *Empire Club Speeches ... 1909–1910*, 105

6 See ibid., especially 107, 113–18, 124; Macphail, *Essays in Politics*, 42. For a cataloguing of masculine qualities ("truthfulness, modesty," etc.), see Macphail, "The Psychology of the Suffragette," 117.

7 Macphail, "The Psychology of the Suffragette," 111; also see 113, 117.

8 Ibid., 116

9 See Mavor to "Mesdames" [Grace Ritchie-England and Anna Scrimger Lyman], 28 March 1914, Macphail Papers.

10 Macphail, "On Certain Aspects of Feminism," *University Magazine* 13 (Feb. 1914): 81

11 Ibid., 84

12 Ibid., 85

13 Ibid., 83

14 Ibid., 86; also see 82.

15 Ibid., 87. Also see 86, and, for several additional highly flavoured comments on the crusade against white slavery, see 89–91.

16 Ibid., 90

17 Ritchie-England and Lyman to Editorial Committee of the *University Magazine*, 20 March 1914, Macphail Papers.

18 Mavor to "Mesdames" [Ritchie-England and Lyman], 28 March 1914, Macphail Papers. Also see Mavor to Macphail, 29 March 1914, Macphail Papers.

19 Frost, *McGill 1*, 286. Also see Griffiths, *The Splendid Vision*, 134n74; Gillett, *We Walked Very Warily*, 109; Cleverdon, *The Woman Suffrage Movement in Canada*, 217; Morgan, ed., *The Canadian Men and Women of the Time*, 1898 edn, 313.

20 See Macphail to "Madam" [presumed Ritchie-England or Lyman], 21 March 1914, MacMechan Papers, DUA. Also see Macphail to MacMechan, 24 April 1914, MacMechan Papers, DUA.

21 Macphail, "On Certain Aspects of Feminism," 82

22 Ibid., 82, 86. Also see 80–3, 87.

23 See ibid., 81, 85, 90, 79; Macphail, "The Cost of Living," *University Magazine* 11 (Dec. 1912): 532–3; Macphail, "Bigotry in Parliament," *Saturday Night*, 9 March 1912.

24 Strong-Boag, "Independent Women, Problematic Men: First- and Second-Wave Anti-Feminism in Canada from Goldwin Smith to Betty Steele," *Histoire sociale/Social History* 29 (May 1996): 1–22

25 Ibid., 22

26 Ibid., 3–6, 9–10.

27 Introductory note to Blackburn, "Hearth and Home: A Memoir," accession 4438, PARO. I thank Professor M. Brook Taylor of Mount Saint Vincent University, who drew Roma Stewart Blackburn to my attention.

28 Blackburn, "Hearth and Home: A Memoir," 43

29 See ibid., 40–1.

30 A reading of Bowker, "Truly Useful Men," 190, would suggest, by inference, that Macphail was less progressive in this respect than the three University of Toronto intellectuals he studied - Mavor, George M. Wrong, and even the arch-Victorian Maurice Hutton: "All three men had gifted daughters whom they encouraged in their careers." Yet Sperdakos, *Dora Mavor Moore*,

47–8, 62–3, 67–8, indicates that Mavor would have been much happier if his daughter had not pursued the independent career she chose.

31   Interview with Mrs Dorothy Lindsay, 10 Sept. 1970

32   Ibid., 9 Sept. 1970

33   Sperdakos, *Dora Mavor Moore*, 47; also see 42, 48.

34   Mavor, *My Windows on the Street of the World*, 2: 167

35   See, for example, the column of Sandra Devlin, Charlottetown *Guardian*, 8 March 1997; there is a defence of Macphail in a letter by Jack Pennock, Charlottetown *Guardian*, 14 March 1997. I thank my late mother and Professor Ian W. Brown, formerly of Prince of Wales College, who initially drew this material to my attention, both in letters dated 15 March 1997; and Katherine Dewar, for subsequently providing me with copies of both the Devlin article and the Pennock letter, and the dates of their appearance.

36   Strong-Boag, "Independent Women, Problematic Men," 2; also see 5.

37   See Sonia Leathes, "Votes for Women," *University Magazine* 13 (Feb. 1914): 68–78; and Macphail, "On Certain Aspects of Feminism," *University Magazine* 13 (Feb. 1914): 79–91. Regarding Leathes, see Bacchi, *Liberation Deferred*, 33, 47, 96.

38   Byrne, "*The University Magazine*: An Inclusive 'Conservative' Periodical," 7. She also refers to a "powerful" pro-suffrage article by McGill administrator Walter Vaughan, which appeared while Macphail was overseas (8). Walton was a strong supporter of female suffrage, and even served as a vice-president of the Montreal Suffrage Association, organized by Ritchie-England in 1913; see Cleverdon, *The Woman Suffrage Movement in Canada*, 222.

39   See Frost, *McGill* 2, 176; Scriver, "Slowly the Doors Opened," 135.

40   Byrne, "*The University Magazine*: An Inclusive 'Conservative' Periodical," 9

41   Ibid., 10

42   Frances Fenwick Williams to Macphail, 6 Sept. 1911, Macphail Papers. She had published "George Eliot's Women," in *University Magazine* 6 (Dec. 1907): 483–94, and her name was given there as Frances de Wolfe Fenwick.

43   I am grateful to Dr Robert Fraser of the *Dictionary of Canadian Biography* for making this connection for me.

44   Williams, *A Soul on Fire*, 50 [original emphasis]

45   Ibid., 130

46   Ibid., 60–1

47   The heroine, or at least the central figure, in Williams, *A Soul on Fire*, is Theodora Carne, the descendant of a witch from the period of Richard Coeur de Lion, and she has inherited some of the characteristics and powers: animals fear her, she faints at the sound of the name of God, people who cross her come to harm, and so forth; on 250 she confesses to practising witchcraft (in contemporary Montreal).

48   See Strong-Boag, "Independent Women, Problematic Men," 6–8.

49   Bottomore, *Social Criticism in North America*, 58

50 This 86-page paper includes also, in full, three shorter pieces published elsewhere in early 1910: "Oxford and Working-Class Education," *University Magazine* 9 (Feb. 1910): 36–50; "An Obverse View of Education," *University Magazine* 9 (April 1910): 192–204; and "Hints of the Progress of Knowledge: An Imperial View of Education," Montreal *World Wide*, 26 March 1910, 268–70. In *Essays in Fallacy* these occupy, respectively, 122–9, 131–47, 150–2; 164–88; 104–5, 107–11, 116–21, 131–2, 152. Except for passages unique to one of the shorter pieces, all page references will be to *Essays in Fallacy*. Over a considerable period, Macphail had been circulating for comment earlier versions of these manuscripts, particularly "Oxford and Working-Class Education." See "W.V." to Macphail, 28 Feb. 1909; Macphail to Strachey, 10 March 1909; Strachey to Macphail, 30 March 1909 (confidential), Macphail Papers.

51 Press cutting from a Charlottetown newspaper, 28 May 1896, Lindsay-Macphail Scrapbooks 1, Macphail Papers

52 Macphail, *Essays in Politics*, 44

53 Macphail, "The Psychology of the Suffragette," 126

54 Macphail, *Essays in Fallacy*, 103

55 Ibid., 105

56 Macphail, "The Education of the People," *Saturday Night*, 21 Aug. 1911

57 See Macphail, *Essays in Fallacy*, 104, 119–20.

58 Ibid., 108

59 Ibid., 108

60 Ibid., 109

61 Ibid., 109–10

62 Ibid., 110

63 See ibid., 109–16.

64 Ibid., 124. The reference was to Stephen Leacock's article, "Literature and Education in America," *University Magazine* 8 (Feb. 1909): 3–17, especially 3. For Macphail's assessment of American medical education in particular, see his article, "The Poor Boy," *Saturday Night*, 21 May 1910.

65 Macphail, *Essays in Fallacy*, 121; see also 120.

66 Ibid., 122; also see Macphail to Strachey, 27 Oct. 1909, Strachey Papers, BL.

67 Macphail, *Essays in Fallacy*, 150

68 See Williams, *Culture and Society*, 317–18, which is particularly illuminating in discussing the social implications of the "ladder" view of education. Also see Macphail, *Essays in Fallacy*, 138, 167–8.

69 Lower, *Canadians in the Making*, 340.

70 See Macphail, *Essays in Fallacy*, 118.

71 Ibid., 116

72 Ibid., 168

73 Ibid., 155. Also see 153–6, 158, 168–9; Macphail, "The Poor Boy," *Saturday Night*, 21 May 1910; Macphail, "The Education of the People," *Saturday Night*, 12 Aug. 1911.

74 Macphail, "The Nine Prophets," *University Magazine* 8 (Oct. 1909): 404.
Also see 403, 405; Macphail, *Essays in Fallacy*, 131, 155–7, 181. The comment
about military drill should not be taken as evidence that Macphail was
a militarist; his emphasis was clearly on the instrumental rather than
intrinsic value of military training. Indeed, in the same essay, he condemned Germany's "system of rigid militarism" (172).

75 Macphail, *Essays in Fallacy*, 174

76 Ibid., 180; also see 163, 176, 131–2, 182.

77 Ibid., 183; also see 180.

78 Ibid., 174

79 Ibid., 174–5. Also see 177–9, 181; Macphail, "The Education of the People"

80 Macphail, *Essays in Fallacy*, 128–9; also see 151, where Macphail paraphrased Matthew Arnold.

81 Macphail, *Essays in Fallacy*, 130

82 Macphail, "Hints of the Progress of Knowledge: An Imperial View of
Education," Montreal *World Wide*, 26 March 1910, 270. Also see Macphail,
"The Poor Boy," *Saturday Night*, 21 May 1910; Macphail, *Essays in Fallacy*,
129–31, 147–9.

83 Macphail, *Essays in Fallacy*, 133; also see 125, 139–42.

84 Ibid., 134

85 Macphail to Strachey, 10 March 1909, Macphail Papers. Strachey, who
with his brother was involved in the movement to bring workers to the
university, disagreed; see Strachey to Macphail, 30 March 1909 (confidential), Macphail Papers.

86 See Macphail, *Essays in Fallacy*, 125, 133–46, 150. McGill's first professor
of education, a former participant in the movement for working-
class education, took a very different view; see J.A. Dale, "Oxford and
Working-Class Education," *University Magazine* 9 (Oct. 1910): 359–76.
The article was not a direct reply to Macphail's essay in the February
number.

87 Macphail, *Essays in Fallacy*, 185; also see 146.

88 Ibid., 187–8. Also see 145; Macphail, "The Education of the People,"
Saturday Night, 12 Aug. 1911.

89 Macphail, *Essays in Fallacy*, 158–9; also see 187–8.

90 See Macphail, "Jonathan Edwards," in Macphail, *Essays in Puritanism*, 3,
12, 16; "The 'American Woman,'" in Macphail, *Essays in Fallacy*, 45–6; "John
Knox in the Church of England," *University Magazine* 6 (Feb. 1907): 18;
"The Dominion and the Spirit," in Macphail, *Essays in Politics*, 49.

91 This essay had originated in an address of the same title ("The Fallacy
in Theology") delivered to an "Inter-denominational Conference of
Ministers" in Montreal on 30 Oct. 1907; see press cutting from Montreal
Gazette, 31 Oct. 1907, Macphail Papers. As published in the book, it
included most of Macphail, "The New Theology," *University Magazine* 9
(Dec. 1910), 683–97.

92 Macphail, *Essays in Fallacy*, 195; also see 220.

93 See Macphail, *Essays in Fallacy*, 195–6; Macphail, "Church and Politics," *Saturday Night*, 4 June 1910.

94 Macphail, *Essays in Fallacy*, 225

95 Ibid., 218; also see 220.

96 Ibid., 225–7, 218–21.

97 Ibid., 310; also see 247–54, 265–79, 288–91, 256, 228–31, 244, 307–9.

98 Ibid., 320

99 Ibid., 321, 325–6; also see 324, 329.

100 Ibid., 326

101 Ibid., 330. Also see 321, 331–8, 341; Macphail, "The New Theology," *University Magazine* 9 (Dec. 1910): 683, 691–2; Macphail to MacMechan, 12 July 1910, MacMechan Papers, DUA.

102 Macphail, *Essays in Fallacy*, 354; also see 353.

103 Ibid., 355

104 Ibid., 333

105 Ibid., 354–5. Also see Macphail, "Unto the Church," *University Magazine* 12 (April 1913): 354–61, 363–4; Macphail, "The Conservative," *University Magazine* 18 (Dec. 1919): 432–3; Macphail, "Conservative – Liberal – Socialist," *University of Toronto Quarterly* 3 (April 1934): 270. In another essay published in 1910, Macphail denounced both Roman Catholic and Protestant clergy for meddling in politics, but his remarks were primarily aimed at the Lord's Day Alliance and attempts to have certain recreations made illegal; see "Church and Politics," *Saturday Night*, 4 June 1910.

106 Macphail, "The New Theology," *University Magazine* 9 (Dec. 1910): 697

107 Macphail, "Unto the Church," *University Magazine* 12 (April 1913): 360; also see 364.

108 Ibid., 354; also see Macphail, "Church and Politics."

109 Macphail, "Unto the Church," 355

110 Ibid., 356

111 Ibid., 359; also see 357.

112 Ibid., 359

113 See Copp, *The Anatomy of Poverty*, 43, 140; and Bradbury, *Working Families*, 99, 116.

114 Macphail, "Conversion," *Proceedings of the American Medico-Psychological Association*, 68th Annual Meeting (1912), 243

115 Macphail, "Unto the Church," 362; also see 363.

116 Ibid., 361–3. In an earlier essay, he had commented that while Protestants had historically defended freedom of thought, "the Catholic Church had always been the champion of freedom of conduct." (Macphail, "Church and Politics," *Saturday Night*, 4 June 1910) Also see Macphail, "Bigotry in Parliament," *Saturday Night*, 9 March 1912, for his praise of the Roman Catholic Church as the bulwark of marriage as a Canadian institution.

117 Review in *New York Times*, 13 Aug. 1910, by H.W. Boynton, Macphail Papers. Also see review in Toronto *Globe*, 13 Aug. 1910; Robert Barr to Macphail, 1 July 1910, Macphail Papers.

118   Review in Milwaukee *Living Church*, 5 Nov. 1910, by "H.O." (sequence altered), Macphail Papers. Also see reviews in *Englishwoman*, Aug. 1910, and *Englishwoman's Review*, 15 July 1910, by "M.A.B.," Macphail Papers.

119   Kipling to Macphail, 9 Oct. 1909, Kipling-Macphail volume, Macphail Papers. Also see Kipling to Macphail, 25 June 1910, Kipling-Macphail volume, Macphail Papers; reviews in *Church Times*, 24 June 1910; Toronto *Globe*, 13 Aug. 1910; *Manchester Guardian*, 27 Sept. 1910; San Francisco *Chronicle*, 3 July 1910, Macphail Papers.

120   Review in New York *Nation*, 1 Sept. 1910, Macphail Papers

121   Review in *Manchester Guardian*, 27 Sept. 1910, Macphail Papers

122   See reviews in *Hartford Courant*, 20 July 1910; *Cleveland Plain Dealer*, Sept. 1910, Macphail Papers; review in *Saturday Night*, 27 Aug. 1910, by Tom Folio.

123   The *New York Sun* of 28 Aug. 1910 published what was ostensibly a seven-column review of *Essays in Fallacy*, but in fact it was a lengthy paraphrased summary of the book's major points; see Macphail Papers.

124   Press cutting from *Montreal Herald*, 8 June 1910, Macphail Papers. Also see press release from the Royal Society of Canada, 10 May 1910; Duncan Campbell Scott to Macphail, n.d. [*ca.* 10 May 1910]; Stacey, "From Meighen to King: The Reversal of Canadian External Policies 1921–1923," 233. Macphail appears to have been called upon rather frequently by the press to give public statements on recently departed notables; see, for example, his comments on Leo Tolstoy and Edward VII in press cutting from *Montreal Herald*, 21 Nov. 1910; press cutting of unknown origin, n.d. [1910], Macphail Papers.

125   Press cutting of unmarked provenance [*Saturday Night*], n.d. [midsummer 1910], Macphail Papers. Also see press cuttings from Charlottetown *Guardian*, 18 June 1910; Toronto *World*, 13 June 1910; *Saint John Evening Times*, 5 July 1910, Macphail Papers; reviews of *Essays in Fallacy* appearing in Toronto *Globe*, 13 Aug. 1910, and *Canadian Magazine*, n.d. [35 (Oct. 1910): 572], Macphail Papers. Finally, review of Macphail, *Essays in Fallacy*, in *Saturday Night*, 27 Aug. 1910, by Tom Folio (not included in Macphail Papers).

126   Press cutting of unknown origin [*The Century?*], n.d. [1910], Macphail Papers

CHAPTER SEVEN

1   Archibald Maclise, "The American Newspaper," *University Magazine* 6 (Oct. 1907): 309

2   See ibid., 310–12; Stephen Leacock, "The Psychology of American Humour," *University Magazine* 6 (Feb. 1907): 57–8, 75; Leacock, "Literature and Education in America," *University Magazine* 8 (Feb. 1909): 3–17, especially 7–9, 16. In the latter essay, Leacock began by explicitly including Canada in "America."

3 Macphail, "Canadian Writers and American Politics," *University Magazine* 9 (Feb. 1910): 3; also see 13. This was the first occasion on which Macphail signed an article in the *University Magazine* "The Editor" rather than with his own name. He did this only in cases where he was contributing twice to the same number. He would sign one article "Andrew Macphail" and the other "The Editor," placing the latter at the first of the number. The one exception to this rule occurred in Oct. 1914, when the piece signed "The Editor" appeared in the second place within the issue, behind a poem by Mary Linda Bradley, "The Women of France" (on the theme of the women of France bringing in the harvest in the absence of their menfolk at war). The use of this title appears to have been a matter of convenience rather than an attempt to imply in certain instances that his words were meant to be more authoritative or consensual than usual. Hence, in reference to articles signed by Macphail as "Editor" I shall simply identify the author in the notes as "Macphail." He also delivered an address to "the Brockville Club" on the theme of this article; the applause was "loud and long." See press cutting of unknown origin, n.d. [1910?], Macphail Papers.

4 Macphail, "Canadian Writers and American Politics," 3, 5

5 Ibid., 6–7; also see 5.

6 Macphail to MacMechan, 14 Feb. 1910, MacMechan Papers, DUA

7 Macphail, "Canadian Writers and American Politics," 6; also see 7–10.

8 Ibid., 11. It may be noted that Macphail's use of the term "race" was often confusing, for in this article, on 11-12, it is unclear whether the "race" in question includes or excludes people of Celtic origin whose mother tongue was English – like himself. The most accurate thing that can probably be said about his usage of the word is that it was imprecise, for on p. 10 he lumps Celts in with "the Orientals, the Slavs, [and] the Latins," but on pp. 12–13 it is clear from the context that he, a person of Celtic origin, identifies with those of English origin.

9 Macphail, *Essays in Politics*, 119. Also see Macphail, "Canadian Writers and American Politics," 26–7.

10 Macphail, "Canadian Writers and American Politics," 16. Also see 14–15, 17; Macphail, *Essays in Politics*, 119.

11 Macphail, "Canadian Writers and American Politics," 12–13

12 Ibid., 17. Despite his reservations about certain types of immigrants, Macphail remained of the opinion that Canada should welcome the English poor and should not require immigrants to have $25 in their possession at the time of landing; see Macphail, "The Manufacturers of Opinion," *Saturday Night*, 9 July 1910.

13 Macphail, "Canadian Writers and American Politics," 3

14 Ibid., 3, 4, 7, 17

15 Kipling to Macphail, 23 Feb. 1910, Kipling-Macphail volume, Macphail Papers

16 Press cutting from *Boston Herald*, 10 Feb. 1910, Macphail Papers

17   Dickinson to Macphail, 13 May 1909, Macphail Papers. Also see Peterson to Dickinson, 19 April 1909, Peterson Letterbooks, vol. 13, 135, MUA; Macphail, "As Others See Us," *University Magazine* 9 (April 1910): 174–5. For Dickinson's account of part of the evening they spent together, see his *Appearances*, 205-7, 210.

18   See Dickinson to Macphail, 1 Dec. 1909, 24 Jan. 1910, Macphail Papers.

19   The material had first appeared in the *English Review*, Nov. 1909 – Jan. 1910, and later in the *Cambridge Review*. It was also to be incorporated in Dickinson's book, *Appearances: Being Notes of Travel*.

20   Cited in Macphail, "As Others See Us," *University Magazine* 9 (April 1910): 167–8; also see 165–6, 173.

21   Ibid., 169; also see 168, 172.

22   Ibid., 174; also see 173.

23   Ibid., 175. Dickinson's prospective fellow commissioner, Kipling, declared his assessment of America to be "horribly true" (Kipling to Macphail, 5 April 1910, Kipling-Macphail volume, Macphail Papers). American response to Dickinson's observations was negative; see Dickinson to Macphail, 24 Jan. 1910, Macphail Papers.

24   Macphail to MacMechan, 14 Feb. 1910, MacMechan Papers, DUA. See "A Canadian" [James White], "The Long Sault Dam," *University Magazine* 9(April 1910): 255–64, especially 255; Arthur V. White, "The Exportation of Electricity," *University Magazine* 9 (Oct. 1910): 460–7. Macphail did express his views on the Long Sault proposal, in "The Past Session," *Saturday Night*, 14 May 1910, and "Shall We Develop or Shall We Exploit?" *Saturday Night*, 11 June 1910.

25   *Canadian Century*, 3 Sept. 1910, 11; also see Macphail to Laurier, 22 March 1910, Laurier Papers, LAC.

26   F.P. Walton, "Divorce in Canada and the United States: A Contrast," *University Magazine* 9 (Dec. 1910): 580; also see 579, 581, 584-6. Macphail cited this statistic in "Bigotry in Parliament," *Saturday Night*, 9 March 1912.

27   See Walton, "Divorce in Canada and the United States," 583, 586–7, 591–6.

28   Macphail, "Certain Varieties of the Apples of Sodom," *University Magazine* 10 (Feb. 1911): 42. Also see press cutting from *Montreal Star*, 6 Jan. 1911; press cutting from Montreal *Gazette*, 20 Oct. 1910; press cutting from *Vancouver World*, 28 Oct. 1910, Macphail Papers. The last two press cuttings concerned an address Macphail delivered on 19 Oct. 1910 to the Nomads' Club of Montreal, on the theme of America as a continent of nomads.

29   Macphail, "Certain Varieties of the Apples of Sodom," 37

30   Ibid., 44.

31   Macphail to Grey, 15 April 1911, Grey Papers, UD [original emphasis]. Also see Grey to Macphail, 30 March 1911, Macphail Papers; Berger, *The Sense of Power*, 162–3.

32   Macphail, "The Psychology of the Suffragette," *Empire Club Speeches ... 1909–1910*, 112

33 Macphail to Grey, 15 April 1911, Grey Papers, UD. Also see Grey to Macphail, 30 March 1911, Macphail Papers; Berger, *The Sense of Power*, 162–3.

34 Macphail, "Certain Varieties of the Apples of Sodom," 42; also see 31, 37–40. For Macphail's ambivalence about democracy, see Macphail, "Government by Party," *Canadian Century*, 15 Oct. 1910; Macphail, "Government by Commission," Charlottetown *Guardian*, 18 Feb. 1911.

35 Macphail, "Certain Varieties of the Apples of Sodom," 41

36 Articulated by Sir Thomas Gresham, a Tudor-era London merchant, it was given the name Gresham's Law in 1857 by the Scottish economist H.D. Macleod, who believed that it had originated with him. See "Sir Thomas Gresham" and "Gresham's Law," in *Encyclopedia Britannica* (1959), 10: 878 and 878–9; and "Henry Dunning Macleod," *Encyclopedia Britannica*, 14: 594. Macleod stated it in more extended form as follows: "The worst form of currency in circulation regulates the value of the whole currency and drives all other forms of currency out of circulation." (10: 878)

37 Macphail, "Certain Varieties of the Apples of Sodom," 46. Also see 38–9; Macphail, "Canadian Writers and American Politics," 6.

38 Macphail to Grey, 8 Jan. 1911, Grey Papers, UD. Also see Macphail, "Certain Varieties of the Apples of Sodom," 45–6.

39 Macphail, "The Past Session," *Saturday Night*, 14 May 1910; also see Macphail's comments on the late Edward VII, in press cutting of unknown origin, n.d. [1910], Macphail Papers. Grey shared Macphail's disgust with the incident and had suggested that he "give the offenders a good lusty crack from your most efficient whip" (Grey to Macphail, 26 April 1910 [private and confidential], Macphail Papers). Macphail returned to the topic during the session of 1910–11; see "The Degradation of Parliaments," *Halifax Chronicle*, 2 Jan. 1911.

40 Macphail, "Confiscatory Legislation," *University Magazine* 10 (April 1911): 206. Also see 195–202 in particular; Macphail, "The Whole Duty of the Canadian Man," 10–11, Macphail Papers; Macphail, "The Peril to Democracy," *Saturday Night*, 5 Aug. 1911; Arthur Levinson, "Ontario's Constitutional Ordeal," *University Magazine* 9 (April 1910): 266–75. The last-cited article complemented Macphail's writings on the Ontario legislation in question.

41 The *Canadian Century* was established in 1910 by Max Aitken, who as Lord Beaverbrook became one of Macphail's closest overseas friends in later years. According to Aitken's biographer, the paper was "a rather ineffective intellectual weekly" (Taylor, *Beaverbrook*, 35).

42 Macphail's articles on the trade question in the *American Review of Reviews* and the *Spectator* had been reprinted, in one case fully, in the other partially, by the Montreal *Gazette*, but this does not appear to have been a frequent occurrence.

43 Macphail, "Shall We Develop or Shall We Exploit?" *Saturday Night*, 11 June 1910. Also see Macphail, "The Poisoning of the People," *Saturday Night*, 29

July 1911; Macphail, "The Manufacture of Opinion," *Saturday Night*, 9 July 1910; Macphail, "Anglo-American Arbitration," Brooklyn *Eagle*, 10 April 1911.

44 Macphail, "Canada's Loyalty," *Saturday Night*, 6 Aug. 1910

45 See Macphail, "British Diplomacy and Canada," *Saturday Night*, 17 Sept. 1910; Macphail, "The Manufacture of Opinion," *Saturday Night*, 9 July 1910; Macphail, "Nation or Empire," *Saturday Night*, 20 Aug. 1910; Macphail, "What Canada Owes to England," *Saturday Night*, 1 Oct. 1910; Macphail, "Lord Grey in Canada," *Canadian Century*, 2 July 1910. The last piece was published before it was known that Grey was to receive a second extension of his term as governor general; for a second assessment by Macphail, see "The Going of the Greys," *Saturday Night*, 30 Sept. 1911.

46 Macphail, "Imperialism: The Problem," *Saturday Night*, 15 July 1911. Also see Macphail, "A Voice from the East," *University Magazine* 9 (Dec. 1910): 522.

47 Macphail, "Imperialism: The Solution," *Saturday Night*, 22 July 1911. Also see Macphail, "Canadian Citizenship," *Saturday Night*, 8 July 1911.

48 For an example of Macphail's continuing assault on protection in these years, see press cutting from Montreal *Standard*, 5 Nov. 1910, Macphail to Editor, n.d., Macphail Papers. Also see MacMechan to Macphail, 15 Nov. 1910, Macphail Papers; Macphail to MacMechan, 17 Nov. 1910, MacMechan Papers, DUA.

49 Cited in Macphail, "Canada and the United States - The Real Danger," *Spectator*, 18 Feb. 1911, 243. Also see 244; Macphail, "Fielding-Taft Reciprocity Agreement," *Montreal Witness*, 21 Feb. 1911; Macphail, "Protection and the Empire," galley proofs of unknown origin, n.d. [1911]; Thomson to W.S. Fielding, 28 March 1911 (private), Macphail Papers; Macphail to Laurier, 27 Jan., 20 July 1911, Laurier Papers, LAC. For reasons that need not concern us, Macphail preferred to avoid using the word "reciprocity" in reference to the Fielding-Taft agreement.

50 Macphail, "Fielding-Taft Reciprocity Agreement," *Montreal Witness*, 21 Feb. 1911. Also see press cutting from Montreal *Standard*, 5 Nov. 1910, Macphail to Editor, n.d.; press cutting from Charlottetown *Guardian*, 22 Nov. 1910, Macphail Papers.

51 See Macphail, "The Cleaning of the Slate," *University Magazine* 10 (April 1911): 187–91. The title had been suggested by Grey, who considered the article "very useful & opportune" (Macphail to Grey, 15 April 1911, Grey Papers, UD; Grey to Macphail, 17 April 1911, Macphail Papers). Also see Macphail, "Anglo-American Arbitration," *Brooklyn Eagle*, 10 April 1911; Macphail, "International Amity," *Saturday Night*, 1 July 1911; Macphail, "Imperialism: The Solution," *Saturday Night*, 22 July 1911; Macphail, "Canada and the United States - The Real Danger," *Spectator*, 18 Feb. 1911, 244; Neary, "Grey, Bryce, and the Settlement of Canadian-American Differences, 1905-1911," *Canadian Historical Review* 49 (Dec. 1968): 357–80.

52 See Macphail, "The Cleaning of the Slate," *University Magazine* 10 (April 1911): 183–4; Macphail, "International Amity," *Saturday Night*, 1 July 1911.

53 Macphail, "Why the Liberals Failed," *University Magazine* 10 (Dec. 1911): 570;

also see 566–9. Grey, for one, was very surprised by the result of the election; see Grey to the Duke of Connaught, 23 Sept. 1911, Grey Papers, LAC.

54   Macphail, "Why the Liberals Failed," 571

55   Ibid., 571–3. The matter of Canadian citizenship had been troubling Macphail prior to the election; see Macphail, "Canadian Citizenship," *Saturday Night*, 8 July 1911.

56   Macphail, "Why the Liberals Failed," 580. Also see Macphail to Grey, 9 Dec. 1911, Grey Papers, UD.

57   Macphail to Grey, 8 Jan. 1911, Grey Papers, UD; also see Grey to Macphail, 17 Dec. 1910 (confidential), Macphail Papers.

58   See Morang to Macphail, 17, 20 Feb. 1911; Macphail to Grey, 8 Jan., 21 Feb. 1911, Grey Papers, UD.

59   See Lawrence J. Burpee, "A Plea for a National Library," *University Magazine* 10 (Feb. 1911): 152–63; John Edward Hoare, "A Plea for a Canadian Theatre," *University Magazine* 10 (April 1911), 239–53; Burpee, "Co-operation in Historical Research," *University Magazine* 7 (Oct. 1908): 360–70.

60   Macphail, "The Going of the Greys," *Saturday Night*, 30 Sept. 1911. Also see Miller, "Albert Henry George Grey, 4th Earl Grey," DCB 14: 441; Macphail to Grey, 18 Aug. 1911, Grey Papers, UD. In the letter, Macphail also noted the beginning of a Canadian opera in Grey's years as governor general.

61   Thomson to Laurier, 11 Nov. 1907 (private), 7 Aug. 1908 (private), Laurier Papers, LAC; Alexander Martin to Macphail, 13 March 1910 (private); press cutting from Charlottetown *Guardian*, 18 June 1910, Macphail Papers.

62   Macphail, untitled address to the University Club, Montreal, n.d. [after 1908], 1st, 2nd, 5th pages, Macphail Papers. Also Macphail, "The Whole Duty of the Canadian Man," 9–10, 15–16, Macphail Papers; Macphail, "Canadian Writers and American Politics," *University Magazine* 9 (Feb. 1910): 7, 14, 17. On the special qualifications of the professor for the role of critic, see Macphail, *Essays in Politics*, 166; also see Macphail, *Essays in Fallacy*, 198. Macphail was contemptuous of the cloistered scholar; see "The Psychology of the Suffragette," *Empire Club Speeches ... 1909–1910*, 115.

63   Macphail, "Why the Liberals Failed," 578

64   Annotation by Macphail, n.d. [mid-1920s?], on Kipling to Macphail, 6 July 1911, Kipling-Macphail volume, Macphail Papers

65   Interview with Mrs Dorothy Lindsay, 30 May 1968. Also see Peterson to Macphail, 7 July 1911, Peterson Letterbooks, vol. 17, 176, MUA; Macphail to Laurier, 20 July 1911, Laurier Papers, LAC.

66   Interviews with Mrs. Dorothy Lindsay, 30 May 1968, 29 Aug., 9 Sept. 1970; letter from Mrs. Dorothy Lindsay to author, dated 14 Aug. [1973]. See Macphail to Mavor, 15 July 1911, 10 Feb. 1914, Mavor Papers, UTRB; Macphail to Grey, 18 Aug. 1911, Grey Papers, UD; Edgar, "Sir Andrew Macphail," *Queen's Quarterly* 54 (Spring 1947): 10; Macphail to MacMechan, 8 Jan. 1921, MacMechan Papers, DUA; MacDermot, "Sir Andrew Macphail," *McGill News* 20 (Winter 1938): 58; Macphail to Thomson, 27 Oct. 1911, Macphail Papers.

CHAPTER EIGHT

1   Thomson to Macphail, 17 Oct. 1911, Macphail Papers. Also see John
    Redpath Dougall to Macphail, 16 Oct. 1911; Thomson to Macphail, 12 Oct.
    1914, 17 Aug. 1915, 12 Feb. 1918, Macphail Papers; Macphail, "The Montreal
    'Witness,'" *Spectator*, 16 Nov. 1912, 808; Macphail, "Personal Tribute" [to John
    Redpath Dougall], *Montreal Witness*, [18 Sept.] 1935; Macphail to Laurier,
    14 Nov. 1907, Laurier Papers, LAC. Thomson appears to have been living in
    Montreal at the time of Georgina Burland Macphail's death, and his letter
    of 12 Feb. 1918 indicates that the disclosure occurred in Tait McKenzie's
    house (McKenzie did not leave McGill for the University of Pennsylvania
    until 1904); see Linda Sheshko, Introduction to Thomson, *Old Man Savarin
    Stories*, xii, xv–xvi.

2   Dougall to Macphail, 16 Oct. 1911, Macphail Papers. Also see Macphail to
    Thomson, 27 Oct. 1911, Macphail Papers.

3   Thomson to Macphail, 17 Oct. 1911, Macphail Papers. Also see Thomson to
    Macphail, 29 Feb. 1912, Macphail Papers.

4   See Macphail, "Why the Liberals Failed," *University Magazine* 10 (Dec. 1911):
    576–7, 579; Macphail, "The Interlude in Politics," *Saturday Night*, 17 Feb.
    1912; Macphail to Grey, 9 Dec. 1911, Grey Papers, UD.

5   Macphail, "The Tariff Commission," *Saturday Night*, 10 Feb. 1912. Also see
    Macphail, "The Tariff Commission," *University Magazine* 11 (Feb. 1912):
    36–40.

6   See Macphail, "The Tariff Commission," *Saturday Night*, 10 Feb. 1912. The
    Liberal majority in the Senate was to defeat the proposal for a Tariff
    Commission; see Brown, "The Political Ideas of Robert Borden," 92.

7   See Macphail, "The Interlude in Politics," *Saturday Night*, 17 Feb. 1912;
    Macphail, "The Appeasement of the Farmer," *Saturday Night*, 24 Feb.
    1912; Macphail, "The Force of Attraction," *Saturday Night*, 2 March 1912;
    Macphail, "The Cost of Living," *University Magazine* 11 (Dec. 1912): 526–7;
    Macphail, "Patriotism and Politics," *University Magazine* 13 (Feb. 1914): 2–3;
    Macphail, "Consequences and Penalties," *University Magazine* 13 (April
    1914): 168. In later years he articulated precisely what Wilson's election had
    signified to him; see Macphail, *Three Persons*, 168–9, 181–2, 190–1.

8   See Peterson to Macphail, 1 Dec. 1911, Peterson Letterbooks, vol. 17, 412–13,
    MUA; Macphail to MacMechan, 12 Dec. 1911, MacMechan Papers, DUA;
    Stephen Leacock, "What Shall We Do About the Navy," *University Magazine*
    10 (Dec. 1911): 535–53.

9   See MacMechan to Macphail, 5, 11, 22 Dec. 1912, Macphail Papers; Macphail
    to MacMechan, 9, 16, 30 Dec. 1912, MacMechan Papers, DUA; Peterson to
    Macphail, 6, 9, 14 Jan. 1913, Peterson Letterbooks, vol. 20, 69, 89–90, 100,
    MUA; Macphail, "The Navy and Politics," *University Magazine* 12 (Feb. 1913):
    1–22; William Peterson, "A Supplement," *University Magazine* 12 (Feb. 1913):

22–9. Pelham Edgar appears to have liked the Macphail article; see Edgar to Macphail, n.d. [mid-Feb. 1913], Macphail Papers. For a modern scholarly account of the development of the naval issue from 1909 to 1914, see Hadley and Sarty, *Tin-Pots and Pirate Ships*, 24–9, 53–75.

10   Macphail to Strachey, n.d. [*ca.* April 1909], Macphail Papers. Also see Thomson to Macphail, 10 Nov. 1909, Macphail Papers; Thomson to Laurier, n.d. "Friday afternoon" [presumed 5 Nov. 1909], Laurier Papers, LAC; Macphail, *Essays in Politics*, 80–1.

11   See Stephen Leacock, "Canada and the Monroe Doctrine," *University Magazine* 8 (Oct. 1909): 351–74; Leacock, "What Shall We Do About the Navy," *University Magazine* 10 (Dec. 1911): 535–53; C. Frederick Hamilton, "The Canadian Navy," *University Magazine* 8 (April 1909): 175–87; C. Frederick Hamilton, "Shall Canada Have a Navy," *University Magazine* 8 (Oct. 1909): 375–97; C. Frederick Hamilton, "Canadian Coast Defence," *University Magazine* 8 (Dec. 1909): 587–602; Francis A. Carman, "The Naval Policy," *University Magazine* 12 (Dec. 1913) 568–77.

12   Macphail to MacMechan, 15 Dec. 1913, MacMechan Papers, DUA

13   See Tucker, *The Canadian Naval Service*, vol. 1, chs. 6–9; Macphail, "The Navy and Politics," *University Magazine* 12 (Feb. 1913): 4, 17–18, 22; Thomson to Macphail, 31 Oct. 1909, Macphail Papers; Thomson to Laurier, n.d. "Friday afternoon" [presumed 5 Nov. 1909]; Laurier to Macphail, 21 March 1910, Laurier Papers, LAC.

14   Macphail, "The Interlude in Politics," *Saturday Night*, 17 Feb. 1912. Also see Macphail, "Our Chief End," *Saturday Night*, 16 March 1912. The phrase "went on the rocks" refers to an accident that befell the HMCS *Niobe*, one of Laurier's two cruisers, in the summer of 1911; see Tucker, *The Canadian Naval Service*, 1: 145–6.

15   Macphail, "The Navy and Politics," 7

16   Cited in ibid., 10 (date of Laurier's statement: 12 Dec. 1912)

17   Ibid., 16. Also see 5–6, 8–10, 17.

18   Macphail to MacMechan, 9 Dec. 1912, MacMechan Papers, DUA. Also see Macphail to MacMechan, 30 Dec. 1912, MacMechan Papers, DUA.

19   Macphail to Wrong, 8 Jan. 1913, George M. Wrong Papers, UTRB. Note his comments on the current state of British institutions in the mother country: Macphail, "The Navy and Politics," 19–21. By this time Thomson was supporting Borden's naval policy; see Thomson to Macphail, n.d. "Wednesday" [presumed Dec. 1912], Macphail Papers.

20   See Macphail to MacMechan, 30 Dec. 1912, MacMechan Papers, DUA; Macphail to Grey, 3 Aug., 20 Oct. 1913, Grey Papers, UD; Macphail, "Patriotism and Politics," *University Magazine* 13 (Feb. 1914): 8.

21   Macphail, "The Hill of Error," *University Magazine* 12 (Dec. 1913): 536–8

22   Ibid., 539

23   MacMechan to Macphail, 12 Dec. 1913, Macphail Papers

24 Macphail to Wrong, 8 Jan. 1913, Wrong Papers, UTRB. Also see Macphail, "Consequences and Penalties," *University Magazine* 13 (April 1914): *passim*, especially 176–7.

25 See Macphail to Thomson, 27 Oct. 1911; Charlottetown *Patriot*, 2, 16 Nov. 1911; Charlottetown *Examiner*, 4, 10 Nov. 1911; Macphail, "Prince Edward Island," *Addresses Delivered before the Canadian Club of Toronto, Season of 1911–12*, 52–3; William Macphail to Macphail, 17 Oct. 1891, Macphail Papers; press cutting from Charlottetown *Examiner*, 2 June 1903, Lindsay-Macphail Scrapbooks 1, Macphail Papers.

26 Macphail, "The End," *Saturday Night*, 6 April 1912. Also see Macphail to Thomas MacNutt, n.d. [1935], Macphail Papers; Macphail to MacMechan, 20, 25 Nov. 1911, MacMechan Papers, DUA; Macphail to Grey, 9 Dec. 1911, Grey Papers, UD; interview with Mrs Dora Campbell and Mrs. Helen Chauvin (daughters of Mathieson), 30 Sept. 1970; Macphail, "Consequences and Penalties," 176.

27 Macphail, "Patriotism and Politics," 2. Also see 3, 5; Macphail, "Consequences and Penalties," 172; Macphail, "Our Chief End," *Saturday Night*, 16 March 1912; Macphail to MacMechan, 24 April 1914, MacMechan Papers, DUA.

28 Macphail, "Consequences and Penalties," 172. Also see 174: "But in the main, the individual Canadian who relied upon himself alone has done well, and is doing well."

29 Macphail, "Patriotism and Politics," 10–11. Also see Stephen Leacock, "The University and Business," *University Magazine* 12 (Dec. 1913): 540–9.

30 Macphail to MacMechan, 12 April [1914], MacMechan Papers, DUA

31 See Macphail to Mavor, 7, 11 May 1914, Mavor Papers, UTRB.

32 See Macphail, "Patriotism and Politics," 5.

33 Ibid., 11

34 Macphail, "Consequences and Penalties," 167–8; also see 173.

35 Ibid., 168. This was not a new posture for Macphail: see "The Nine Prophets," *University Magazine* 8 (Oct. 1909): 398–406; *Essays in Fallacy*, vi; "Church and Politics," *Saturday Night*, 4 June 1910; "The End," *Saturday Night*, 6 April 1912.

36 Macphail, "The Tariff Commission," *University Magazine* 9 (Feb. 1912): 27. Also see Macphail, "Prince Edward Island," *Addresses Delivered before the Canadian Club of Toronto ... 1911–12*, 58–9; Macphail, "Patriotism and Politics," 3; Macphail, "The Cost of Living," 536, 539, 543.

37 Macphail, "The Cost of Living," 540. Also see 538, 528, 542–3; Macphail, "The End," *Saturday Night*, 6 April 1912; Macphail, "On Certain Aspects of Feminism," *University Magazine* 13 (Feb. 1914): 79.

38 Macphail, "The Cost of Living," 540. Also see 526, 538; Macphail, *Essays in Politics*, 101; Macphail, "The Nine Prophets," *The University Magazine* 8 (Oct. 1909): 406; Macphail, "Government by Commission," Charlottetown *Guardian*, 18 Feb. 1911; Macphail, "The Tariff Commission," *University*

Magazine 11 (Feb. 1912): 30, 34–6; Macphail, "Patriotism and Politics," 7; Macphail, "Consequences and Penalties," 169–71. A number of his examples had come from Montreal; for information that clarifies some of the allusions, see Cooper, *Montreal*, 130, 132–4.

39 Macphail, "The Cost of Living," 541

40 Ibid., 542

41 Ibid.

42 Ibid., 539

43 Macphail, "The Tariff Commission," *University Magazine* 11 (Feb. 1912): 27; also see 28–36.

44 Macphail, "Theory and Practice," *University Magazine* 12 (Oct. 1913): 381. "Theory and Practice" was not published in the *Papers and Proceedings* of the cpsa, because it was already scheduled to appear in the *University Magazine*. In the Macphail Papers there is a typescript report of the address to the cpsa that differs somewhat from the *University Magazine* essay. Yet the points are substantially the same.

45 Macphail, "Theory and Practice," 380–1

46 Ibid., 381

47 Ibid., 395; also see 384.

48 Ibid., 390

49 Ibid.

50 Ibid., 392

51 Ibid., 391. Also see Macphail, "The Cost of Living," 531–2.

52 Macphail, "Theory and Practice," 394

53 Ibid., 383; also see 381–2. What B.C. Parekh has written of Burke applies equally to Macphail: "Though Burke is opposed to 'theories,' he is not opposed to the introduction of 'principles' in political life; and seems to believe that faith in the providential arrangement of human history is of immense value both to rulers and subjects" (Parekh, "The Nature of Political Philosophy," 193 n. 1). For Macphail's comments on the emasculation of the British House of Lords by the Asquith government, see Macphail, "The Tariff Commission," *University Magazine* 11 (Feb. 1912): 32.

54 See Macphail to MacMechan, 15 Dec. 1913, MacMechan Papers, dua; C.E.A. Simonds to Macphail, 23 Dec. 1913, Macphail Papers.

55 Macphail to MacMechan, 23 March 1914, MacMechan Papers, dua

56 Macphail, "Patriotism and Politics," 2

57 See Macphail, "Consequences and Penalties," 168; Macphail, "Theory and Practice," 386–7.

58 See Porter, comp., *Canadian Social Structure*, 44, table A2. For more statistical data on what Macphail interpreted as the economic and demographic effects of the National Policy infrastructure on Prince Edward Island, see Macphail, "A Voice from the East," *University Magazine* 9 (Dec. 1910): 521–2. He continued to be interested in this subject as long as he lived. After reading Grant, "Population Shifts in the Maritime Provinces," *Dalhousie Review*

17 (1937–38), 282–94, in which a young scholar (according to the journal, a Dalhousie undergraduate) pondered the causes and effects of the decline in population of the region relative to other parts of Canada and the shift in rural-urban balance, and the relationship of the two phenomena (concluding on a cautiously optimistic note), Macphail pronounced the article to be "a rare piece of work." (*Montreal Star*, 30 Nov. 1937) The author - "J.W. Grant" - was John Webster Grant, future historian of religion in Canada; born 27 June 1919, he was still a teenager when this sophisticated article appears to have been published.

59 See Macphail to MacMechan, 16 April 1913, MacMechan Papers, DUA.

60 Macphail, "A Voice from the East," *University Magazine* 9 (Dec. 1910): 519. Also see Macphail, "Prince Edward Island," *Addresses Delivered before the Canadian Club of Toronto ... 1911–12*, 49.

61 This is a reference to a dominion by-election in Quebec on 3 Nov. 1910 in which the Nationalists of Bourassa and the Quebec Conservatives combined to defeat Laurier's candidate in a Liberal stronghold, following a campaign that turned upon the naval issue. The Quebec Conservatives had distanced themselves from the rest of their party on this matter, and the result represented a victory for Bourassa's point of view.

62 Macphail, "A Voice from the East," 518, 520; also see 522. For examples of Macphail's wit at the expense of the nationalists, see 517–18.

63 Macphail, "The Atlantic Provinces in the Dominion: Introduction," in Shortt and Doughty, eds., *Canada and Its Provinces*, 13: 6; also see 3–5.

64 Ibid., 7

65 Ibid., 8. The publication in 1967 of Charles Tupper's minutes of the Charlottetown Conference confirmed that the Maritime union plan had evoked more sustained interest than Canadian historians had commonly acknowledged. Discussion of this alternative was not laid to rest until 16 Sept. 1864, nine days later than the earlier accepted date. See Smith, ed., "Charles Tupper's Minutes of the Charlottetown Conference," 101–12, especially 102–5.

66 Macphail, "The Atlantic Provinces in the Dominion," 10–11; also see 9.

67 Macphail, "The History of Prince Edward Island," in Shortt and Doughty, eds., *Canada and Its Provinces*, 13: 370; also see 363.

68 Ibid., 370. Also see 371–3; R.R. Fitzgerald to Macphail, 19 Jan. 1912, Macphail Papers. For a more vehement presentation of this view, see Captain Joseph Read, "Trade and Commerce of Prince Edward Island," 99–108.

69 Macphail, "Why the Liberals Failed," 578

70 Macphail, "The History of Prince Edward Island," 359. For a modern scholarly account of the Prince Edward Island Loyalists and how they became a factor in the colony (really as a stalking horse for the predatory governor who imported them), see Bumsted, *Land, Settlement, and Politics on Eighteenth-Century Prince Edward Island*, especially chs. 7 and 8.

71   See Macphail, "The History of Prince Edward Island," 374. Also see 305–6;
     Clark, *Three Centuries and the Island*, 210. One school inspector calculated
     that no less than 88 percent of the emigrants from school districts under
     his surveillance found homes in the United States; see Macphail, "Prince
     Edward Island," *Addresses Delivered before the Canadian Club of Toronto ...*
     1911–12, 52. Macphail's journal had published two articles on the contem-
     porary plight of PEI: C.F. Deacon, "The Two Islands: A Contrast," *University
     Magazine* 8 (Feb. 1909): 77–86, and J.E.B. McCready, "A Tragedy of the
     Census," *University Magazine* 10 (Dec. 1911): 581–8.

72   Macphail, "The History of Prince Edward Island," 323; also see 329. For an
     excellent modern analysis, see Earle Lockerby, "The Deportation of the
     Acadians from Île St.-Jean," *Acadiensis* 27 (Spring 1998): 45–94. The same
     author has published a briefer version: "Deportation of the Acadians from
     Île St.-Jean," *Island Magazine* 46 (Fall/Winter 1999): 17–25.

73   Macphail, "The History of Prince Edward Island," 324; also see 317.
     Lockerby, "The Deportation of the Acadians from Île St.-Jean," 72, refutes
     this accusation by Macphail.

74   D.C. Harvey to MacMechan, 25 Feb. 1913, MacMechan Papers, DUA. Also see
     MacMechan to Macphail, 4 Oct. 1912, 23 Feb. 1913, Macphail Papers; Harvey,
     The French Régime in Prince Edward Island. Harvey's two articles were "The
     Rhodes Scholar," *University Magazine* 11 (Dec. 1912): 602–15, and "La leçon
     du Canada," *University Magazine* 12 (Dec. 1913): 609–21.

75   Bumsted, "Historical Writing in English," 354. For criticism of Macphail's
     portrait of the state of the colony prior to Confederation, see Hatvany,
     "Tenant, Landlord, and Historian: A Thematic Review of the 'Polarization'
     Process in the Writing of Nineteenth-Century Prince Edward Island
     History," 121–2; in his view, "Macphail's comments about the Island's pre-
     industrial isolation, self-sufficiency, prosperity and contentment owed
     more to nostalgia than to fact." (122)

76   Macphail, "A Voice from the East," 522

77   Macphail, "The Dominion and the Provinces," *University Magazine* 12
     (Dec. 1913): 561. Under the heading "Premier of Canada Has More Power
     Than a King, Declares Prof. Macphail," this article was reprinted in part
     by the *Montreal Herald*, 17 Dec. 1913; see press cutting in McGill University
     Scrapbooks 3, 261, MUA. Also see 557, 559 of the *University Magazine* version;
     Grey to Strachey, 17 Feb. 1909, Strachey Papers, BL; Macphail, "Prince Edward
     Island," *Addresses Delivered before the Canadian Club of Toronto ... 1911–12*, 53.

78   Macphail, "The Dominion and the Provinces," 567. Also see 565–6;
     Macphail to Grey, 9 Dec. 1911, Grey Papers, UD.

79   Macphail, "The Dominion and the Provinces," 557–8; also see 559.

80   Macphail, "Town and Country," *Saturday Night*, 23 March 1912

81   See Macphail, "The Dominion and the Provinces," 554.

82   Ibid.

83   This play was published as an 82-page booklet in 1914: Macphail, *The Land:*
     A Play of Character, in One Act with Five Scenes. The first scene was pub-
     lished as "The Land" in the *University Magazine* 13 (April 1914): 275–91. Page
     references to scene 1 will be to the version appearing in Macphail's journal.
84   See www.canadianshakespeares.ca/a_theland.cfm (accessed 25 July 2004).
     I owe this reference to Prof. M. Brook Taylor of Mount Saint Vincent
     University. The project also lists, as a Canadian adaptation of Shakespeare,
     a work by Macphail's mentor from his undergraduate days at McGill,
     Professor Charles E. Moyse, writing under the pseudonym of Belgrave
     Titmarsh: *Shakspere's Skull and Falstaff's Nose: A Fancy in Three Acts* (1889).
     Rather than an actual adaptation of a specific play, it is a satire on an aspect
     of Shakespeare scholarship in the latter part of the nineteenth century, the
     "authorship controversy." Moyse used the same pseudonym when he pub-
     lished a short story, "House-Hunting," in the *McGill University Magazine* 3
     (Dec. 1903): 83–95.
85   Macphail, "The Land," 275
86   Ibid., 276
87   Ibid., 278
88   Macphail, *The Land,* 42
89   See Thomson to Macphail, 11 Feb., 4 March 1913, Macphail Papers.
90   Macphail to MacMechan, 30 Oct. 1912, MacMechan Papers, DUA
91   Macphail, "Prince Edward Island," press cutting from a PEI newspaper,
     n.d. [Oct. 1912], Burland-Macphail Scrapbook, Macphail Papers. The essay
     was solicited by an Island promoter for a "Patriotic Poetry, Prose and
     Photography" competition. Macphail's submission was to be marked "not
     for competition" and published along with the winners (H.T. Holman
     to author, 7 Aug. 1973, in author's possession; W.S. Louson to Macphail,
     1 Oct. 1912, Macphail Papers).
92   Macphail, "Prince Edward Island," press cutting from a PEI newspaper, n.d.
     [Oct. 1912], Burland-Macphail Scrapbook, Macphail Papers
93   See Macphail, "Town and Country," *Saturday Night,* 23 March 1912;
     Macphail, "The Cost of Living," 537, 543; Macphail, "The Atlantic Provinces
     in the Dominion," 11; Macphail, "The History of Prince Edward Island,"
     374–5; Macphail, *The Land, passim.*
94   Macphail, "The Cost of Living ," 535
95   Ibid., 537. Also see, for example, Macphail, "Patriotism and Politics," 3;
     Macphail, *The Land, passim.*
96   Macphail, "Patriotism and Politics," 3
97   Berger, *The Sense of Power,* 193 (word sequence altered)
98   Macphail to MacMechan, 24 Dec. 1913, MacMechan Papers, DUA. Also see
     Macphail to MacMechan, 30 Jan., 23 March 1914, MacMechan Papers, DUA;
     Macphail to Grey, 14 Feb. 1912, Grey Papers, UD; Macphail, "The Church
     and the Theatre," *Saturday Night,* 30 March 1912; John Edward Hoare, "A
     Plea for a Canadian Theatre," *University Magazine* 10 (April 1911): 239–53;

Macphail to D.S. Walker, 16 Oct. 1913; Pickthall to Macphail, 12 Oct., 1
Nov. 1912; Macphail to Pickthall,12 Nov. 1912, 24 March 1913; Macphail to
Morang, 19 Nov. 1912, Macphail Papers. The *University Magazine* published
a rather critical review of Pickthall's volume by Grey's son-in-law; see
Laurence E. Jones, "The Drift of Pinions," *University Magazine* 12 (Dec. 1913):
660–4.

99   MacMechan to Macphail, 13 Jan. 1911, Macphail Papers. MacMechan
began another letter to Macphail thus: "O man-of-many-Concerns, who
multipliest irons in various fires ..." (MacMechan to Macphail, 23 March
1912, Macphail Papers). Also see William Wood to Macphail, 30 Jan., 14
Feb. 1912, Macphail Papers; Macphail, "What Is the News," *Saturday Night*,
18 June 1910; Macphail to Grey, 18 Aug. 1911, Grey Papers, UD; Macphail
to MacMechan, 25 Nov., 1, 12, 26 Dec. 1911, 17 Jan., 7 Feb., 1 March 1912,
MacMechan Papers, DUA; Spadoni, "The Publishers Press of Montreal,"
38–50.

100 MacMechan to Macphail, 18 Aug. 1910, Macphail Papers

101 Macphail, "The Dominion and the Provinces," 556–7

102 Press cutting from a PEI newspaper, n.d. [*ca.* 1910], Burland-Macphail
Scrapbook, Macphail Papers. Beginning in 1912, Alexander (who had
married two years earlier) occupied a separate house, a fraction of a mile
from the family home; see Macphail to Dorothy Macphail, 13 April 1912,
Burland-Macphail Scrapbook, Macphail Papers. For its location, see *Atlas
of Province of Prince Edward Island Canada and the World*, 75. According to
Orwell W.I. [Women's Institute], *Orwell: Good Days* ..., the second house
was purchased in 1903 by Andrew Macphail for overflow guests; see photo
of "Alan Stanley" house. Almost exactly a century later, the house was
acquired by the new Prince Edward Island Agricultural Museum, which is
adjacent to what had been Alexander's property.

103 Press cutting from a PEI newspaper, n.d. [*ca.* 1 Sept. 1909], Burland-
Macphail Scrapbook, Macphail Papers.

104 Ibid.

105 Ibid.

106 See Charlottetown *Patriot*, 8 July 1905.

107 See press cutting from Charlottetown *Patriot*, 14 Oct. 1910; press cutting
from Charlottetown *Guardian*, 29 Nov. 1910, Macphail Papers; Macphail to
MacMechan, 15 June 1912, MacMechan Papers, DUA; interviews with Mrs
Dorothy Lindsay, 30 May 1968, 21 July, 7 Sept. 1970; Earl Ings, 6 Sept. 1968;
Percy MacLeod, 4 Sept. 1969; Mr and Mrs Malcolm "Mackie" MacLeod, 4
Sept. 1969; Katherine Dewar Interviews, interview with Marguerite (Meg)
Stanley, granddaughter (audio tape), 18 July 1990. For a critical view by
"M.W." (a potato grower) of Macphail's methods of potato growing, see
press cutting of unknown origin, n.d. [1910], Burland-Macphail Scrapbook,
Macphail Papers. Little has been written about the history of the seed
potato industry on the Island, and one lengthy article on the subject,

in the Summerside *Journal*, 20 June 1923, does not mention Macphail.
Regarding the "Katherine Dewar Interviews," see pp. 264, 396, below.

108   Interview with Mrs Dorothy Lindsay, 21 July 1970; Katherine Dewar
Interviews, interview with Katie Martin (audio tape), 23 July 1990

109   Kipling to Macphail, 21 Oct. 1911, Kipling-Macphail volume, Macphail
Papers [original emphasis]

110   See [Macphail], unpublished manuscript entitled "Island Tobacco," n.d.
[1912], 1st page, Macphail Papers; interview with Earl Ings, 6 Sept. 1968.

111   Interview with Mr and Mrs Malcolm "Mackie" MacLeod, 4 Sept. 1969;
Fitzgerald to Macphail, 12, 19 Jan., 14 Feb. 1912; Mathieson to Macphail, 25
Nov. 1912, Macphail Papers. Although Macphail appears to have complied
with the request for contributions to the "Exhibition" pamphlet, I have
been unable to locate a copy to confirm this.

112   [Macphail], unpublished manuscript entitled "Island Tobacco," n.d. [1912],
1st and 2nd pages, Macphail Papers. Macphail had other suggestions, such
as the development of cooperative institutions; see "Prince Edward Island,"
Addresses Delivered before the Canadian Club of Toronto … 1911–12, 55–6. He
did not consistently advocate the cooperative approach.

113   See Gordy McCarville to the author, electronic mail, 22 Dec. 2004. Mr
McCarville has kindly provided me with photocopies of a number of
documents relevant to the beginnings of tobacco cultivation on the Island.
One of them is a report in the Charlottetown *Examiner*, 30 Nov. 1912,
which mentions Macphail's experiments with tobacco. Mr McCarville
initially developed his interest in the history of the Prince Edward Island
tobacco industry when, as a young person, he worked as a tobacconist;
he was part of the third generation of his family to work in a particular
Charlottetown tobacco factory and had started there with a summer job at
age twelve in 1962. He commenced formal study of the subject as a university student ten years later.

114   McCarville to the author, electronic mail, 17 Jan. 2005; also 22 Dec. 2004.
An article in the Charlottetown *Guardian*, 26 May 1959, regarding the
rebirth of tobacco cultivation on the Island states that Nicholson commenced growing in 1910, but McCarville is "sure that 1910 date is incorrect";
McCarville to the author, electronic mail, 22 Jan. 2005.

115   McCarville to the author, electronic mail, 11 Feb. 2005.

116   The building is often referred to as the Macdonald-Workman Engineering
Building, and there is a photograph of it dated 1893 in Frost, *McGill 1*, 275.
Frost, *McGill 2*, 4, states that the building had an annex, "the excellently
equipped Workman technical shops." Another photograph of the building, next to two other "Macdonald" buildings on the McGill campus,
can be found in Gournay and Vanlaethem, eds., *Montreal Metropolis*,
86. The "Macdonald" was of course the Montreal tycoon Sir William
Macdonald, a native of Prince Edward Island; the "Workman" was Thomas
Workman, another major benefactor of McGill. See a modern study of

Macdonald, Fong, *Sir William C. Macdonald: A Biography*, especially 165–71. The "Macphail pillars" are shown with maximum clarity in "Macdonald Technical Building, Montreal," a sketch by architect Andrew Thomas Taylor, dated 1890, part of the permanent collection of the National Gallery, Ottawa, "Royal Canadian Academy of Arts diploma work, deposited by the architect, Montreal, 1890, no. 240." Concerning Taylor, see Gersovitz, "Sir Andrew Thomas Taylor," *The Canadian Encyclopedia*, 2nd edn (1988), 4: 2114.

117 See Cincinnati Bell Foundry Co. to Macphail, 11 Aug. 1909, 17, 28 Feb. 1910; S.M. Martin to Macphail, 3 Feb. 1910, Macphail Papers. Both the pillars and the bell remain in place, although, with the restoration of Macphail's house in the 1990s, the entranceway to the property was, inexplicably, rerouted, more or less sidelining the pillars, one of the most prominent features of the site. The bell can be seen in the foreground in a photograph of the house in Porter, "Architectural Treasures," 95. The replacement bell is no longer in Valleyfield either; in 1971 the Valleyfield church was moved to the neighbouring town of Montague. Another gift Macphail gave in memory of his family was a stained-glass window for the church at Orwell Head; several family members, including his parents, are buried in the adjacent cemetery. The United Church of Canada closed the church (and four others in the area) in 1967 as part of a church consolidation movement, and it is now apparently impossible to determine where the window went after the structure was demolished. See Orwell W.I. [Women's Institute], *Orwell: Good Days in Orwell*, 22; Marian Bruce to the author, electronic mail, 16 Jan., 13 Feb. 2008.

118 Alexander Macphail to Macphail, 26 May 1909, Macphail Papers. Also see Thomson to Macphail, 12 Sept. 1912, 19 Jan. 1914, Macphail Papers; Laurier to Thomson, 11 Sept. 1912, with pencilled addendum, n.d. [12 Sept. 1912], from Thomson to Macphail, Macphail Papers; Macphail to MacMechan, 28 April 1911, MacMechan Papers, DUA.

119 Interview with Mr and Mrs Malcolm "Mackie" MacLeod, 4 Sept. 1969. Within the memory of the present writer the road was so narrow that the higher boughs of trees from either side almost touched.

120 Interviews with Mrs W.E. MacKinnon, 26 June 1970; Miss Goldie McInnis and Miss Mary Martin, 6 Sept. 1969; Katherine Dewar Interviews, interview with the Rev. Harvey Bishop (audio tape), 6 Aug. 1990.

121 For accounts of incidents from Grey's trip to Orwell in 1910, which was part of a much larger tour, see John Macnaughton, "Some Personal Impressions of the Late Earl Grey," *University Magazine* 16 (Oct. 1917): 350; Macphail, "John McCrae: An Essay in Character," in McCrae, *In Flanders Fields and Other Poems*, 128–9; Macphail, *The Master's Wife*, 88–90; Hinds, "A Governor-General Goes North," 53; Rubio and Waterston, eds., *The Selected Journals of L.M. Montgomery*, 2: 12–16, 402–3.

122   Untitled sonnet by MacMechan, dated 6 Nov. 1912, enclosed in a letter
      of the same date from MacMechan to Macphail, Macphail Papers. Also
      see MacMechan to Macphail, 27 Oct. 1912, Macphail Papers; Macphail to
      MacMechan, 30 Oct., 29 Nov. 1912, MacMechan Papers, DUA.

123   See Archibald MacMechan, "A Portrait," *University Magazine* 17 (April 1918):
      196. It also appeared with the title "Andrew Macphail" in MacMechan's
      posthumously published *Late Harvest*, 51.

124   Thomson to MacMechan, 20 Dec. 1919, MacMechan Papers, DUA

CHAPTER NINE

1   Macphail to Borden, 28 Sept. 1914, Sir Robert Borden Papers, LAC. His only
    previous direct contact with the Borden government had been through
    participation in a successful effort to obtain the release of an Islander
    convicted of murdering his wife. See Macphail, *The Master's Wife*, 197–200;
    Alexander Martin to Macphail, 26 March, 28 Dec. 1912, 8 Dec. 1913, 27
    Feb., 25[?] April 1914; C.J. Doherty to Macphail, 4 April 1912, 3 Dec. 1913;
    Macphail to Doherty, 6 April 1912, 25 Oct., 2 Dec. 1913, 9 Feb., 2, 30 April
    1914; Macphail to Alexander Martin, 6 April 1912, 4 Dec. 1913; Mathieson
    to Doherty, 16 Aug. 1913; Macphail to Mathieson, 4 Dec. 1913; Mathieson to
    Macphail, 8 Dec. 1913; Under-Secretary of State to Macphail, 18 May 1914,
    Macphail Papers.

2   Macphail, *The Master's Wife*, 208. Also see 228–40; Macphail to Mavor, 31
    Aug. 1914, Mavor Papers, UTRB; Macphail to Kipling, 4–5 Jan. 1919; "D.G.M.S."
    [director-general of medical services] to Macphail, 19 Sept. 1914 (telegram);
    "A.D.M.S." [assistant director of medical services] to Macphail, 3 Oct. 1914
    (telegram), Macphail Papers; entry for 4 Aug. 1916, War Diaries 2, Macphail
    Papers; entry for 4 Oct. 1915, War Diaries 1, Macphail Papers; Peterson to
    Macphail, 26 Sept. 1914, Peterson Letterbooks, vol. 23, 226, MUA; Borden to
    Macphail, 28 Sept. 1914 (telegram).

3   Macphail, "The Day of Wrath," *University Magazine* 13 (Oct. 1914): 346. Also
    see Macphail to Peterson, 13 April 1915, Peterson Papers, MUA; Peterson to
    Grey, 6 March 1915, Peterson Letterbooks, vol. 23, 381-2, MUA.

4   Macphail, "The Day of Wrath," 348. As early as 1908 he had written, "To-day,
    German science and learning have surrendered themselves to the vin-
    dication of brute force over moral ideals" (Macphail, "The Dominion
    and the Spirit," *University Magazine* 7 [Feb. 1908]: 14). This sentence did
    not appear in the version that was incorporated into *Essays in Politics* the
    following year.

5   Macphail, "The Day of Wrath," 353. Also see 344; for more in the same
    vein, although in somewhat different form and with an air of great solem-
    nity, see Macphail, "Lessons Proper for 1914–15," *University Magazine* 14
    (Feb. 1915): 1–9.

6   Macphail, "The Day of Wrath," 356-7

7   Macphail, "Val Cartier Camp," *University Magazine* 13 (Oct. 1914): 362. Also
    see Alexander Macphail to Macphail, 27 Aug., 30 Sept. 1914, War Letters 1,
    Macphail Papers.

8   Macphail, "Val Cartier Camp," 365

9   Macphail, "The Day of Wrath," 358; also see 357.

10 Ibid., 344–5.

11 Macphail to Mavor, 22 March 1915, Mavor Papers, UTRB. Also see Macphail
    to Mavor, 8 March 1915, Mavor Papers, UTRB; Macphail to Dorothy
    Macphail, 21 April 1915, War Letters 4, Macphail Papers; Macphail to
    MacMechan, 17 Nov. 1914, MacMechan Papers, DUA.

12 See entries for 3 Oct. 1914, 9 Jan. 1915, Pen and Pencil Club Minutes, vol. 3,
    17–19, 38–9, MMCH.

13 Macphail to Dorothy Macphail, 9 May 1915, War Letters 4, Macphail Papers

14 Macphail to Dorothy Macphail, 18 April 1915, War Letters 4,
    Macphail Papers

15 Entry for 18 Sept. 1915, War Diaries 1, Macphail Papers; also see entry for
    16 Sept. 1915, War Diaries 1, Macphail Papers.

16 Macphail's war diaries and war letters during this period were a major
    source for a Canadian Broadcasting Corporation *Ideas* program on medi-
    cine in wartime, entitled "Crosses, Row on Row." The program was prepared
    for Remembrance Day 1989 and initially broadcast on 10 Nov. 1989. It won
    two important radio awards: in May 1990 the program was presented with
    the Canadian Nurses' Association Media Award of Excellence for Radio;
    in June 1990 ACTRA (the Association of Canadian Cinema, Television, and
    Radio Artists) named the program "Best Radio Program of the Year, Public
    Radio." "Crosses, Row on Row" has been rebroadcast many times.

17 Campbell, "I Would Not Have Missed It for the World: Sir Andrew
    Macphail's War," 4. For a perceptive summary of Macphail's wartime ser-
    vice, see 2–10; and Campbell, "I Would Not Have Missed It for the World:
    Sir Andrew Macphail's War, Part 2," 2–9.

18 Bourne, *Who's Who in World War One*, 3

19 Entry for 8 Feb. 1916, War Diaries 2, Macphail Papers

20 Entry for 14 Oct. 1916, War Diaries 2, Macphail Papers; also see entry for
    9 Oct. 1916, War Diaries 2, Macphail Papers.

21 Entry for 23 March 1916, War Diaries 2, Macphail Papers

22 Macphail to Peterson, 23 Oct. 1915, Peterson Papers, MUA. Also see Jeffrey
    Macphail to Macphail, 31 Oct. 1914, War Letters 1, Macphail Papers; press
    cutting of unknown origin, n.d. [early Jan. 1918]; Macphail to Dorothy
    Macphail, 8 Sept. 1916, Burland-Macphail Scrapbook, Macphail Papers;
    Macphail to Mavor, 12 Nov. 1915, Mavor Papers, UTRB; entry for 29 Oct.
    1915, War Diaries 1, Macphail Papers; entry for 16 Dec. 1916, War Diaries 3,
    Macphail Papers; entry for 8 Aug. 1916, War Diaries 2, Macphail Papers;
    Macphail, "The War: A Wet Night," *British Medical Journal*, 7 Dec. 1918, 637;
    Macphail, *The Master's Wife*, 236–7; Macphail to MacMechan, 24 May 1917,

MacMechan Papers, DUA; Alexander Macphail to Macphail, 21 April 1918; Macphail to Borden, n.d. [Nov. or Dec. 1917] Macphail Papers.

23	Macphail to [J.B.] Fitzmaurice, 23 Nov. 1915, Pen and Pencil Club Papers, MMCH

24	Entry for 29 June 1916, War Diaries 2, Macphail Papers. Also see entries for 30 Jan., 4 June 1916, War Diaries 2, Macphail Papers; entries for 31 March, 22 Oct., 11 Dec. 1915, War Diaries 1, Macphail Papers; Kipling to Macphail, 5 Oct. 1914, 15 June 1916, Kipling-Macphail volume, Macphail Papers; Jeffrey Macphail to Macphail, 15 Jan. 1915; Alexander Macphail to Macphail, 8 Feb. 1915, War Letters 2, Macphail Papers; Dorothy Macphail to Macphail, 26 Nov. 1916, Macphail Papers. Alexander had already met Aitken and had found him quite congenial; see Macphail to Jeffrey Macphail, 18 May 1915, War Letters 4, Macphail Papers.

25	Entry for 28 Sept. 1916, War Diaries 2, Macphail Papers. See Grant, "Charles William Gordon," 474–6; Allen, The Social Passion, 7, 32–4; Gordon, "The New State and the New Church," 192–8.

26	Entries for 22, 29, Nov., 25 Dec. 1916, War Diaries 3, Macphail Papers

27	See Campbell, "I Would Not Have Missed It for the World: Sir Andrew Macphail's War, Part 2," 6.

28	Entry for 1 Jan. 1917, War Diaries 3, Macphail Papers

29	Entry for 27 Jan. 1917, War Diaries 3, Macphail Papers

30	Entry for 16 March 1917, War Diaries 3, Macphail Papers

31	See the entries for 15 Aug. 1916, War Diaries 2, and 22 Nov. 1916, War Diaries 3, Macphail Papers.

32	Entry for 13 Nov. 1916, War Diaries 3, Macphail Papers

33	Entry for 26 May 1917, War Diaries 3, Macphail Papers

34	Entry for 29 April 1917, War Diaries 3, Macphail Papers; also see entry for 29 May 1917, War Diaries 3, Macphail Papers.

35	See entries for 15 Sept. 1915, War Diaries 1, and 16 Sept. 1916, War Diaries 2, Macphail Papers; Macphail to Dorothy Macphail, 22 April 1915, War Letters 4, Macphail Papers; Macphail to Peterson, 26 Sept. 1916, Peterson Papers, MUA.

36	Entry for 14 Feb. 1916, War Diaries 2, Macphail Papers

37	See entries for 9 April, 18, 29 Oct. 1916, War Diaries 2, Macphail Papers; entries for 27 Jan., 3 Feb. 1917, War Diaries 3, Macphail Papers; interviews with Mrs Dorothy Lindsay, 30 May 1968, 9 Sept. 1970; admission cards dated 3, 13 Dec. 1890 for executions to be carried out 12, 19 Dec. 1890; untitled draft manuscript, n.d. [1891 or 1892] (89 loose and unnumbered pages), Macphail Papers; Macphail, The Master's Wife, 198; Morton, "The Supreme Penalty: Canadian Deaths by Firing Squad in the First World War," 345–52. For concrete examples of Macphail's compassion in dealing with men of the lower ranks, see Campbell, "I Would Not Have Missed It for the World: Sir Andrew Macphail's War," 7–8.

38 Entry for 9 July 1916, War Diaries 2, Macphail Papers; also see entry for 26 Feb. 1916, War Diaries 2, Macphail Papers.
39 Entry for 23 Nov. 1916, War Diaries 3, Macphail Papers
40 Macphail, *The Master's Wife*, 204–9
41 Entry for 19 April 1917, War Diaries 3, Macphail Papers. Also see entry for 25 April 1917, War Diaries 3, Macphail Papers.
42 See entries for 23 Nov. 1916, 13 Feb., 24 April, 21, 29 May 1917, War Diaries 3, Macphail Papers; entries for 30 May, 9, 14 Oct. 1916, War Diaries 2, Macphail Papers; Macphail to Dorothy Macphail, 19 Jan. 1917; Macphail to Catherine Macphail, 13 July 1917; press cutting from *Montreal Star*, 2 Jan. 1918, Burland-Macphail Scrapbook, Macphail Papers; Macphail to MacMechan, 3 Feb. 1916, MacMechan Papers, DUA; Thomson to Macphail, 9 Aug. 1917; Alexander Macphail to Macphail, 11 June, 22 July 1917, Macphail Papers; Macphail, *The Master's Wife*, 242–4.
43 Macphail to MacMechan, 31 Jan. 1918, MacMechan Papers, DUA. Thomson had been for some time urging Borden to have Macphail included on an honours list. See Thomson to Macphail, 23 July, 27 Aug. 1917, Macphail Papers; Thomson to Borden, 26 July 1917 (private); Borden to Thomson, 2 Aug. 1917, Borden Papers, LAC.
44 Press cutting of unknown origin, n.d. [early Jan. 1918], Burland-Macphail Scrapbook, Macphail Papers. The conferment took place on 23 March; see entry for 23 March 1918, War Diaries 3, Macphail Papers.
45 MacMechan to Macphail, 20 Aug. 1916, Macphail Papers. For references to other, unpublished poems by Macphail, see Thomson to Macphail, 13 May 1915, 10 Nov. 1920, Macphail Papers.
46 Macphail, ed., *The Book of Sorrow*, Preface, v. Also see Macphail, untitled manuscript on "Best Work and Why," n.d. [1929], Macphail Papers, in which he reiterated this assertion. Macphail's poems, no. 157, "Illusion," and no. 316, "The Marriage Feast," were Petrarchan sonnets. He also translated three poems from French (nos. 98, 228, 235). For extensive and mildly critical reviews, see review in *Times Literary Supplement*, n.d., pasted to the inside back cover of the copy belonging to the Osler Library, McGill University; review in *Saturday Review*, 23 Sept. 1916, Macphail Papers. The former reviewer detected both in the anthology as a whole and in Macphail's own poem "Illusion" "a solemn pensiveness which ... is characteristically Victorian."
47 Macphail, "A Day's Work," offprint from *Lancet*, 30 June 1917, 20. Also see Macphail to Dorothy Macphail, 9 Jan. 1916, War Letters 4, Macphail Papers; entries for 10 Jan., 25 Sept. 1916, War Diaries 1, Macphail Papers; entry for 17 July 1916, War Diaries 2, Macphail Papers; Thomson to Macphail, 6 June, 27 Aug. 1917; William M. Macphail to Macphail, 6 Oct. 1917, Macphail Papers; press cutting of unknown origin, n.d. [early Jan. 1918], Burland-Macphail Scrapbook, Macphail Papers. J.T. Fotheringham, a prewar friend of Macphail from Toronto, also with the medical services, had declined

an invitation to give the lecture and suggested him as a substitute; see Fotheringham to Macphail, 23 March [1917], Macphail Papers. Alexander Macphail appears to have been less hopeful than Andrew about the probable results of the war; see Alexander Macphail to Macphail, 23 Sept. 1917, Macphail Papers.

48 Macphail, "A Day's Work," offprint from *Lancet*, 30 June 1917, 21. Also see 19; entry for 17 May 1917, War Diaries 3, Macphail Papers.

49 Macphail, "Val Cartier Camp," 369–70; also see 372.

50 See Macphail, "The Day of Wrath," 345; Macphail to MacMechan, 1 Oct. 1914, MacMechan Papers, DUA.

51 See entry for 28 Oct. 1915, War Diaries 1, Macphail Papers; entry for 2 Nov. 1916, War Diaries 2, Macphail Papers; entries for 22 Jan., 13 May 1917, War Diaries 3, Macphail Papers. One occasion on which Macphail did publicly criticize the military service occurred very early in the war; see Macphail, "Val Cartier Camp," 366–8.

52 See Macphail, "An Ambulance at Rest," *University Magazine* 16 (Oct. 1917): 330–7; Macphail, "The War: A Wet Night," *British Medical Journal*, 7 Dec. 1918, 636–8; Macphail, "The Bridge-head," *British Medical Journal*, 15 Feb. 1919, 189–91.

53 Falconer to Macphail, 7 May 1919, Falconer Papers, UTA; Macphail, "John McCrae: An Essay in Character," in McCrae, *In Flanders Fields and Other Poems*, especially 50–3, 59, 84, 91–6, 113; Janet McCrae to Macphail, 24 Nov. 1918, Macphail Papers; Kipling to Macphail, 23 June 1918, undated annotation by Macphail, Kipling-Macphail volume, Macphail Papers; Macphail, *The Master's Wife*, 16; Macphail to Kipling, 12 Nov. 1918, Burland-Macphail Scrapbook, Macphail Papers.

54 Macphail to Mavor, 29 Nov. 1917, Mavor Papers, UTRB. Also see Borden to Macphail, 30 Oct., 5 (confidential), 19 (personal) Nov. 1917; Alexander Martin to Macphail, 6 Oct. 1917; Macphail to Borden, 15 Dec. 1917; Mavor to Macphail, 3 Dec. 1917, Macphail Papers; 22 Dec. "Note," 23 Dec. "Note," 1917, War Diaries 3, Macphail Papers; Macphail, "War and Business," *Addresses Delivered before the Canadian Club of Toronto, Season of 1917–18*, 98–105.

55 Press cutting from Montreal *Gazette*, 7 Dec. 1917, McGill University Scrapbooks, vol. 4, 78, MUA

56 Macphail to Borden, 15 Dec. 1917, Macphail Papers. Also see Macphail, "Val Cartier Camp," 365; Macphail to Borden, 28 Sept. 1914, Borden Papers, LAC. Macphail appears to have been quite orthodox in his attitude towards demands for "conscription of wealth"; see memorandum from Macphail to Lord Atholstan (Sir Hugh Graham), 3 Dec. 1917, Macphail Papers.

57 Macphail, "In This Our Necessity," *University Magazine*, 16 (Dec. 1917): 476

58 Ibid., 480; also see 478–9. These pre-election words seem rather restrained when compared with the readiness for civil war which an English Canadian military and naval historian (a resident of Quebec City)

expressed in a letter to Macphail; see Wood to Macphail, 13 Dec. 1917, Macphail Papers.

59   Macphail to MacMechan, 21 Dec. 1917, MacMechan Papers, DUA. The Liberals also obtained a majority of the popular vote (50.2%) in Prince Edward Island; for this, the Island became known in some circles as "Little Quebec." See Beck, *Pendulum of Power*, 148; Harvey, *The French Régime in Prince Edward Island*, Preface, ix.

60   Macphail to McKenzie, 12 June 1918, R. Tait McKenzie Papers, UPA; also see Macphail McKenzie, 21 Nov. 1918, McKenzie Papers, UPA.

61   Kipling to Aitken, 9 Nov. 1916 [original emphasis], in Pinney, ed., *The Letters of Rudyard Kipling, vol. 4, 1911–19*, 416; "your Armies" because of Aitken's role as propagandist for the Canadian Expeditionary Force.

62   See pp. 211–12, below.

63   Entry for 1 Jan. 1917, War Diaries 3, Macphail Papers

64   Entry for 23 Sept. 1916, War Diaries 2, Macphail Papers; also see entry for 1 Nov. 1916, War Diaries 2, Macphail Papers.

CHAPTER TEN

1   Interview with Mrs Dorothy Lindsay, 5 Dec. 1968; entries for 7 June, 30 Oct. 1916, War Diaries 2, Macphail Papers; entries for 27, 30 April 1917, War Diaries 3, Macphail Papers; Alexander Macphail to Macphail, 8 July 1915, War Letters 3, Macphail Papers; Janet McCrae to Macphail, 24 Nov. 1918; Macphail to Sir Thomas White, 9 April 1919, Macphail Papers; Macphail to Dorothy Macphail, 13 April 1912; "Certificate of Service," dated 18 Nov. 1919, Burland-Macphail Scrapbook, Macphail Papers; Macphail to Borden, 29 May 1919, Borden Papers, LAC; Macphail to Falconer, 6 May 1919 (personal), Falconer Papers, UTA. His problems did not prevent him from becoming involved in a defence of the reputation of the medical services. See Sir George Perley to Borden, 3 April 1919; Prime Minister's Secretary [George W. Yates] to Macphail, 4, 7 April 1919; White to Perley, 30 April 1919 (telegram), Borden Papers, LAC; memorandum [by Macphail], n.d. [late March or early April 1919], on the charges made by Brig. Gen. C.A. Smart; memorandum by Macphail, 5 April 1919; White to Macphail, 8, 11 April 1919; Macphail to White, 9 April 1919; G.L. Foster to Macphail, 21 April 1919, Macphail Papers.

2   Entry for 31 Dec. 1916, War Diaries 3, Macphail Papers

3   See entry for 29 May 1917, War Diaries 3, Macphail Papers; Macphail, "War and Business," *Addresses Delivered before the Canadian Club of Toronto ... 1917–18*, 417; Macphail, "In This Our Necessity," *University Magazine* 16 (Dec. 1917): 477.

4   Macphail, "Val Cartier Camp," *University Magazine* 13 (Oct. 1914): 365

5   Macphail, "Sir Henry Wilson," *Quarterly Review* 251 (July 1928): 23; also see 22, 24–5 [emphasis added].

6 See Peterson to Walton, 11 May 1914, Peterson Letterbooks, vol. 23, 42–3, MUA; Peterson to Walton, 9 Dec. 1914, Peterson Letterbooks, vol. 24, 25–6, MUA; Macphail to Peterson, 13 April 1915, Peterson Papers, MUA.

7 See Peterson to Macphail, 13 March 1908, Peterson Letterbooks, vol. 12, 254, MUA; Peterson to Macphail, 24 Oct. 1911, Peterson Letterbooks, vo. 27, 275, MUA; Peterson to Grey, 6 March 1915, Peterson Letterbooks, vol. 24, 381, MUA; Peterson to Macphail, 18 Dec. 1918, Peterson Letterbooks, vol. 31, 301–2, MUA. Although Macphail allowed the first "Topics ..." to appear in the April 1915 number, he retained complete control over the rest of the content. See Peterson to Leacock, 18 March 1915, Peterson Letterbooks, vol. 24, 428, MUA; Peterson to Hickson, 4, 30 Jan. 1915, Peterson Letterbooks, vol. 24, 97, 226, MUA; Peterson to Macphail, 14 April 1915, Peterson Letterbooks, vol. 25, 30, MUA; Peterson to Hickson, 16 April 1915 (private), Peterson Letterbooks, vol. 25, 39, MUA; Macphail to Peterson, 29 Jan. 1915, Peterson Papers, MUA.

8 See Macphail to Peterson, 30 Jan. 1915, Peterson Papers, MUA; Peterson to Macphail, 3 Feb. 1915 (private), Peterson Letterbooks, vol. 24, 251, MUA; Peterson to Macphail, 28 Feb., 29 April 1918, Peterson Letterbooks, vol. 30, 213, 412, MUA; Peterson to Arthur E. Darby, 13 Nov. 1918 (private), Peterson Letterbooks, vol. 31, 167, MUA; Peterson to Thomson, 2 Sept. 1915, Peterson Letterbooks, vol. 25, 328, MUA; Peterson to W.D. LeSueur, 9 Oct. 1915, Peterson Letterbooks, vol. 25, 406, MUA; Peterson to Edgar, 28 Feb., 27 March 1916, Peterson Letterbooks, vol. 36, 410, 503, MUA; Peterson to Lafleur, 29 June 1917, Peterson Letterbooks, vol. 29, 112, MUA; Peterson to Grey, 6 March 1915, Peterson Letterbooks, vol. 24, 381, MUA; Peterson to Edgar, 9 March 1918, Peterson Letterbooks, vol. 30, 262, MUA; Peterson to MacMechan, 8 Nov. 1918, MacMechan Papers, DUA. The *University Magazine* had formerly averaged about 700 pages in bulk per volume.

9 Peterson to Macphail, 28 Feb. 1918, Peterson Letterbooks, vol. 30, 213, MUA. Also see Peterson to Mavor, 15 Jan., 11 (private), 21, 22 Feb., 1 March 1916, Peterson Letterbooks, vol. 26, 239, 351, 389, 393–4, 431, MUA; Peterson to Mavor, 31 March, 5 April 1916, Peterson Letterbooks, vol. 27, 10–11, 27, MUA; Peterson to Macphail, 7 April 1916, Peterson Letterbooks, vol. 27, 39–40, MUA; Peterson to Alexander, 13 April 1916, Peterson Letterbooks, vol. 27, 67, MUA; Peterson to Edgar, 12 Dec. 1916, Peterson Letterbooks, vol. 27, 479, MUA; Peterson to Edgar, 15, 25 Jan. 1917, Peterson Letterbooks, vol. 28, 86, 121, MUA; Mavor to Peterson, 19 (draft), 25 Feb., 3 April 1916; Mavor to Macphail, n.d. [early 1916] (draft); Macphail to Mavor, 16 April 1916, Mavor Papers, UTRB.

10 See Peterson to Leacock, 14 Feb. 1916, Peterson Letterbooks, vol. 26, 358, MUA; interview with Mrs Dorothy Lindsay, 5 Dec. 1968; Forsey, *A Life on the Fringe*, 24.

11 Leacock, "Andrew Macphail," *Queen's Quarterly* 45 (Winter 1938), 447. Also see Macnaughton to Macphail, 18 Sept. 1917, Macphail Papers; Peterson to Macphail, 29 April 1918, Peterson Letterbooks, vol. 30, 412, MUA; Collard,

ed., *The McGill You Knew*, 63–6, as follows: Herbert Stewart Everett, "Professors before Students...," 63; Col. Paul P. Hutchison, "... And Senior Professors before Junior," 63; Dr Laurence C. Tombs, "Acknowledged with a Slight Smile," 63–4; Mrs W.E. Baldwin (Alice Sharples), "'Polly' Lafleur – Funny, Marvellous Little Man," 64–6.

12 See Peterson to Macphail, 28 Feb., 14, 23 March, 29 April, 1 May 1918, Peterson Letterbooks, vol. 30, 213, 288, 317, 411–12, 426, MUA; Peterson to Macphail, 18 Dec. 1918, Peterson Letterbooks, vol. 31, 301–2, MUA; M.D. Field (Peterson's secretary) to Lafleur, 4 June 1918, Peterson Letterbooks, vol. 31, 2, MUA; Peterson to Colby, 21 April 1919, Peterson Letterbooks, vol. 31, 427, MUA; Peterson to Edgar, 21 Oct. 1918, Peterson Letterbooks, vol. 31, 78, MUA; Peterson to Cappon, 24 Dec. 1918, Peterson Letterbooks, vol. 31, 330, MUA; Peterson to MacMechan, 8 Nov. 1918, MacMechan Papers, DUA.

13 Falconer to Macphail, 7 May 1919, Falconer Papers, UTA. Also see Macphail to Falconer, 6 May 1919 (personal); Falconer to Macphail, 10 May 1919, Falconer Papers, UTA; Peterson to Macphail, 28 Feb., 29 April 1918, Peterson Letterbooks, vol. 30, 213, 411–12, MUA; Peterson to Edgar, 8, 16 April 1918, Peterson Letterbooks, vol. 30, 344–5, 376, MUA; Peterson to Cappon, 24 Dec. 1918, Peterson Letterbooks, vol. 31, 330, MUA. Bowker, "Truly Useful Men," 40, reports that the University of Toronto accumulated $1,300,000 in deficits between 1918 and 1921.

14 See Macphail to Mavor, 2 Nov., 23 Sept. 1919, Mavor Papers, UTRB; Macphail to Falconer, 6 May 1919 (personal), Falconer Papers, UTA; "To Readers," *University Magazine* 19 (Feb. 1920), inside cover.

15 Macphail to Kipling, 4–5 Jan. 1919, Macphail Papers. Also see Macphail, "The Day of Wrath," *University Magazine* 13 (Oct. 1914): 344, 346; "Staff Officer" [Macphail], "The Last Days," *University Magazine* 18 (Oct. 1919): 334, 340–1; entry for 26 Feb. 1916, War Diaries 2, Macphail Papers. The "better right" of Kipling presumably arose from his having lost his son John in the war.

16 Macphail, "The Peace and Its Consequence," *University Magazine* 19 (April 1920): 129–31. Also see Macphail to Mavor, 31 Jan. 1920, Mavor Papers, UTRB.

17 Macphail, "The Peace and Its Consequence," 132; also see 131.

18 Macphail, "Article Nineteen," *University Magazine* 18 (Oct. 1919): 314; also see 312–13, 315, 326.

19 Ibid., 326; also see 324.

20 Ibid., 324–6.

21 Borden to Macphail, 26 June 1918 (confidential), Macphail Papers. Also see "Private Memorandum" from Macphail to Borden, n.d. [*ca.* 7 July 1918] (this memorandum formed the basis for Macphail's "Article Nineteen" essay); Macphail to MacMechan, 17 Nov. 1919, MacMechan Papers, DUA; press cutting from Montreal *Gazette*, 19 Nov. 1919, McGill University Scrapbooks 4, 215, MUA; Macphail to Borden, 24 June, 6 Oct. 1918, Borden

Papers, LAC; Borden and Macquarrie, eds., *Robert Laird Borden: His Memoirs*, 2: 164; interviews with Mrs Dorothy Lindsay, 15, 16 June 1969. The idea appears to have struck Macphail in the period before American entry into the war; see entries for 9 Nov. 1916, 17 Jan. 1917, War Diaries 3, Macphail Papers.

22 Macphail to Borden, 7 July 1918, Borden Papers, LAC

23 Macphail, "The Peace and Its Consequence," 131

24 Ibid., 132. For Macphail's wartime fears that the war would not consolidate the empire, see entries for 11 Nov. 1916, 23 April, 6, 13 May 1917, War Diaries 3, Macphail Papers. These premonitions were based on his observations of the interaction of Canadian and British officers.

25 Macphail, "The Conservative," *University Magazine* 18 (Dec. 1919): 419. Also see press cuttings from Montreal *Gazette*, 11 Nov., 17 Dec. 1919, 10 Jan. 1920, McGill University Scrapbooks 4, 213, 222, 227, MUA.

26 Macphail, "The Conservative," 420–1

27 Ibid., 422. Also see Thomson to Macphail, 9 Aug. 1917, Macphail Papers; Macphail, Postscript to Belcourt, "French in Ontario," *University Magazine* 11 (Dec. 1912): 561; entry for 20 Dec. 1916, War Diaries 3, Macphail Papers.

28 Macphail, "The Conservative," 427-8; also see 422, 424, 434.

29 Ibid., 434. Also see 428–9, 432–3; *Canadian Annual Review* 19 (1919): 680; entry for 10 Jan. 1915, War Diaries 1, Macphail Papers.

30 See p. 56, above.

31 Macphail, "The Conservative," 422. Also see Macphail, "The Immigrant," *University Magazine* 19 (April 1920): 138–9.

32 Macphail, "The Conservative," 427; also see 423–4, 426.

33 Ibid., 430

34 Ibid., 430; Sellar, *The Tragedy of Quebec*, with Introduction by Hill; Hill, "Robert Sellar," DCB 14: 919-21.

35 Press cutting from Montreal *Gazette*, 11 Nov. 1919, McGill University Scrapbooks 4: 213, MUA.

36 See Macphail, "The Conservative," 434–44. The actual end of the article came with a political *non sequitur*, which indicated the frailty of his hopes for regeneration: a plea for the gathering of conservative forces behind Borden and Sir Lomer Gouin (444). Also see Macphail to Borden, 1 March 1918, Macphail Papers.

37 Macphail, "Women in Democracy," *University Magazine* 19 (Feb. 1920): 1; also see 5–6. This essay grew out of an address to the Women's Art Society in Montreal, which was later also delivered at the University of Toronto. See press cuttings from Montreal *Gazette*, 19 Nov. 1919, 12 Jan. 1920, McGill University Scrapbooks 4, 217, 227, MUA; Macphail to Mavor, 9, 11 Dec. 1919, Mavor Papers, UTRB.

38 Macphail, "Women in Democracy," 2; also see 3.

39 Ibid., 5.

40 Ibid., 4; also see 12; Maggie Macphail Jenkins to Macphail, 5 Dec. 1916, Macphail Papers.
41 Macphail, "Women in Democracy," 5
42 Press cutting from Charlottetown *Patriot*, 12 July 1920, Macphail Papers
43 Macphail, "Women in Democracy," 6, 8; also see 7.
44 Macphail, "The Immigrant," *University Magazine* 19 (April 1920): 158–9
45 Ibid., 149–50, 157. Also see Borden and Macquarrie, eds., *Robert Laird Borden: His Memoirs*, 2: 164.
46 Macphail, "The Immigrant," 157; also see 150–2.
47 Ibid., 153
48 Ibid., 157–8; also see 153–4, 156.
49 Ibid., 154.
50 See Alexander Macphail to Macphail, 29 June 1915, War Letters 2, Macphail Papers; Alexander Macphail to Macphail, 3 July 1915; Jeffrey Macphail to Dorothy Macphail, 16 Aug. 1915; Jeffrey Macphail to Macphail, 22 Aug. 1915, War Letters 3, Macphail Papers; Dorothy Macphail to Macphail, 22 July, 1 Aug. 1915, Macphail Papers.
51 Macphail, "The Immigrant," 151. Also see 150; Macphail, "The Farmer," *Empire Club of Canada: Addresses Delivered to the Members during the Year 1920*, 119–21.
52 Macphail, "The Immigrant," 157. Also see Macphail, "The Farmer," *Empire Club of Canada: Addresses ... 1920*, 116, 121.
53 Macphail, "The Immigrant," 148–9
54 See Macphail, "The Education of Graduates," *British Medical Journal*, 30 Aug. 1919, 261; Macphail, "The Conservative," 423–4; press cutting from *Montreal Herald*, 14 Jan. 1920, McGill University Scrapbooks 4, 228, MUA; Macphail, "The Immigrant," 149, 157, 161, 162; Macphail, "The Farmer," *Empire Club of Canada: Addresses ... 1920*, 118; Kipling to Macphail, 14 Feb. 1919, Kipling-Macphail volume, Macphail Papers.
55 Macphail, "The Immigrant," 161
56 Ibid., 162. Also see 143, 146–7, 160–1; Macphail, "The Farmer," *Empire Club of Canada: Addresses ... 1920*, 113–15, 120, 123-4; Macphail, "The Immigrant," *Addresses Delivered before the Canadian Club of Ottawa, 1919–1920*, 170, 173-4, 176–7; press cutting from Montreal *Gazette*, 31 Jan. 1920, McGill University Scrapbooks 4, 231, MUA; "Staff Officer" [Macphail], "The Last Days," *University Magazine* 18 (Oct. 1919): 328–9.
57 "To Readers," *University Magazine* 19 (Feb. 1920), inside cover. Also see Macphail to Falconer, 6 May 1919 (personal), Falconer Papers, UTA; Macphail to Mavor, 2 Nov. 1919, Mavor Papers, UTRB.
58 Macphail to Mavor, 3 Oct. 1920, Mavor Papers, UTRB. Also see Macphail to MacMechan, 4 Oct. 1920, 8 Jan. 1921, MacMechan Papers, DUA; Thomson to Macphail, 10 Nov. 1920, Macphail Papers; Peterson to Edgar, 6 March 1919, Peterson Letterbooks vol. 26, 503, MUA; Macphail to Falconer, 6 May 1919 (personal), Falconer Papers, UTA.

59 *Canadian Forum*, editorial, 1 (Nov. 1920): 36. The *Canadian Forum* was unable to pay its contributors.

60 *Canadian Forum*, editorial, 1 (Nov. 1920): 37

61 Edgar, "Sir Andrew Macphail," *Queen's Quarterly* 54 (Spring 1947): 9. Also see Macphail to MacMechan, 4 Oct. 1920, MacMechan Papers, DUA; Macphail to Mavor, 3 Oct. 1920, Mavor Papers, UTRB; Pickthall to Macphail, 23 Sept. 1920; Thomson to Macphail, 10 Nov. 1920; William E. Marshall to Macphail, 26 Oct., 1 Nov. 1920, Macphail Papers.

62 The only other Macphail articles to exceed 20 pp. were "British Diplomacy and Canada," *University Magazine* 8 (April 1909) (27 pp.), and "The Navy and Politics," *University Magazine* 12 (Feb. 1913) (22 pp.).

63 Macphail to Alexander Macphail, "Queen's Birthday" [21 May] 1920, Sir Arthur Currie Papers, LAC. Also see Alexander Macphail to Currie, 27 May 1920, Currie Papers, LAC; Alexander Macphail to Macphail, 20 May 1920, Macphail Papers. In later years, and in print, Macphail extended his comments on McGill; see Macphail, "Sir Arthur Currie: The Value of a Degree," *Queen's Quarterly* 41 (Spring 1934): 2–3, 10.

64 Macphail to McKenzie, 21 Nov. 1918, McKenzie Papers, UPA. Also see Macphail to MacMechan, 19 Oct. 1918, MacMechan Papers, DUA; Macphail, "The Immigrant," *University Magazine* 19 (April 1920): 157; Macphail, "The Immigrant," *Addresses Delivered before the Canadian Club of Ottawa, 1919–1920*, 176.

65 In fact Macphail loved buttermilk. More than a half-century after his death, Louise Macqueen Colpitts recalled that on Tuesdays he could be counted on to show up at her family homestead to get his buttermilk, since he knew that her aunts churned on that day. Katherine Dewar Interviews, interview with Ruth MacLeod VanIderstine and Louise Macqueen Colpitts (audio tape), 20 July 1990.

66 Leacock, "Andrew Macphail," 451. According to Alan Bowker, Leacock's most candid account of his own boyhood on a farm was penned in the last year of his life; see Bowker, ed., *On the Front Line of Life: Stephen Leacock*, 18, and "Life on the Old Farm," in ibid., 47-73.

CHAPTER ELEVEN

1 There are only two brief references to this controversy in his published works, and neither appeared in a place where one would seek informed commentary on Canadian politics; I have been unable to locate any mention of it in his private correspondence. See Macphail, "American Methods in Medical Education," offprint from *British Medical Journal*, 3 Sept. 1927, 10; Macphail, "The Freedom of England," *Quarterly Review* 255 (July 1930): 2.

2 Macphail to Mavor, 9 Dec. 1919, Mavor Papers, UTRB. Also see Macphail, "The Conservative," *University Magazine* 18 (Dec. 1919): 442.

3 Macphail to Mavor, 23 Jan. 1925, Mavor Papers, UTRB. Also see Macphail to Beaverbrook, 30 Aug. 1921, Beaverbrook Papers, BL.

4 See Macphail to MacMechan, 27 March 1926, MacMechan Papers, DUA; MacMechan to Macphail, 30 March 1926, Macphail Papers; interviews with Mrs Dorothy Lindsay, 15, 16 June 1969; Miss Goldie McInnis and Miss Mary Martin, 6 Sept. 1969; Mrs W.E. MacKinnon, 26 June 1970.

5 Interview with Mrs Dorothy Lindsay, 30 May 1968; Macphail to MacMechan, "1925," 16 [?], 19 Jan. 1926, MacMechan Papers, DUA; Jeffrey Macphail to Macphail, 27 Aug. 1929, Macphail Papers

6 Interview with Mrs Dorothy Lindsay, 13 March 1970. Also interviews with Mrs Dorothy Lindsay, 21 July, 29 Nov. 1970. For a sense of her alarm at the time, see Mrs Dorothy Lindsay to Howard Murray, 11 Aug. [1931], Macphail-Murray Scrapbooks 1, Macphail Papers; Mrs Dorothy Lindsay to Currie, 11 Aug. [1931], McGill Principals' Papers, MUA.

7 Macphail to Beaverbrook, 28 Oct., 13 Nov. 1931, Beaverbrook Papers, BL.

8 Press cutting from *Montreal Star*, n.d. [*ca.* 15 Nov. 1921], Lindsay-Macphail Scrapbooks 2, Macphail Papers

9 *Canadian Medical Association Journal* 39 (1938): 508.

10 Press cutting from *Montreal Star*, n.d. [*ca.* 15 Nov. 1921], Lindsay-Macphail Scrapbooks 2, Macphail Papers. Over the years the area where Macphail lived changed in character, for a bootlegger was reported to have an operation nearby; interview with John A. Stevenson, 19 May 1968.

11 Prefatory annotation by Macphail, n.d., to Kipling to Macphail, 26 March 1922, Kipling-Macphail volume, Macphail Papers

12 Press cutting from *Montreal Star*, n.d. [*ca.* 15 Nov. 1921], Lindsay-Macphail Scrapbooks 2, Macphail Papers.

13 Kipling to Macphail, 26 March 1922, annotation by Macphail, Kipling-Macphail volume, Macphail Papers; interview with Mrs Dorothy Lindsay, 27 Sept. 1970

14 Macphail to McKenzie, 30 Sept. 1926, McKenzie Papers, UPA. Also see Macphail to MacMechan, 5 Dec. 1921, MacMechan Papers, DUA

15 Macphail to McKenzie, 30 Sept. 1926, McKenzie Papers, UPA

16 Leacock, "Andrew Macphail," *Queen's Quarterly* 45 (Winter 1938): 450. Also interview with Mrs Dorothy Lindsay, 15 Sept. 1970.

17 Mrs Helen Chauvin, interview with her and with her sister Mrs Dora Campbell, 30 Sept. 1970. They were daughters of his longtime friend from Prince of Wales College days, John A. Mathieson, who was chief justice of the Supreme Court of Prince Edward Island during the interwar period.

18 Interviews with Mrs Dorothy Lindsay, 5 Dec. 1968, 23 Sept. 1970; Frank MacKinnon, 27 Dec. 1967; Sally MacKinnon, 26 June 1970; Mrs Dora Campbell and Mrs Helen Chauvin, 30 Sept. 1970; W.E.C. and Elizabeth Harrison, 7 June 1973; Katherine Dewar Interviews, interview with Sally MacKinnon (audio tape), 7 Sept. 1990; also see Edgar, "Sir Andrew Macphail," *Queen's Quarterly* 54 (Spring 1947): 9–10; Leacock, "Andrew

Macphail," *Queen's Quarterly* 45 (Winter 1938): 448; Sir Dawson Williams to Macphail, 26 July 1925; William M. Macphail to Macphail, 27 April 1930, Macphail Papers; prefatory annotation by Macphail, n.d., to Kipling to Macphail, 26 March 1922, Kipling-Macphail volume, Macphail Papers.

19   Interviews with Mrs Dorothy Lindsay, 21, 31 July 1970

20   See Macphail, *Official History*; Macphail, *Three Persons*; Macphail, *The Master's Wife*; C.J. S— ? [name illegible] (assistant provincial secretary, Province of Quebec) to Macphail, 30 April 1926, Macphail Papers; Macphail to Lorne Pierce, 13 May 1930, Lorne Pierce Papers, QUL; press cutting from Montreal *Gazette*, 21 May 1930, McGill University Scrapbooks 7, 120, MUA.

21   Macphail, untitled manuscript on "Best Work and Why," n.d. [1929], Macphail Papers

22   Wilfrid Bovey, "Macphail's Book," *McGill News* 6 (Sept. 1925), 8–10. Also see Kipling to Macphail, 17 Jan. 1917 (private), Kipling-Macphail volume, Macphail Papers; A. Fortescue Duguid, preface to Macphail, *Official History*,·v.

23   Cook, *Clio's Warriors*, 55

24   See Hyatt, "Official History in Canada," 89; Cook, *Clio's Warriors*, 44–5.

25   Macphail to MacMechan, 4 Oct. 1923, MacMechan Papers, DUA. Also see Macphail to MacMechan, 2 Oct. 1922, MacMechan Papers, DUA; Macphail to Mavor, 4 Oct. 1921, Mavor Papers, UTRB; Macphail to Beaverbrook, 7 Sept. 1922, Beaverbrook Papers, BL; Macphail to J.H. MacBrien, 30 Jan. 1923 (draft letter); Williams to Macphail, 26 July 1926, Macphail Papers; Macphail to Pierce, 28 Oct., 9 Nov. 1923, Pierce Papers, QUL; Macphail to Currie, 24 March 1933, Currie Papers, LAC; Stevenson, "Sir Andrew Macphail," *Canadian Defence Quarterly* 16 (Jan. 1939): 208.

26   See Cook, *Clio's Warriors*, 192n19.

27   Macphail, *Official History*, 6; also see 98, 402.

28   Ibid., 1; also see 12, 14, and (concerning Hughes, for example), 17–24. Macphail had already made his views on the accomplishments of the Canadian medical services a matter of public record, and his wartime opinion of Hughes is clear from his diaries. See Macphail, "A Day's Work," offprint from *Lancet*, 30 June 1917, 11, 14; Macphail, "In This Our Necessity," *University Magazine* 16 (Dec. 1917): 477; Macphail, "War and Business," *Addresses Delivered before the Canadian Club of Toronto, Season of 1917–18*, 103–4; Macphail, "John McCrae: An Essay in Character," in McCrae, *In Flanders Fields and Other Poems*, 131; and, for example, entry for 25 Aug. 1915, War Diaries 1, Macphail Papers.

29   See Cook, "The Madman and the Butcher: Sir Sam Hughes, Sir Arthur Currie, and Their War of Reputations," 693–719.

30   See Macphail, *Official History*, 4, 1, 287–94, 276–8.

31   Morton, *When Your Number's Up*, 200. For a classic study of the stripping away of sexual inhibition and restraint in wartime, both at the front

and in civilian life, see Hirschfeld, *The Sexual History of the World War*. A sampling of the chapter titles indicates the contents: "The Release of Sexual Restraints," "Eroticism of Nurses," "Sensuality in the Trenches," "Prostitution Behind the Lines," "Lust in the Conquered Areas," and "Civilian Debauchery Back Home." I am grateful to Professor Modris Eksteins of the University of Toronto at Scarborough for this reference.

32 See entry for 26 March 1916, War Diaries 2, Macphail Papers. Regarding the state of psychiatric knowledge on this problem during the war years and the impact that dealing with it had on the psychiatric profession (new status, power, and legitimacy), see Brown, "Shell Shock in the Canadian Expeditionary Force, 1914–1918: Canadian Psychiatry in the Great War," 308–32. For the different types of disorder to which this term referred, see 313–14.

33 See Macphail, *Three Persons*, 150.

34 Cited in obituary to Macphail in Charlottetown *Patriot*, 28 Sept. 1938

35 Review in the *Times* of London, 20 Aug. 1925, Macphail Papers. Also see, for examples, reviews in *Calgary Daily Herald*, 29 June 1925; *Montreal Witness*, 15 July 1925; *Brockville Recorder and Times*, 11 July 1925, all in Macphail Papers.

36 Review in *Canada Lancet and Practitioner*, Sept. 1925, Macphail Papers. For more in a similar vein, see H.A. Bruce, *Varied Operations*, 90. Although not in such an *ad hominem* manner, highly critical views were also expressed by both editor and reviewer in *Willisons Monthly* 1 (Aug. 1925): 81, and 1 (Sept. 1925): 130–2. The reviewer at least conceded that "no [political] party can gain any advantage from this amazing volume" (130). For the contrary view concerning Macphail's partiality or impartiality, see reviews in Toronto *Globe*, 11 July 1925, and *Canadian Medical Association Journal*, Nov. 1925, Macphail Papers.

37 Press cutting from *Manitoba Free Press*, 4 Jan. 1926, Macphail Papers. Also see press cuttings from Montreal *Gazette*, 16 July 1925; *Montreal Star*, 17 July 1925, McGill University Scrapbooks 6, 40, MUA; Wilfrid Bovey, "Macphail's Book," *McGill News* 6 (Sept. 1925): 8–10.

38 *Canadian Historical Review* 6 (Sept. 1925): 261 (sequence altered), review by Ryerson. Also see 260, 262.

39 Bumsted, "Historical Writing in English," 353

40 Humphries, "The Horror at Home: The Canadian Military and the 'Great' Influenza Pandemic of 1918," 239. Humphries's conclusion is that the Canadian pandemic can be accounted for initially by contact with American soldiers heading overseas late in the war, and then by the movement of Canadian soldiers across the country in support of the intervention in Siberia.

41 Vance, *Death So Noble*, 75

42 Cook, *Clio's Warriors*, 8, 55

43 Campbell, "Politics, Polemics, and the Boundaries of Personal Experience," 6

44 Ibid., 6-7

45 Cook has also noted the contrast between the approaches of the two men.
    Thus, as well as Campbell (e.g., 7, 15n17), see Cook "'Literary Memorials':
    The Great War Regimental Histories, 1919–1939," 173n26.

46 See Campbell, "Politics, Polemics, and the Boundaries of Personal
    Experience," 7–8, 11.

47 See ibid., 2, 11; Higham, ed., *Official Histories*; A. Fortescue Duguid, preface
    to Macphail, *Official History*, v.

48 Campbell, "Politics, Polemics, and the Boundaries of Personal Experience,"
    17–31

49 Macphail to Currie, 24 March 1933, Currie Papers, LAC. Or, in Macphail,
    "The Reading of History," offprint from *Canadian Medical Association
    Journal* 29 (Dec. 1933): 664–71, pp. 1–2: "Soldiers and politicians make cam-
    paigns; but it is the historians who make the history of them."

50 Macphail, *Three Persons*, Preface to the third edition, 8. All page references
    are to this edition.

51 John Murray to Macphail, 19, 25 Feb., 1 March 1929, Macphail Papers. The
    Lawrence essay was also to have appeared in the *Quarterly Review*, but once
    Murray had accepted the book for publication he persuaded Macphail
    to withdraw it in order to preserve the freshness of the collection. See Sir
    John Murray to Macphail, 4 July 1928; Macphail to Sir John Murray, 15 Aug.
    1928, Sir John Murray (1884–1967) Papers (in private possession). There
    were two "Sir John Murrays" in the twentieth century; their dates were
    1851–1928 and 1884–1967. The younger was known as Col. John Murray at
    this time and will be referred to simply as "John Murray"; except where
    otherwise specified, "Sir John Murray" refers to the elder. The publishing
    house was established in 1768 and folded into a large publishing group in
    2002; information courtesy of Virginia Murray (via fax), 7 March 2005.

52 Although Keith Jeffery, the author of the most recent (2006) study of
    Wilson, *Field Marshal Sir Henry Wilson: A Political Soldier*, is sympathetic to
    his subject, the subtitle is significant.

53 Macphail, *Three Persons*, 135. Also see 54, 147; Macphail, "Sir Henry Wilson,"
    Quarterly Review 251 (July 1928): 20–1, 24–33, 38–9, 45–8. The essay that
    appeared in the book was a revised and expanded version of the *Quarterly
    Review* article.

54 Macphail, *Three Persons*, 143. Also see 144–5; Macphail, "Sir Henry Wilson,"
    Quarterly Review 251 (July 1928): 22, 36–41, 44–6, 48.

55 Ibid., 41

56 See Macphail, *Three Persons*, 62–3; Macphail, "The Goat and the Vine,"
    *Empire Club of Canada: Addresses Delivered to the Members during the Year
    1934–35*, 164.

57 Macphail, "Sir Henry Wilson," *Quarterly Review* 251 (July 1928): 50, 45; also
    see 51.

58 Ibid., 48; also see 46, 47, 49, 50.

59 Beaverbrook to Macphail, 25 July 1928, Beaverbrook Papers, BL. Borden was

another who had formed an extremely unflattering impression of Wilson's character and capacities; see Borden and Macquarrie, eds., *Robert Laird Borden: His Memoirs*, 2: 13–40.

60   See Kipling to Macphail, 9 June 1930, Kipling-Macphail volume, Macphail Papers.

61   Press cutting from *New York Times*, n.d. [July 1928], Sir John Murray (1884–1967) Papers.

62   See Macphail, "Sir Henry Wilson," *Quarterly Review* 251 (July 1928): 23–6, 45–9; Macphail, *Three Persons*, 32–7, 61–4, 94, 116–17; Macphail, "Hindenburg," *Queen's Quarterly* 41 (Winter 1934–35): 442.

63   Macphail to Beaverbrook, 15 Aug. 1928, Beaverbrook Papers, BL. Beaverbrook's candid opinions of Lawrence and House appear in his reply to Macphail, 27 Aug. 1928, Beaverbrook Papers, BL.

64   Macphail, *Three Persons*, 162; also see 277.

65   Ibid., 163–4, 169–70; also see 171–4, 219–20, 240–1, 245, 247.

66   Ibid., 286; also see 290–300, 306–10.

67   Ibid., 321

68   Ibid., 309, 326, 328–9

69   Ibid., 310. Also see Macphail to Beaverbrook, 20 Nov. 1934, Beaverbrook Papers, BL.

70   See Macphail, *Three Persons*, 328–36, 316–17.

71   Macphail to Beaverbrook, 3 July 1932, Beaverbrook Papers, BL. See Edgar, "Sir Andrew Macphail (1864–1938)," *Transactions* of the Royal Society of Canada, 3rd series, 33 (1939): 147, 149; the comments by the British press cited in obituary to Macphail, Charlottetown *Patriot*, 24 Sept. 1938.

72   See Macphail, "Sir Arthur Currie: The Value of a Degree," *Queen's Quarterly* 41 (Spring 1934): 1–19; Macphail, "Hindenburg," *Queen's Quarterly* 41 (Winter 1934–35), 433–52; Macphail, "Robert Edward Lee," *Queen's Quarterly* 45 (Spring 1938): 1–10.

73   The reviews are in *Canadian Defence Quarterly* 9 (Jan. 1932): 282–3; *McGill News* 18 (Winter 1936): 34–5. Also see Macphail's obituary to Currie in *Transactions* of the Royal Society of Canada, 3rd series, 28 (1934): 12–14; Macphail, "Armistice Day 1933," *McGill News* 15 (Dec. 1933): 39–42.

74   Stevenson, "Sir Andrew Macphail," *Canadian Defence Quarterly* 16 (Jan. 1939): 208

75   Berger, *The Sense of Power*, 47

76   See Macphail to Strachey, 10 March 1909, Macphail Papers.

77   See entry for 14 Dec. 1915, War Diaries 1, Macphail Papers; entry for 25 Sept. 1917, War Diaries 3, Macphail Papers.

78   Macphail, "Sir Arthur Currie: The Value of a Degree," 14–15. Also see Macphail, untitled manuscript on "Best Work and Why," n.d. [1929], Macphail Papers. At one point Macphail expressed the desire to write a *Quarterly Review* essay on Rawlinson, but John Murray dissuaded him on the grounds of the subject's unimportance. See Macphail to John Murray,

1 March 1929, Sir John Murray (1884–1967) Papers; John Murray to Macphail, 14 March 1929, Macphail Papers.

79　Macphail, "Robert Edward Lee," 3; also see 2, 6, 7, 10.

80　See Macphail, "Sir Arthur Currie: The Value of a Degree," 11–14.

81　Stevenson, "Sir Andrew Macphail," *Canadian Defence Quarterly* 16 (Jan. 1939): 208. It is possible that Stevenson's misconception arose in part from his being a considerably younger man, who would have known Macphail better after than before the war; yet they had been at least acquainted as early as 1911, since they were allies on the reciprocity issue. See Macphail to Grey, 15 April 1911, Grey Papers, UD; Stevenson to Macphail, 28 July 1911, Macphail Papers; interview with Stevenson, 19 May 1968.

82　See Macphail, "The Navy and Politics," *University Magazine* 12 (Feb. 1913): 1–22; Macphail, *Three Persons*, Preface, 5, 8; Macphail, "Sir Arthur Currie: The Value of a Degree," 1–2; Macphail, "The Goat and the Vine," *Empire Club of Canada: Addresses ... 1934–35*, 161–72; Macphail, "Woman of Moscow," *Saturday Night*, 5 Oct. 1935; Beaverbrook to Macphail, 25 Dec. 1934; Macphail to Beaverbrook, 14 Jan. 1935, Macphail Papers.

83　Macphail, "Conservative – Liberal – Socialist," *University of Toronto Quarterly* 3 (April 1934): 263

84　Ibid., 281; also see 265.

85　Ibid., 283. Also see 267–8; Macphail, "Government by Party," *Canadian Century*, 15 Oct. 1910, 16.

86　Macphail, "Conservative – Liberal – Socialist," 269 [original emphasis]; also see 268, 278.

87　Ibid., 284–5

88　Ibid., 281.

89　Macphail to McKenzie, 5 June 1935, McKenzie Papers, UPA [original emphasis]

90　Macphail, "Woman of Moscow," *Saturday Night*, 5 Oct. 1935

91　Ibid. Also see interview with Macphail, press cutting from London *Daily Express*, 24 July 1935; Macphail to Howard Murray, 7 July 1935, Macphail-Murray Scrapbooks 1, Macphail Papers; Macphail to Mrs Dorothy Lindsay, 7 July 1935, Lindsay-Macphail Scrapbooks 2, Macphail Papers.

92　Macphail, "Woman of Leningrad," *Saturday Night*, 24 Aug. 1935

93　Ibid. Also see Macphail to Howard Murray, 7 July 1935, Macphail-Murray Scrapbooks 1, Macphail Papers.

94　See Macphail, "Woman of Moscow."

95　Macphail to Howard Murray, 7 July 1935, Macphail-Murray Scrapbooks 1, Macphail Papers. Also see Macphail to Mrs Dorothy Lindsay, 7 July 1935, Lindsay-Macphail Scrapbooks 2, Macphail Papers.

96　Interview with Macphail, press cutting from London *Daily Express*, 24 July 1935, Macphail-Murray Scrapbooks 1, Macphail Papers. This interview provoked intemperate criticism; see Meriel Buchanan, "The Peregrinations of a Professor," *Saturday Review* [London], 10 Aug. 1935, 9–10.

97 "Beth" [Bethune] to "Pony" [Marian Scott], 8 Oct. 1935, "Bethune Material, 1924-42," OL. Cited with the permission of Dr Norman Bethune Allan.

98 Press cutting from Montreal *Gazette*, 19 Feb. 1936, McGill University Scrapbooks 8, 362, MUA

99 Macphail, "Woman of Leningrad." Also see Macphail, *The Bible in Scotland*, 125; Macphail, "Women in Democracy," *University Magazine* 19 (Feb. 1920): 7–8; Macphail, "Art in Democracy," *Dalhousie Review* 4 (July 1924): 172; Laqueur, *The Fate of the Revolution*, 8–12, 60–1. Although a letter of intro-duction on Macphail's behalf to the American minister in St Petersburg, dated 6 April 1891, survives in Lindsay-Macphail Scrapbooks 1, Macphail Papers, there is no indication that he used it on his world trip of that year; and in no other part of the Papers is there any suggestion of a trip to Russia before 1935.

100 Macphail, "Woman of Moscow." Also see Macphail, "Woman of Leningrad."

101 Macphail, "In Retrospect: Armistice Day," an address delivered to the Maritime Officers' Reunion in Saint John, NB, 11 Nov. 1936, 8. Also see Macphail, "Woman of Moscow"; interview with Macphail, press cutting from *Montreal Star*, 6 Aug. 1935, Lindsay-Macphail Scrapbooks 2, Macphail Papers.

102 Interview with Macphail, press cutting from London *Daily Express*, 24 July 1935, Macphail-Murray Scrapbooks 1, Macphail Papers. Also see Stevenson, "Sir Andrew Macphail," *Canadian Defence Quarterly* 16 (Jan. 1939): 209.

103 Alexander Macphail to Macphail, 2 Aug. 1935, Macphail Papers. Also see Alexander Macphail to Macphail, 10 Aug. 1935. For a similar response to Russia in the same year by a distinguished British intellectual with a value system much like that of Macphail, see Moran, "Wittgenstein and Russia," 85–96.

104 See, for example, the writings of Horowitz: "Conservatism, Liberalism, and Socialism in Canada: An Interpretation," 158–9, and "Tories, Socialists, and the Demise of Canada," 12–15.

105 See Leacock, *The Unsolved Riddle of Social Justice*; King, *Industry and Humanity*; and Ferns, "The Ideas of Mackenzie King," 11.

106 Shortt, *The Search for an Ideal*, 29–30

107 See, for example, Macphail, "Family and Society," *Quarterly Review* 268 (April 1937): 220–1, 224; Macphail, "The Inward Light," unpublished frag-ment, n.d. [*ca.* 1908], 5, Macphail Papers: "A duty to the state which would injure the family is not a duty."

108 Leacock, "Andrew Macphail," *Queen's Quarterly* 45 (Winter 1938): 452

CHAPTER TWELVE

1 Sisler, *Passionate Spirits*, 87. Also see 163. For a portrait of Dyonnet, *ca.* 1922, by G. Horne Russell, also a member of the Pen and Pencil Club and an ally of Dyonnet, which conveys well his personality as described by Sisler, see Hill, *The Group of Seven*, 131; also see 307.

2   See entries for 8 Jan. 1921, 9 Dec. 1922, Pen and Pencil Club Minutes, vol. 3, 197, 227, MMCH. Regarding the Arts Club, see Cox, *Portrait of a Club*.

3   See entry for 13 Oct. 1928, Pen and Pencil Club Minutes, vol. 3, 290, MMCH.

4   Entry for 13 Dec. 1919, 170

5   See entries for 27 Dec. 1919, 20 March 1920, 172, 182–3.

6   See entries for 5, 19 Feb. 1927, 278–9.

7   Macphail to Sinclair Ross, 27 Jan. 1936, Sinclair Ross Papers, LAC

8   It is not known whether the controversial menu cards survive. There is a menu card for 1924, M982.525.15, at the MMCH, with an illustration featuring a clam digger, and it appears unlikely, on the face of it, that this caused contention. In some instances more than one menu card for the same year survive; for example, different menu cards for 1908 can be found at the MMCH and in the Confederation Centre Art Gallery, Charlottetown.

9   Regarding Nobbs's temperament, see the following in Collard, ed., *The McGill You Knew*, 213–14: J. Kenneth Nesbitt, "Percy Nobbs: A Genius but Irascible," 213; John Bland, "Percy Nobbs: Superb but So Explosive," 213–14 (the quotation comes from Bland and appears on 213); see also Wagg, *Percy Erskine Nobbs*, 23–4.

10 See entries for 3 May, 1 Nov., 20 Dec. 1924, Pen and Pencil Club Minutes, vol. 3, 250, 251, 253–4, MMCH.

11 See Macphail, "Design," *Queen's Quarterly* 44 (Spring 1937): 28–35; Macphail, "Origins," *Quarterly Review* 265 (Oct. 1935): 189–98; Macphail, "Family and Society," *Quarterly Review* 268 (April 1937): 214–24; Macphail, "A History of the Idea of Evolution," *Dalhousie Review* 5 (April 1925): 22–32.

12 See Macphail, "Sir William Van Horne," *Canadian Bookman*, new series, 3 (June 1921): 30–2; Macphail, "Sir Sandford Fleming," *Queen's Quarterly* 36 (Spring 1929): 185–204.

13 Leacock, "Andrew Macphail," *Queen's Quarterly* 45 (Winter 1938): 447. See Macphail, *The Bible in Scotland*; Macphail, "The Bible in Scotland," *Quarterly Review* 257 (July 1931), 15–36. As an alternative to publication of the book, Macphail had suggested a collection of four of his *Quarterly Review* essays under the title "Four Quarters." Besides "The Bible in Scotland" and the Boswell article, it would have included "The Freedom of England," *Quarterly Review* 255 (July 1930): 1–16, and "The Burden of the Stuarts," *Quarterly Review* 255 (April 1930): 218–29. The last mentioned was a medical history of the Stuart family. See Macphail to John Murray, 2, 25 March 1931; John Murray to Macphail, 13 March, 8 April (letter and cable of the same date) 1931, Sir John Murray (1884-1967) Papers. Another idea for a book that did not materialize is contained in Macphail to Pierce, 28 Oct. 1923, Pierce Papers, QUL.

14 Macphail to John Murray, 8 April 1931, Sir John Murray (1884–1967) Papers

15 Macphail, "The Bible in Scotland," *Quarterly Review* 257 (July 1931): 25, 35. Also see, for example, 16, 22, 24; Macphail to John Murray, 16 Dec. 1930, Sir John Murray (1884-1967) Papers.

16 Macphail to John Murray, 10 March 1932, Sir John Murray (1884–1967) Papers. Also see John Murray to Macphail, 8 April 1931 (letter), 19 Feb., 21 March 1932, Sir John Murray (1884–1967) Papers. Throughout *The Bible in Scotland*, Macphail argued from precisely the theological position he had developed in "The Fallacy in Theology." The book was reviewed favourably in the Edinburgh *Evening News*, 6 [or 8] Dec. 1931, and unfavourably in the Edinburgh *Scotsman*, 23 Nov. 1931; *Times Literary Supplement*, 10 Dec. 1931; Montreal *Gazette*, 24 Oct. 1931, by "J.S." A response by a teacher who had used the syllabus appeared in the *Scottish Educational Journal*, 6 Nov. 1931, p. 1215: "The 'Syllabus' in Use: A Defence," by J.A. Russell (press cutting in Macphail Papers).

17 Macphail, untitled manuscript on "Best Work and Why," n.d. [1929], Macphail Papers

18 Macphail, "Johnson's Life of Boswell," *Quarterly Review* 253 (July 1929): 43–4; also see 56, 59–60.

19 Ibid., 54; also see 53, 56, 61–2.

20 Ibid., 58; also see 56–7.

21 Ibid., 57

22 Ibid., 43, 54, 61, 63-5, 67-73. Not all Boswell scholars were won over by Macphail's defence; see Macphail to Howard Murray, 6 Oct. 1930, Macphail-Murray Scrapbooks 1, Macphail Papers.

23 Edgar, "Sir Andrew Macphail," *Queen's Quarterly* 54 (Spring 1947): 8. Also see Macphail, "The American Novel," Montreal *Gazette*, 17 Nov. 1922.

24 Edgar, "Sir Andrew Macphail," 8

25 Macphail, "Sir Gilbert Parker: An Appraisal," *Transactions* of the Royal Society of Canada, 3rd series, 33, section 2 (1939): 123; also see 127. Although not published until after Macphail's death, this essay was to have appeared in the early 1920s as an introduction to a reprint of Parker's *Pierre and His People*, a plan that aborted. In 1909 he had taken a similar position; see *Essays in Politics*, 245–6.

26 Macphail, "In Memoriam: William E. Marshall," *Dalhousie Review* 3 (July 1923): 153. Also see 152; Macphail, "Introduction" to Crichton, *A Vista*, v; Macphail, "News-Value in Literature," *Montreal Star*, 1 Nov. 1930; Macphail, "Our Canadian Speech," *McGill News* 14 (Dec. 1932): 28.

27 Interview with Mrs Dorothy Lindsay, 28 Aug. 1970

28 See press cutting from Montreal *Gazette*, 21 May 1931, Macphail Papers; Macphail to Cyrus Macmillan, 16 May 1932, Cyrus Macmillan Papers, MUA. For both of these plays, see bound volume of plays, mostly unpublished, in Macphail Papers.

29 See Macphail, "The Last Rising: A Melodrama," *Queen's Quarterly* 37 (Spring 1930): 246–58; *cf.* Macphail, *The Master's Wife*, 228 ff. The other two acts are contained in the bound volume of plays in the Macphail Papers; the wartime developments in Acts 2 and 3 are imaginary. Also *cf. The Master's Wife*, 189 ff., and Macphail, "The New House," *Saturday Night*, 12 June 1937.

30 See bound volume of plays, Macphail Papers; Macphail, "Our Canadian Speech," *McGill News* 14 (Dec. 1932): 28.

31 For example, cf. Macphail, "The Four Musicians," *Saturday Night*, 1 Feb. 1936, and Macphail, *The Master's Wife*, 210 ff. Macphail's dark thoughts on the contemporary state of the genre are in "The Short Story," *Quarterly Review* 258 (July 1934): 16–28. His brother Alexander fully agreed; see Alexander Macphail to Macphail, n.d. [1934], Macphail Papers.

32 Macphail, "The Graduate," *Queen's Quarterly* 39 (Aug. 1932): 377–91. Earlier drafts, entitled "The Moonshiner" and "The Drunkard," are in the Macphail Papers. For one of Macphail's best received short stories, see "A Pair of Brogues," *Saturday Night*, 21 Dec. 1935.

33 Macphail, "The Hand or the Book," *Dalhousie Review* 6 (July 1926): 218; also see 219.

34 Ibid., 219

35 Ibid., 220

36 Macphail to McKenzie, 26 May 1933, McKenzie Papers, UPA. The Canadian Guild of Crafts Quebec has now moved to Sherbrooke St West, almost as far west as Guy/Cote des Neiges, but as late as February 2000 it could still be found on Peel Street more or less directly across from where Macphail had resided.

37 Macphail, "Art in Democracy," *Dalhousie Review* 4 (July 1924): 173; also see 174.

38 Ibid., 172. Also see 173, 177, 178; Macphail, "The American Novel," Montreal *Gazette*, 17 Nov. 1922; Macphail, "The Short Story," *Quarterly Review* 263 (July 1934): 19.

39 Macphail, "Art in Democracy," 175; also see 179.

40 See Macphail, "Women in Democracy," *University Magazine* 19 (Feb. 1920): 8–10.

41 Macphail, "Art in Democracy," 176

42 Press cutting from Charlottetown *Patriot*, n.d. [*ca.* 18 July 1938], Macphail-Murray Scrapbooks 2, Macphail Papers. Also see Leacock, "Andrew Macphail," *Queen's Quarterly* 45 (Winter 1938): 451–2; obituaries to Macphail in Charlottetown *Guardian*, 24 Sept. 1938, and Charlottetown *Patriot*, 24 Sept. 1938.

43 Interview with Mrs Dorothy Lindsay, 30 May 1968; Macphail, *The Master's Wife*, 108

44 An address on weaving by Mrs Dorothy Lindsay to the Women's Institute in Orwell, PEI, *ca.* 1927, 10, in personal possession of the author.

45 Mrs Dorothy Lindsay to the author, 17 Nov. 1979, in personal possession of the author

46 Macphail, "Our Canadian Speech," *McGill News* 14 (Dec. 1932): 28

47 See Macphail, "Our Canadian Speech," *Saturday Night*, 29 June 1935. According to John A. Stevenson, Macphail would allow no radio in his house; see "Sir Andrew Macphail," *Canadian Defence Quarterly* 16 (Jan.

1939): 210. In Macphail's posthumously published memoir he acknowledged one use for the radio: to "turn [it] on ... when ... visitors threaten to become tiresome" (Macphail, *The Master's Wife*, 60).

48 Macphail, "A History of the Idea of Evolution," *Dalhousie Review* 5 (April 1925): 27

49 Macphail, "The Senses and the Mind," draft radio address, intended for broadcast 24 Nov. 1933, first page, in personal possession of author. This draft, with erratic page numbering and some pages in fragments, survived in the Macphail Papers and came to light in 1974. The copy used for the present study was provided through the courtesy of Mrs Dorothy Lindsay. Also see press cutting from *McGill Daily*, 27 Nov. 1933, Macphail Papers.

50 Macphail, "Art in Democracy," 174; also interview with Mrs Dorothy Lindsay, 26 July 1970.

51 The way he had put it on one occasion was: "I find my French quite adequate for all ordinary purposes." Entry for 1 Nov. 1916, War Diaries 2, Macphail Papers. But also see Macphail, "Our Canadian Speech," *McGill News* 14 (Dec. 1932): 27; Macphail, "Woman of Danzig," *Saturday Night*, 17 Aug. 1935.

52 Entry for 8 Jan. 1921, Pen and Pencil Club Minutes, vol. 3, 197, MMCH

53 Macphail to MacMechan, 8 Jan. 1921, MacMechan Papers, DUA

54 Louis Hémon, *Maria Chapdelaine: A Romance of French Canada* [trans. Macphail], 211; also see 107, 207, 212, 213.

55 Macphail, "Art in Democracy," 174.

56 See Hamer, "William Hume Blake"; Macphail to M.J. Montgomery, 11 Jan. 1938, Macphail Papers.

57 See Boivin, "Louis Hémon, *DCB* 14: 475. Since 1984 the permanent collection of the National Gallery of Canada has contained a bust of *Maria Chapdelaine* (1925) by Suzor-Coté.

58 See the Pearce Photographic Albums, MP-1994.64.1 and MP-1994.64.2, MMCH. I thank Senior Cataloguer Nora Hague for bringing these to my attention.

59 For an account of the failed collaboration and the complicated publication history, which involved questions of confused copyright, see Whiteman, "The Publication of *Maria Chapdelaine* in English," 52–9. Also see "Statement of Account," 12 June 1924, between Macphail and A.T. Chapman, the publisher of his translation, Macphail Papers; Surveyer, "Maria Chapdelaine"; and two anonymous articles: "The Three Sisters Chapdelaine," *Canadian Bookman*, new series, 4 (Dec. 1921): 7–8, and "The Two Translations and the Original," *Canadian Bookman*, new series, 4 (Dec. 1921): 8–10.

60 Macphail to Beaverbrook, 30 May 1921, Beaverbrook Papers, BL.

61 Toker, *The Church of Notre-Dame in Montreal*, 59

62 See Lambert, "Foreword," in Gournay and Vanlaethem, eds., *Montreal Metropolis*, 6–7. This was about ten minutes' walk southeast from Beaver

Hall Terrace, where Macphail had his first lodgings in Montreal. As Lambert observes, the competition between religion and commerce was also played out on Dominion Square (named as such in 1872 but renamed Dorchester Square in 1987).

63　Linteau, "Factors in the Development of Montreal," 27

64　Notes taken at the "Montréal Métropole, 1880–1930" exhibition, National Gallery of Canada, Ottawa, 21 Jan. 1999.

65　For a graphic reminder of how great the change from earlier years was, note the dominance of Notre Dame Church in two sketches by William Henry Bartlett, drawn from the perspectives of the St Lawrence River and of Mount Royal, in 1838; [Campbell and Tyrwhitt], *Bartlett's Canada*, 176–7. Bartlett's Montreal has one great building distinguishing the skyline, and by the early twentieth century that church was almost lost among the towers of commerce.

66　Macphail, "American Methods in Medical Education," offprint from *British Medical Journal*, 3 Sept. 1927, 10. Also see 1–8, 19, 21; Macphail, "The Poor Boy," *Saturday Night*, 21 May 1910; Macphail, "The Healing of a Wound," *Quarterly Review* 262 (Jan. 1934): 123.

67　Macphail, "American Methods in Medical Education," 11

68　Ibid., 8

69　Ibid., 9; also see 4, 12–14.

70　Ibid., 3–4. For a more positive reading of the Flexner Report in relation to Dalhousie, and an understanding of the background, see Waite, *The Lives of Dalhousie University*, vol. 1, 164–8, 202–03, and *The Lives of Dalhousie University*, vol. 2, 23–4.

71　Press cutting from Kingston *Standard*, 20 Nov. 1926, Macphail Papers. Connell clearly shared Macphail's perspective. Upon reading a draft of the "American Methods" address, he stated that on one point Macphail had mistakenly given too much credit to American influences: "Our natural development was really arrested by the foreign inspection." "J.C.C." [Connell] to Macphail, n.d. [*ca.* 1926], Macphail Papers.

72　Macphail, "American Methods in Medical Education," 22; also see 1.

73　Ibid., 18, 21-2.

74　Macphail to C.F. Martin, 18 Nov. 1926, McGill Principals' Papers, MUA

75　Blackader to Macphail, 3 March 1927, Macphail Papers. Also see Blackader to Macphail, 14 Nov. 1926; C.F. Martin to Macphail, 17, 19 Nov., 4 Dec. 1926; Macphail to C.F. Martin, 18 Nov. 1926; J.[?]C. Simpson to Macphail, 7 Dec. 1926; L. Lang to Macphail, 14 Feb. 1927, Macphail Papers. Whatever offence Macphail may have given to the Congress could not have been overwhelming, for its director general thanked him in writing for his "big part" in making the meeting a success; see Franklin H. Martin to Macphail, 8 Nov. 1926, Macphail Papers.

76　Mathieson to Macphail, 22 Oct. 1927, Macphail Papers. Also see Williams to Macphail, 17 Aug., 1 Sept. 1927; and, for example, William Boyd to

Macphail, 5 Oct. 1927; John Tait to Macphail, 7 Oct. 1927; H.S. Birkett to Macphail, 7 Oct. 1927, Macphail Papers.

77 Frost, *McGill* 2, 58n40

78 Ibid., 138n25

79 Ibid., 30

80 See, for example, C.F. Martin to Currie, 17 Nov. 1926, enclosing a copy of his letter of the same date to Macphail, McGill Principals' Papers, MUA.

81 See Macphail, "Sir Arthur Currie: The Value of a Degree," *Queen's Quarterly* 41 (Spring 1934): 1–19.

82 [McMurray] to "Mr. [J.W.] McConnell," 12 April 1934, McGill Principals' Papers, MUA. Regarding Dorothy McMurray, see her *Four Principals of McGill*.

83 See [McMurray], "A Defence of the Currie Principalship with Particular Reference to an Article by Sir Andrew Macphail in the Queen's Quarterly Magazine, Spring 1934," n.d. [1934]; [McMurray], "McGill during Sir Arthur Currie's Principalship, August 1920 to November 1933," n.d. [1934], McGill Principals' Papers, MUA. "A Defense ..." (9 pp.) seems to be a first draft; "McGill during ..." (14 pp.) is marked "2nd draft" and is more sharply worded.

84 McMurray to George C. McDonald, 24 April 1934, McGill Principals' Papers, MUA

85 McMurray to Macphail, 23 April 1934, McGill Principals' Papers, MUA

86 See [McMurray], "McGill during Sir Arthur Currie's Principalship, August 1920 to November 1933," n.d. [1934], 1; also see McMurray to McDonald, 28 April 1934, McGill Principals' Papers, MUA.

87 Frost, *McGill* 2, 119. Frost notes that Macphail had made somewhat similar comments concerning McGill during the era of Sir William Peterson's principalship (1895–1919); see *McGill* 2, 138n25, 58n40.

88 Frost, *McGill* 2, 138n25

89 See "Principal's Secretary" [McMurray] to E.W. Beatty, 7 April 1934; [McMurray] to McConnell, 12 April 1934; McMurray to McDonald, 24, 28 April 1934; McDonald to McMurray, 27 April 1934, McGill Principals' Papers, MUA.

90 McDonald to McMurray, 27 April 1934, McGill Principals' Papers, MUA

91 Macphail, "Sir Arthur Currie: The Value of a Degree," 10

92 Extract from *Canadian Forum*, Sept. 1934, retyped, McGill Principals' Papers, MUA

93 See press cutting from Montreal *Gazette*, 15 April 1937, Macphail-Murray Scrapbooks 2, Macphail Papers; press cutting from *Montreal Star*, 14 April 1937, Macphail Papers.

94 Lewis W. Douglas to Macphail, 25 March 1938; unsigned comment, n.d. [25 March 1938 or later in 1938], McGill Principals' Papers, MUA

95 Leacock, "Andrew Macphail," *Queen's Quarterly* 45 (Winter 1938): 452

96   Stevenson, "Sir Andrew Macphail," *Canadian Defence Quarterly* 16 (Jan.
     1939): 209
97   Katherine Dewar Interviews, interview with the Rev. Harvey Bishop (audio
     tape), 6 Aug. 1990
98   Interview with Mrs Dorothy Lindsay, 26 July 1970; Macphail to McKenzie,
     3, 14, 21 Feb., 3 March, 6 April 1933, McKenzie Papers, UPA.
99   Samuel Morgan-Powell in *The Cue* 8 (Oct. 1938): 2 in Macphail-Murray
     Scrapbooks 2, Macphail Papers. The same critic published a brief poem
     honouring Macphail's memory shortly after his death. It appeared in
     the *Montreal Star*, 26 Sept. 1938; found inside a specially bound copy of
     Macphail, *The Master's Wife*, in Macphail Papers. See Hathorn, "Samuel
     Morgan-Powell," 348–9.
100 Whittaker, *Setting the Stage*, 74
101 Whittaker, "Montreal Repertory Theatre," 346. Also see Whittaker, *Setting
     the Stage*, 74.
102 As cited in Whittaker, *Setting the Stage*, 147.
103 Macphail to Ross, 27 Jan. 1936, Ross Papers, LAC
104 Macphail to Ross, 10 Feb. 1936, Ross Papers, LAC
105 See John W. Garvin to Macphail, 3, 15 Feb. 1923, 15 Nov. 1926, Macphail
     Papers.
106 See Macphail, "Sir Gilbert Parker: An Appraisal," *Transactions* of the Royal
     Society of Canada, 3rd series, 33, section 2 (1939): 123–35.
107 See Pierce to Macphail, 29 Sept. 1923, 8, 13 Feb. 1924; Macphail to Pierce, 10
     Feb. 1924, Macphail Papers; Macphail to Pierce, 28 Oct. 1923, 12 Jan., 14, 26
     Feb. 1924, Pierce Papers, QUL.
108 Macphail to C.F. Martin, 19 Aug. 1938, C.F. Martin Papers, OL. Also letter
     from Mrs Dorothy Lindsay to author, dated 14 Aug. [1973], in author's pos-
     session.
109 The house at 216 Peel Street has long since disappeared. It was renumbered
     2016 while Macphail was still living, the new number being a compromise
     after his protests over the initial plan which, as part of a general scheme for
     renumbering addresses, would have given it a number totally dissimilar
     to the old one. The Lindsay family rented it out until they sold it after the
     Second World War. Interviews with Mrs Dorothy Lindsay, 10, 21 July 1970.
110 Leacock, "Andrew Macphail," *Queen's Quarterly* 45 (Winter 1938): 452
111 Interview with Mrs Dorothy Lindsay, 9 Sept. 1970

CHAPTER THIRTEEN

1   Macphail, *The Master's Wife*, 20
2   Ibid., 48
3   Ibid., 204
4   Katherine Dewar Interviews, interview with Katie Martin (audio tape), 23
     July 1990, in private possession

5   Katherine Dewar Interviews, interview with Marguerite (Meg) Stanley, granddaughter (audio tape), 18 July 1990
6   Macphail, *The Master's Wife*, 212
7   Ibid., 102
8   Ibid., 3
9   Macqueen to Macphail, 16 Feb. 1933, Macphail Papers
10 The peddlers would probably have been Lebanese; see Weale, *A Stream Out of Lebanon*.
11 Macphail, *The Master's Wife*, 2
12 *Le Devoir*, 3 Feb. 1940: "This book contains an entire philosophy of life. It would be relatively easy to extract from it a whole series of profound thoughts which reads as maxims. One feels that the author has condensed in it the results of his experience of the world and of men."
13 Macphail, *The Master's Wife*, 105–6. Johannes Vermeer, a seventeenth-century Dutch painter, was a perfectionist who had a limited output; but almost all of his works were masterpieces.
14 Macphail, *The Master's Wife*, 206
15 Ibid., 202
16 Ibid., 49-51. In 1970 the present author found in the Macphail Papers an unpublished short story on the murder, which was published later with an introduction by himself: Macphail, "The Traveller," *Island Magazine*, 3 (Fall–Winter 1977), 26–7 (introduction by Robertson) and 27–30 (text). It is a semi-fictional first-person account about a traveller who learns of the murder when passing through Orwell on a Sabbath a number of years after the event. The local family that invites the stranger to share the midday meal is clearly that of Andrew's parents. Also see Campbell and Campbell, "The Murder at Goblin Hollow," 32–5. The Campbells write that the murder, which occurred in 1859, "has haunted [the] community for over a hundred years" (34). A previously unpublished ballad – "The Ballad of Ann Beaton" – by Donald Lamont of Orwell Rear refers to the victim, apparently an unwed mother about forty-one years of age, as follows: "light was her way" (32; the six stanzas of five lines each are reproduced on this page, transcribed based on oral tradition). Macphail's mother was known to comment that Beaton was "no better than she should have been"; interview with Mrs Dorothy Lindsay, 30 June 1970. Both Murdoch Lamont (brother of Donald, the author of an article on the murder published in 1902), and the Campbells thought it most likely that the perpetrator was "a jealous wife," angry because of a liaison with her husband (35). As the Campbells remark, "The uncertainty generated by the knowledge that a murderer lurked in the settlement created a great uneasiness among the people" (34).
17 Macphail, *The Master's Wife*, 49
18 Ibid., 160
19 Ibid., 167

20   Ibid., 179

21   Ibid., 181

22   Ibid., 186

23   Macphail to McKenzie, 10 March 1927, McKenzie Papers, UPA. In the published book Macphail refers to McKenzie as "a companion, yet inseparable" (Macphail, *The Master's Wife*, 188). McKenzie had visited him in Orwell in the company of Jongers. One calculation in the text indicates that 1927 was the date of a draft: he writes that his paternal grandfather, who passed away in 1852, "died seventy-five years ago" (Macphail, *The Master's Wife*, 26).

24   Macphail to McKenzie, 1 Feb. 1927, McKenzie Papers, UPA. The bust was exhibited at a meeting of the Pen and Pencil Club on 5 March 1927 and is now part of the collection of the Confederation Centre Art Gallery and Museum, Charlottetown. See entry for 5 March 1927, Pen and Pencil Club Minutes, 3, 279, MMCH. An excellent photograph of the bust is included in the catalogue resulting from an exhibition of Hébert's works at the Musée du Québec, Quebec City, 5 Oct. 2000 – 7 Jan. 2001; see Brooke, *Henri Hébert, 1884–1950*, 164–6.

25   Montreal *Gazette*, 3 Oct. 1945, as quoted in MacDonald, *A Dictionary of Canadian Artists*, 3: 580. Jongers's portrait of Macphail was donated to the Macphail Homestead historic site, Orwell, PEI, in July 2000. The group was closely interrelated; in 1926 Hébert had shown Pen and Pencil members photographs of a bust of Jongers that he had recently completed and that is now part of the collection of the National Gallery of Canada, Ottawa. See entry for 9 Jan. 1926, Pen and Pencil Club Minutes, vol. 3, 266–7, MMCH. A striking photograph of the Jongers bust is included in Brooke, *Henri Hébert, 1884–1950*, 147.

26   Macphail, untitled manuscript on "Best Work and Why," n.d. [1929], Macphail Papers

27   Interview with Mrs. Dorothy Lindsay, 30 May 1968; also see Macphail, *The Master's Wife*, 139, 246.

28   Interview with Mrs Dorothy Lindsay, 21 July 1970

29   [Macphail], "Style in Medical Writing," *Canadian Medical Association Journal* 1 (Jan. 1911): 70

30   Macphail, *The Master's Wife*, 25; also see 66–7, 72, 116–17

31   Interview with W.M. Martin, 17 Feb. 2000

32   Macphail, *The Master's Wife*, 170

33   Ibid., 186

34   Leacock, "Andrew Macphail," *Queen's Quarterly* 45 (Winter 1938): 452

35   See, for example, Fingard, "The 1880s: Paradoxes of Progress," 107, and Davies, "Maritimes, Writing in the: 4," 736, both of whom describe the book as a "novel"; or "Macphail, Sir John Andrew," in New, ed., *Encyclopedia of Literature in Canada*, 696, where *The Master's Wife* is referred to as the work of Macphail "as a novelist"; or MacDonald, *If You're Stronghearted*, 47, where the book is described as "thinly fictionalized." The

standard definition of "novel" begins with the words "Fictitious prose narrative" (*The Concise Oxford Dictionary of Current English*, 6th edn. [1976], 746) or "an invented prose narrative" (*Webster's New Collegiate Dictionary* [1975], 786). The words "fictitious," "invented," and synonyms of them are intrinsic to the concept of a novel, and *The Master's Wife* is neither fictitious nor invented.

36 Macphail, *The Master's Wife*, 65
37 Kulyk Keefer, *Under Eastern Eyes*, 52–3
38 Harvey, review of *The Master's Wife*, in *Dalhousie Review* 20 (April 1940): 125
39 Edgar, "Sir Andrew Macphail (1864-1938)," *Transactions* of the Royal Society of Canada, 3rd series, 33 (1939): 148
40 The typescripts in the William Macphail Family Papers, PARO (actually copies passed down through the family of William Matheson Macphail, a younger brother of Andrew) reveal that the broadcasts occurred on Tuesdays between 10:30 and 10:45 PM, EST, on 26 October and 7 and 21 December 1937. They were "Canadian National Broadcasts" in the *I Remember* series. They appeared in the following places: "The Old School," in Charlottetown *Patriot*, 28 Dec. 1937, and *Saturday Night*, 1 Jan. 1938; "The Old College" in *Patriot*, 3 Jan. 1938, and *Saturday Night*, 14 May 1938; "The Old University" in *McGill News* 19 (Spring 1938): 27–9, 67.
41 See Edgar, "Sir Andrew Macphail," *Queen's Quarterly* 54 (1947): 8–22. There was the occasional appreciation of it in the press; see, for example, Wilfrid Eggleston in the *Winnipeg Free Press*, 9 Sept. 1950, citing it as "classical Canadian regional literature" (press cutting in Wilfrid Eggleston Papers, LAC).
42 See Mrs Dorothy Lindsay to the author, n.d. [1970, postmarked 16 Dec.], 17 Jan., 29 March, 24 April 1971, 28 July, 17, 28 Oct., 6, 9 Dec. 1974, 1 Jan., 5 June 1975; Malcolm Ross to Mrs Dorothy Lindsay, 2 March, 1 April 1971; the author to Mrs Dorothy Lindsay, 21 Dec. 1974, 2 June 1975; the author to Ross, 15 Sept. 1975; Ross to the author, 4 Dec. 1975, in personal possession of the author. Macphail's son, Jeffrey Burland, had died in 1947.
43 See the author to Mrs Dorothy Lindsay, 6, 21 March, 11, 16 July, 12 Nov. 1977; Mrs Dorothy Lindsay to the author, 15 March, 8 April, 22 July 1977; the author to Linda McKnight of McClelland & Stewart (M&S), 16 June 1977; McKnight to the author, 5 July 1977, in personal possession of the author. The second printing occurred in 1981 after (1) the book had become unavailable (although M&S refused to admit that it was out of print), and, perhaps equally importantly, (2) another publishing house, the fledgling Ragweed Press, led by the dynamic and very capable Harry Baglole and Libby Oughton, had expressed serious interest in acquiring the rights to reprint. See the author to Mrs Dorothy Lindsay, 3, 17 Nov. 1980, 18 Feb., 17 May, 17 Sept., 18 Oct. 1981; Mrs Dorothy Lindsay to the author, 12 Nov. 1980, 2 March, 23 Sept. 1981 (with résumé, dated 23 Sept. 1981, of her contacts with M&S, 29 Jan. – 1 Sept. 1981); David McGill of M&S to Mrs Dorothy

Lindsay, 9 Feb. 1981; Mrs Dorothy Lindsay to McGill, 2 March 1981, in personal possession of the author. As though to add insult to injury, M&S, in changing the front cover, put there a photograph of a couple with no relationship to the book – an elderly couple from British Columbia! – despite the fact that relevant photographs were easily available. A third edition, in 1994, by a different publisher (but led by Baglole) placed a photograph of Macphail's mother on the cover. M&S had initially expressed interest in *The Master's Wife* in 1940; see Dorothy Macphail Lindsay to William Matheson Macphail, 28 March 1940, William Macphail Family Papers, PARO.

44 On Kulyk Keefer, a writer, and how she came to write the book, see Sanderson, "Janice Kulyk Keefer," 610–11.

45 Kulyk Keefer, *Under Eastern Eyes*, 52

46 Ibid., 268n33

47 Ibid., 49

48 Ibid., 53

49 See, for example, ibid., 37. Regarding the "Golden Age," see Robertson, "Maritimes 'Golden Age,'" 391.

50 Kulyk Keefer, *Under Eastern Eyes*, 48

51 Macphail, *The Master's Wife*, 65

52 Reid, *Six Crucial Decades*, 165. The out-migrants would of course include a disproportionate number of people in their most productive years, in terms of both economic output and fertility.

53 Kulyk Keefer, *Under Eastern Eyes*, 48, 54

54 Ibid., 49

55 Bumsted, "Historical Writing in English," 353

56 MacKinnon, "Technique in *The Master's Wife*," 68

57 MacLaine, "Crooked Signs and Shining Things: The Magic of Books in the Literature of Atlantic Canadian Islands," 37–50

58 Peter Hay, "Appreciating The Master's Wife from the Other Side of the Planet," Charlottetown *Guardian*, 18 Jan. 2002; press cutting courtesy of Professor W.M. Martin. Also see Hay, *Vandiemonian Essays*, 120. Harry Baglole, founding director of the Institute of Island Studies at the University of Prince Edward Island, brought this reference to my attention.

59 MacKinnon, "Technique in *The Master's Wife*," 71

60 Kulyk Keefer, *Under Eastern Eyes*, 49

61 MacKinnon, "Technique in *The Master's Wife*," 67

62 Ibid.

63 Jeffrey Burland Lindsay, "The Spirit," in Macphail, *The Master's Wife*, 3rd edn., viii; Harry Baglole, "Preface to the Third Edition," in Macphail, *The Master's Wife*, 3rd edn., ix–x

64 Robertson, "Sir Andrew Macphail and Orwell," *Island Magazine* 1 (Fall–Winter 1976): 4–8

65 *"Island Scotch ...": A Medley from the Scottish Tradition in Prince Edward Island*, produced by Wayne MacKinnon and others for the Caledonian Club Prince Edward Island, 1976

66 David Weale, review, *Island Magazine* 2 (Spring-Summer 1977): 47

67 They had not visited Orwell as a family since 1941, for two reasons, according to Mrs Dorothy Lindsay, Macphail's daughter: first because of the Second World War and then because the grown-up age of the Lindsay children (six in number, born at two-year intervals from 1922 to 1932) interfered; interview with Mrs Dorothy Lindsay, 13 March 1970.

68 See, for example, the author to Mrs Dorothy Lindsay, 6 June 1968, 8 Oct. 1970, 25 June 1972, 4 July 1976, 17 Feb. 1979; Mrs Dorothy Lindsay to the author, 30 July 1973, 8 July 1976, 31 March 1979; Abegweit Research Group, "Historic Resources Study of Selected Sites on Prince Edward Island," March 1976, 2–5, 18, 21–34; Sheila Larmer to the author, 22 June 1976; "The Intent of a Park Master Plan" [Sept. 1976]; all items are in personal possession of the author. The conditions of the 1961 donation are included as appendix 1 to "The Intent of a Park Master Plan"; they had not been met, as the Abegweit Research Group, commissioned by the government, concluded, and as Mrs. Lindsay reminded government planners in 1976 ("Historic Resources Study of Selected Sites on Prince Edward Island," 18; Mrs Dorothy Lindsay to the author, 8 July 1976).

69 Mrs Dorothy Lindsay to the author, 31 March 1979, in personal possession of the author

70 One of the most vocal was Etta B. Ehrlich, a summer resident who, during the late 1980s, wrote letters to politicians, civil servants, and others, and even published a poem in Macphail's honour (entitled "Save Our Pride") in the Charlottetown *Guardian* in August 1986. She displayed exceptional energy for a period and encountered much political and bureaucratic inertia and buck-passing. In the summer of 1993 Ehrlich conveyed to the present writer a substantial, albeit idiosyncratic, file of material concerning her activities on the matter. It includes a 5-page personal account, untitled, covering the years 1986–92. From the beginning, she wrote, she "was struck by the beauty, as well as the rampant decay, of the place" (1). In her words, "I began nagging everyone who would listen" (2). This file will be referred to as the Ehrlich Papers.

71 For alarm at the state of the property as expressed by one of Macphail's nieces, see Catherine Lockhart to Ehrlich, 4 Aug. 1986, Ehrlich Papers, in personal possession of the author.

72 Press cutting from Charlottetown *Guardian*, 17 [?] Aug. 1988, Ehrlich Papers

73 Press cutting from Charlottetown *Guardian*, n.d. [1988], Ehrlich Papers

74 One of the newspaper cuttings, n.d. [Oct. 1988], Ehrlich Papers, provides a list of the materials needed for repairs to be done on their planned "Helping Hand Day" of 22 Oct. 1988.

75 Press cuttings from Charlottetown *Guardian*, 9 May, 25 July, 3 Aug. 1989, Ehrlich Papers

76 The agenda was outlined in the document "Sir Andrew Macphail Heritage Property, Development Plan, Summary," n.d. [15 Jan. 1991],"

attached as appendix B to the Indenture of Lease between Government of Prince Edward Island as represented by the Minister of Transportation and Public Works, Lessor, and Sir Andrew Macphail (of Orwell, PEI) Foundation Inc., Lessee, 15 Aug. 1991, copy in personal possession of the author. Appendix C to the same Indenture of Lease specifies the purposes of the foundation. The copy of the indenture, with appendices, and copies of several other documents concerning the property were provided through the kindness of Jean Macphail Weber.

77 This judgment, first published in Robertson, "Introduction" to Macphail, *The Master's Wife*, 3rd edn., xxviii, has subsequently been repeated by several authors. See, for example, McQuaid, "Island Culture," 68, or the poet Joe Sherman, "Poets on the Half Shell," *The Buzz* (Charlottetown), Jan. 2001.

78 The commercialization has continued unabated. See, for example, the articles by Carolyn Drake in the Charlottetown *Guardian*, 24 Aug. 2004: "The Business of Anne" and "Protecting Anne's Image." As Drake remarks in the former article, "It's a name that sells, it's an image that makes money." "Anne" is an anchor of the PEI tourism industry, and "millions of dollars change hands every year because of her." Viewed from a marketing perspective, the unique claim of the Island to Anne – through Montgomery's authorship and the setting of the story – is an important factor differentiating it from competing tourism destinations. Yet an industry spokesperson is quoted acknowledging that a common complaint among Islanders is that they are "Anned to death." It is a fact that the Cavendish area, where the "Anne industry" is centred, has for several decades had a feel about it that is alien to some Islanders, who studiously avoid it. At the other end of the spectrum, the attitude of the beneficiaries is akin to a statement known to be made by owners of industrial-scale hog farms in response to complaints about noxious odours: "That's the smell of money."

79 See *The Prince Edward Island Guide* ([Charlottetown], 2007), 88–135.

80 Charlottetown *Patriot*, 4 Oct. 1924. I am grateful to Marian Bruce for providing me with a copy of this report, on 30 Nov. 2004. Macphail's views regarding tourism also appeared in the Summerside *Journal*, 8 Oct. 1924; see Bruce to the author, electronic mail, 19 Oct. 2004.

81 "H.B." [Harry Baglole], "The Island and Confederation" [24 Oct. 1973], in Baglole and Weale, eds., *Cornelius Howatt: Superstar!*, 181. Also see Weale and Baglole, *The Island and Confederation*. For a review article on the spate of material that appeared in 1973, see Robertson, "Recent Island History," *Acadiensis* 4 (Spring 1975): 111–18.

82 See "D.W." [David Weale], "Tourism – The Big Sell" [15 Aug. 1973], in Baglole and Weale, eds., *Cornelius Howatt: Superstar!*, 151–3.

83 For a study of this phenomenon, see O'Connor, "The Brothers and Sisters of Cornelius Howatt: Protest, 'Progress,' and the Island Way of Life."

84 See *The Prince Edward Island Guide* (2007), 7, for the remarkable assertion, without qualification, that "at Green Gables, you see the house where Anne grew up." Buried much deeper in the 216-page booklet is the more sober and accurate statement that "Green Gables is the original site that inspired the famous author to write the novel *Anne of Green Gables*" (92).

85 See Indenture of Lease between Government of Prince Edward Island as represented by the Minister of Transportation and Public Works, Lessor, and Sir Andrew Macphail (of Orwell, PEI) Foundation Inc., Lessee, 15 Aug. 1991, provision no. 1, copy in personal possession of the author.

86 Jean Macphail Weber to Patrick G. Binns, 30 July 2003, copy in personal possession of the author. Also see copy, electronic mail, of Shirlee Hogan (president of the Macphail Foundation) to Binns, 1 Aug. 2003, in personal possession of the author.

87 See Grant from the Province of Prince Edward Island to the Estate of Mrs Dorothy Lindsay, 22 Nov. 1990, copy in personal possession of the author.

88 Deed of Conveyance from Mrs Dorothy Lindsay to Her Majesty the Queen in the right of the Province of Prince Edward Island, 14 June 1961, conditions nos. 14, 15, copy in personal possession of the author.

89 See Deed of Conveyance, from Executors of the Estate of Mrs Dorothy Lindsay, and four children of Mrs Lindsay (acting as one party), to the Government of Prince Edward Island, 15 Aug. 1991, copy in personal possession of the author; and Release Agreement between Executors of the Estate of Mrs Dorothy Lindsay, and four children of Mrs. Lindsay (acting as one party), and the Government of Prince Edward Island, 15 Aug. 1991, copy in personal possession of the author. The conditions from which the Government has been released are appended in Schedule B; these are the same conditions – verbatim – embodied in the Deed of Conveyance from Mrs Dorothy Lindsay to the provincial government in 1961. The sole limitation on the government's freedom of action is an unnumbered provision in the 1991 Deed of Conveyance giving the grantors a five-year period in which to demand reconveyance of the property if ten specified conditions were not met; but those provisions explicitly recognized the right of the government to sell the property, and the right of the grantors to seek redress expired in 1996.

90 Interview with Jean Macphail Weber and Katherine Dewar, 28 Aug. 2004

91 Parts of this story were covered in the Prince Edward Island news media in the spring and summer of 2004.

92 Deed of Conveyance, from Executors of the Estate of Mrs Dorothy Lindsay, and four children of Mrs Lindsay (acting as one party), to the Government of Prince Edward Island, 15 Aug. 1991, provision no. 10, copy in personal possession of the author. A recent transaction involving a nearby property suggests that the amount potentially involved would be substantial, probably several hundreds of thousands of dollars.

93 Katherine Dewar, personal communication, 28 May 1990

94 For example, Katherine Dewar Interviews, interview with Christine MacLeod (audio tape), 29 Sept. 1990. Subsequently, Dewar lectured in Charlottetown and Montague about the Macphail who emerged from these interviews. She also lectured in Malpeque about Macphail during his time in Malpeque (Katherine Dewar, telephone conversation with author, 20 Aug. 2003).

95 Katherine Dewar Interviews, interview with Wolcott MacPherson (audio tape), 26 July 1990

96 See Edgar, "Sir Andrew Macphail," Queen's Quarterly 54 (1947): 9–10.

97 Katherine Dewar Interviews, interview with Marguerite (Meg) Stanley, granddaughter of Macphail (audio tape), 18 July 1990

98 Katherine Dewar Interviews, interview with Wolcott MacPherson (audio tape), 26 July 1990

99 Katherine Dewar Interviews, interview with Katie Martin (audio tape), 23 July 1990. Martin reported that Macphail was "very displeased" about the snake's death and tried in vain to discover who had killed it.

100 Katherine Dewar Interviews, interview with Wolcott MacPherson (audio tape), 26 July 1990. Probably because of Macphail's prominence, there was apparently quite a bit of mimicry of his voice, etc., by local people; Katherine Dewar Interviews, interview with Ruth MacLeod VanIderstine (audio tape), 20 July 1990. What Archibald MacMechan described in his poem honouring Macphail as his "humorous whine" when speaking probably also provided fodder for mimicry; see poem on p. 175, above.

101 Katherine Dewar Interviews, Dewar's summary, 7 Nov. 1990, of undated interview with Everett MacLeod

102 Katherine Dewar Interviews, interview with Wolcott MacPherson (audio tape), 26 July 1990

103 Katherine Dewar Interviews, interview with Marguerite (Meg) Stanley, granddaughter of Macphail (audio tape), 18 July 1990

104 Katherine Dewar Interviews, interviews with Stanwood MacLeod (audio tape), 30 July 1990, with Katie Martin (audio tape), 23 July 1990, and with Wolcott MacPherson (audio tape), 26 July 1990

105 Katherine Dewar Interviews, interviews with Wolcott MacPherson (audio tape), 26 July 1990, with Stanwood MacLeod (audio tape), 30 July 1990, and with Ruth MacLeod VanIderstine (audio tape), 20 July 1990

106 Interview with Mrs Dorothy Lindsay, 26 July 1970

107 W.M. Martin, "The Four Brothers," personal communication, 13 Feb. 2000, 5, in personal possession of the author. Professor Martin's essay "The Four Brothers" is 21 single-spaced pages in length and includes evocative portraits of (James) Alexander (12–16), William Matheson (16–18), and John Goodwill (18–21), the three brothers in whose company he saw (John) Andrew. Eighty years of age at the time of the interview, he remembered how, as a teenager, he had been in awe of these uncles – "real powerhouses,"

he stated more than once. Finlay Smith was the only son without a university degree and, in Martin's view, was "marginalized"; interview with W.M. Martin, 17 Feb. 2000. Finlay was blind from about the age of fifty, that is, around 1912; Macphail family stories, as told by family members at the Sir Andrew Macphail Heritage Days, at the Macphail Homestead, Orwell, 10 Aug. 2002.

108 Interview with Miss Anne Haley, 23 July 1970

109 Katherine Dewar Interviews, interview with Stanwood MacLeod (audio tape), 30 July 1990

110 Katherine Dewar Interviews, interview with Wolcott MacPherson (audio tape), 26 July 1990. The informant may well have known this from family experience, for he related that in 1932 or 1933 his father's store had burned down, and he had had to rebuild. His father already had a special relationship with Macphail, taking telephone messages for him at his store – as Macphail himself would have no telephone in his home. Since the building had two storeys, Macphail could see it from his study, and the arrangement was that if there had been a call for him, MacPherson's father was to fly a white flag from the store; the store was about a mile away.

111 Interview with W.M. Martin, 17 Feb. 2000; also W.M. Martin, "The Four Brothers," 12, personal communication. Professor Martin, who died on 12 Feb. 2005, was the youngest child of Catherine, or "Katie," youngest daughter in the family of William Macphail and Catherine Smith.

112 C.F. Martin, obituary article on Macphail, in *Canadian Medical Association Journal* 39 (Nov. 1938): 509

113 Interview with W.M. Martin, 17 Feb. 2000; W.M. Martin, "The Four Brothers," 12, personal communication; interviews with Mrs Dorothy Lindsay, 30 June, 22 July 1970, and Sally MacKinnon, 26 June 1970; Katherine Dewar Interviews, interviews with Sally MacKinnon (audio tape), 7 Sept. 1990, and with Stanwood MacLeod (audio tape), 30 July 1990; Edgar, "Sir Andrew Macphail (1864–1938)," *Transactions* of the Royal Society of Canada, 1939, 149; Francis, obituary article on Macphail, *Bulletin of the History of Medicine* 7 (1939): 800; Stewart, "Address Delivered during the Unveiling of a Memorial to Sir Andrew Macphail, Kt ... in Prince of Wales College, Charlottetown 8.00 p.m. Monday, July 11th, 1955," 6, in personal possession of the author; Whittaker, *Setting the Stage*, 74.

114 Katherine Dewar Interviews, interview with the Rev. Harvey Bishop (audio tape), 6 Aug. 1990. One informant gave detailed information on the ritual of drawing water from the well as she remembered it from her early twenties: At 11 a.m. she would go to the well-house, where she was to draw two buckets of water, empty the first one, and use the second for Macphail, placing it in a glass water jug, as it would be colder than the first. He would then have that water with whisky – and give her some. Katherine Dewar Interviews, interview with Sally MacKinnon (audio tape), 7 Sept. 1990. Macphail was vocal in his praise for the water drawn this way from

his well – "The water in that well was better than anywhere else, he said"; Katherine Dewar Interviews, interview with Christine MacLeod (audio tape), 29 Sept. 1990.

115 Interview with the Rev. Harvey Bishop, 27 Aug. 2003

116 See Macphail to Mathieson, 16 Aug. 1923, John A. Mathieson Papers, PARO. The Orwell neighbours would not be among those invited to dinner at Macphail's home; Katherine Dewar Interviews, interviews with Sally MacKinnon (audio tape), 7 Sept. 1990, and with Katie MacLeod, (audio tape), 30 July 1990. His most important interactions with local people, aside from bringing them occasional gifts of wine or tea, seem to have been when hiring and employing individuals, making purchases, attending church, and, when disasters occurred, offering aid. There were, of course, random encounters in the general stores, at the railway station, and so on.

117 Interview with Frank MacKinnon, 27 Dec. 1967

118 Macphail family stories, as told by family members at the Sir Andrew Macphail Heritage Days, at the Macphail Homestead, Orwell, 29 July 2000. One of Dewar's informants, who had initially worked for Macphail's daughter in Montreal and married a Prince Edward Islander, reported that some people in the district were rather annoyed about his bringing in alcohol during Prohibition; Katherine Dewar Interviews, interview with Sally MacKinnon (audio tape), 7 Sept. 1990. Another recounted Macphail advising his father, a carpenter, that alcohol was on the sideboard and that he should help himself at any time when working around the premises, but that since his father was a teetotaller he did not avail himself of the standing offer; Katherine Dewar Interviews, interview with Stanwood MacLeod (audio tape), 30 July 1990.

119 Katherine Dewar Interviews, interview with Christine MacLeod (audio tape), 29 Sept. 1990. Information concerning the showering routine (which seems to have been widely known and much talked about) also came out in interviews with Miss Goldie McInnis and Miss Mary Martin, 6 Sept. 1969 and with Sally MacKinnon, 26 June 1970.

120 Interview with Mrs Dorothy Lindsay, 28 May 1977

121 Interview with Sally MacKinnon, 26 June 1970. Also Macphail family stories, as told by family members at the Sir Andrew Macphail Heritage Days, at the Macphail Homestead, Orwell, 29 July 2000; Katherine Dewar Interviews, interview with Sally MacKinnon (audio tape), 7 Sept. 1990.

122 Katherine Dewar Interviews, interview with Christine MacLeod (audio tape), 29 Sept. 1990.

123 See, for example, Katherine Dewar Interviews, interviews with Christine MacLeod (audio tape), 29 Sept. 1990, and with Stanwood MacLeod (audio tape), 30 July 1990.

124 Interview with Miss Anne Haley, 23 July 1970

125 See, for example, McQuaid, "Island Culture," 68; Porter, "Architectural

Treasures," 162; McAskill and MacQuarrie, *Nature Trails of Prince Edward Island*, 76, 86–9; *Canada: Ulysses Travel Guide* (Montreal, 1998), 116–17; *Lonely Planet Canada*, 8th edn. (Melbourne, 2002), 514.

CHAPTER FOURTEEN

1 See Robertson, "Andrew Macphail," in Chevalier, ed., *Encyclopedia of the Essay*, 512–13.

2 See Connor, "Canadian Essay (English)," 144.

3 See K. MacKinnon, "Technique in *The Master's Wife*," 65–74; Kulyk Keefer, *Under Eastern Eyes, passim*; MacLaine, "Crooked Signs and Shining Things: The Magic of Books in the Literature of Atlantic Canadian Islands," 37–50; Peter Hay, "Appreciating The Master's Wife from the other side of the planet," Charlottetown *Guardian*, 18 Jan. 2002.

4 See McBrine, "The Development of the Familiar Essay in English Canadian Literature from 1900 to 1920," iii.

5 As an example, see Sonia Leathes, "Votes for Women," *University Magazine* 13 (Feb. 1914): 67–78.

6 Macphail made 43 contributions, and was followed by Marjorie Pickthall with 21 and MacMechan with 19.

7 See Leacock, "Andrew Macphail," *Queen's Quarterly* 45 (Winter 1938): 449–50; Edgar, "Sir Andrew Macphail," *Queen's Quarterly* 54 (Spring 1947): 9; MacMechan, *Head-waters of Canadian Literature*, 201–4.

8 St Pierre, "Andrew Macphail," 227

9 Gross, *The Rise and Fall of the Man of Letters*, Foreword, xiii. In the Canadian milieu the only possible rival to Macphail as an example of the man of letters would be the English-born and -educated Goldwin Smith.

10 This point concerning the periodicals was suggested by Professor Peter McNally of McGill University.

11 Gross, *The Rise and Fall of the Man of Letters*, 227; also see 81–2.

12 See speech by Greenshields in proposing a toast to the health of Macphail at the University Club, Montreal, 10 March 1909, 13–14; Strachey to Macphail, 27 Nov. 1908 (confidential), Macphail Papers; Gross, *The Rise and Fall of the Man of Letters*, 2, 6–7.

13 See Williams, *Culture and Society 1780–1950*, ch. 7, especially 140, 145–7, 158–9; also see 165, 200–2, 256–7.

14 Macphail, "The Senses and the Mind," draft radio address, intended for broadcast 24 Nov. 1933, in personal possession of author

15 Shortt, *The Search for an Ideal*, 36. The two articles are: "Sir Andrew Macphail: Physician, Philosopher, Founding Editor of CMAJ," *Canadian Medical Association Journal*, 4 Feb. 1978, 323–6, and "Essayist, Editor, and Physician: The Career of Sir Andrew Macphail, 1864–1938," *Canadian Literature* 96 (Spring 1983): 49–58. The point of Shortt's two articles on Macphail appears to be the highlighting of his diverse areas of

achievement. But despite Shortt's combination of credentials by the time
the articles appeared (a PH D in intellectual history and an MD), the two
pieces are strangely uninformative regarding the interaction between
the literary and scientific spheres of his life. They explain neither the
distinctive qualities evident in his activities nor how each sphere affected
the other, amounting, rather, to simple listings. See Robertson, "Andrew
Macphail: A Holistic Approach," *Canadian Literature* 107 (Winter 1985):
179–86.

16   See Shortt, *The Search for an Ideal*, 3.
17   See the following reviews of Shortt, *The Search for an Ideal*: by Allan Smith,
     in *Histoire Sociale/Social History* 20 (Nov. 1977): 464–5; by J.M. Bumsted,
     in "Canadian Intellectual History and the 'Buzzing Factuality,'" *Acadiensis*
     7 (Autumn 1977): 119; by Barry Cooper, in *Canadian Journal of Political
     Science* 11 (June 1978): 469; by F.W. Watt, review in *Canadian Historical
     Review* 59 (Sept. 1978): 396.
18   For example, on the opening page of Shortt's chapter on Macphail he has
     the grandfather's family shipwrecked on Prince Edward Island, whereas
     Macphail himself states explicitly in *The Master's Wife* that it was Nova
     Scotia. On the next page Shortt affirms that the father had taught at
     Fanning Grammar School in Malpeque (where Andrew spent two and
     one-half formative years), whereas there is no known evidence that he did
     so, and Macphail states explicitly, again in *The Master's Wife*, that his own
     first teaching job, *before* Malpeque, was in a district where his father and
     grandfather had taught previously. The district was Melville. Compare
     Shortt, *The Search for an Ideal*, 13–14, with Macphail, *The Master's Wife*, 31, 181.
19   Shortt, *The Search for an Ideal*, 13
20   See ibid., 197; Alexander Macphail, "The Sonnets," *University Magazine* 18
     (Oct. 1919): 358.
21   See, for example, chapter 3 in the present study.
22   Shortt, *The Search for an Ideal*, 29
23   Macphail, "The Peace and its Consequence," *University Magazine* 19 (April
     1920): 121
24   Janet E. Baker finds similar weaknesses in Shortt's treatment of
     MacMechan, which she characterizes both reductive and tending towards
     exaggeration, to the extent of attributing to him views "that are actually
     quite alien to MacMechan." Shortt's presentation of some works by
     MacMechan represents a misreading that "is to parody what actually hap-
     pens in [them]" (Baker, *Archibald MacMechan*, 174; also see 172–3).
25   The task of assessing whether Shortt's statements about Macphail's views
     correspond with what Macphail actually wrote is complicated by his
     footnoting practices: "The present study adopts the device of cumulative
     notes on the assumption that only by viewing a number of sources taken
     together is a particular idea clearly documented." (Shortt, *The Search for an*

Ideal, 151n30). This unorthodox method may also mask the lack of appropriate documentation. Nor is the clarity of Shortt's work enhanced by a
writing style that seems at times to lend itself to evasiveness. For example,
Shortt states that of the six intellectuals he is studying in his book, "none ...
was a systematic philosopher (except, perhaps, Andrew Macphail)" (Shortt,
The Search for an Ideal, 10). The reader is left to wonder: was he or was
he not?

26 "Ruralism" and "agrarianism" are used by such writers as G. Ramsay
Cook, Michel Brunet, and Pierre-Elliott Trudeau in dealing with certain
aspects of French Canadian intellectual history. See Cook, *Canada and
the French-Canadian Question*, 85–7; Brunet, *La présence anglaise and les
Canadiens*, 85–7; Trudeau, "La Province de Québec au moment de la grève,"
in Trudeau, ed., *La grève de l'amiante*, 17–18, 27–9.

27 See *The Grain Growers' Guide*, 21 Feb. 1912; Partridge, *A War on Poverty*,
44–6, 87.

28 It might be added as a common-sense observation that this condition of
non-interference from the outside world was dependent upon peace and
relative security from external threats.

29 See in particular Macphail, *Essays in Politics*, 38–9; Macphail, "Prince
Edward Island," press cutting from a PEI newspaper, n.d. [Oct. 1912],
Burland-Macphail Scrapbook, Macphail Papers; Macphail, "The Cost
of Living," *University Magazine* 11 (Dec. 1912): 537; Macphail, "The
Conservative," *University Magazine* 18 (Dec. 1919): 421; Macphail, "The
Immigrant," *University Magazine* 19 (April 1920): 149–50, 157.

30 Cf. D.H. Lawrence's condemnation of the industrial ethic as the "forcing
of all human energy into a competition of mere acquisition," which
Raymond Williams cites as "the common element in all the diverse interpretations of which the [romantic, anti-industrial] tradition is composed"
(Williams, *Culture and Society, 1780-1950*, 202; also see 200).

31 See Macpherson, *Democracy in Alberta*, especially 222.

32 This is not to suggest that Macphail and the organized farmers had no contact whatever. See the comments by J.J. Morrison, secretary of the United
Farmers of Ontario, after Macphail's address on "The Farmer," *Empire Club
of Canada: Addresses ... during the Year 1920*, 124–5; Morrison to Macphail,
17 Jan. 1923, Macphail Papers.

33 See F. MacKinnon, *The Government of Prince Edward Island*, ch. 5; Bumsted,
Land, Settlement, and Politics on Eighteenth-Century Prince Edward Island;
Bittermann, *Rural Protest on Prince Edward Island*; Robertson, *The Tenant
League of Prince Edward Island*. That Macphail understood the impor-
tance of the land question in Island history is evident from "The History
of Prince Edward Island," in Shortt and Doughty, eds., *Canada and Its
Provinces* 13: 363; Macphail, "The God in the Machine," n.d., p. 12, Macphail
Papers; Macphail to Beaverbrook, 6 Jan. 1932, Macphail Papers.

34 See Bittermann and McCallum, "Upholding the Land Legislation of a 'Communistic and Socialist Assembly': The Benefits of Confederation for Prince Edward Island," 1–28.

35 Macphail, *The Master's Wife*, 18. On the matter of debt and its perceived importance within the community of Macphail's childhood, see Macphail, *The Master's Wife*, 51, 55. On the prevalence and significance of rent arrears, see Robertson, *The Tenant League of Prince Edward Island*, 22–3, 41–2, 322n49.

36 See Robertson, *The Tenant League of Prince Edward Island*, xvii, 7–8, 43, 76, 280.

37 Macpherson, *The Political Theory of Possessive Individualism*, 51. Also see 46–61; Sweezy, *The Theory of Capitalist Development*, 23, 57, 243.

38 Macphail, "The Conservative," *University Magazine* 18 (Dec. 1919): 421

39 I owe this insight to Professor Paul Potter of the University of Western Ontario, a scholarly authority on Hippocrates. For an example of Macphail's own emphasis on understanding the patient as an interrelated whole, see "American Methods in Medical Education," offprint from *British Medical Journal*, 3 Sept. 1927, 11.

40 See Berger, "The Other Mr. Leacock," 23–40; Bowker, "Introduction" to Bowker, ed., *The Social Criticism of Stephen Leacock*, ix–xlviii; Cook, "Stephen Leacock and the Age of Plutocracy, 1903–1921," 163–81; Watt, "Critic or Entertainer: Leacock and the Growth of Materialism," 33–42; Levitt, "Henri Bourassa and Modern Industrial Society, 1900–1914," 37–50, and *Henri Bourassa and the Golden Calf*. Despite the invitation to join that the Pen and Pencil Club extended to Bourassa in 1906 (an invitation that Macphail supported), there is no evidence that Macphail was personally acquainted with Bourassa or any other leading member of the Nationalist League (see p.60, above).

41 A contributing factor was the impassable condition of the roads for more than one-half of the year; business simply had to be transacted within one's own community. These roads also assured the end of the first experiment with rural consolidated schools. See Croteau, *Cradled in the Waves*, 11–12; interview with Earl Ings, 8 Sept. 1968. In an interview on 13 Jan. 1967 the Acadian historian J-Henri Blanchard (1881–1968), longtime Professor of French at Prince of Wales College, then retired, stated that he had noticed no significant change in Island society until about 1950.

42 Macphail, *The Master's Wife*, 41

43 See Leacock, *Sunshine Sketches of a Little Town*.

44 See Watt, "Critic or Entertainer: Leacock and the Growth of Materialism," 40.

45 Leacock, "Andrew Macphail," *Queen's Quarterly* 45 (Winter 1938): 451–2; also see 446.

46 Moore, *Social Origins of Dictatorship and Democracy*, 490–3. For some parallels to Macphail drawn from German intellectual history, see Stern, *The Politics of Cultural Despair*.

47 See Berger, *The Sense of Power, passim*.

48 Shortt, *The Search for an Ideal*, 36, suggests that Macphail had "a rigid adherence to the idea of laissez-faire"; also see 27, 29.

49 Macphail, "The Farmer," *Empire Club of Canada: Addresses ... 1920*, 120. Also see Macphail, "The Freedom of England," *Quarterly Review* 255 (July 1930): 1, 6–16. Beaverbrook, who was then campaigning for "Imperial Free Trade" in general (or tariffs against all but the dominions), was able to put the article to considerable use. See Beaverbrook to Macphail, 28 Aug. 1930; Macphail to Beaverbrook, 23 Oct. 1930, 6 Jan. 1932, Macphail Papers; Macphail to Beaverbrook, 11 Aug. 1930, Beaverbrook Papers, BL.

50 Macphail, "The Freedom of England," *Quarterly Review* 255 (July 1930): 15

51 Ibid., 7, 10. He did not explain why food would be cheaper. Also see Macphail to Beaverbrook, 12 April, 10 June 1930, Beaverbrook Papers, BL; Macphail to Howard Murray, 22 July 1930, Macphail-Murray Scrapbooks 1, Macphail Papers; interview with Macphail, press cutting from London *Sunday Express*, 27 April 1930; Macphail to Beaverbrook, 6 Jan. 1932, Macphail Papers.

52 Macphail, *Essays in Puritanism*, 79

53 See Macphail, "The Immigrant," *Addresses Delivered before the Canadian Club of Ottawa, 1919–1920*, 176.

54 Other examples of this tradition are Grant, "An Ethic of Community," 3–26, and Taylor, "The Agony of Economic Man," 221–35. B.C. Parekh writes that a "philosophical understanding of an activity ... points to its essential and permanent features, and offers criteria for evaluating relevant practical proposals and actions – not, of course, in their specificity but in their general assumptions and orientation" (Parekh, "The Nature of Political Philosophy," 181).

Short Chronology of Macphail's Life

1864　Birth of Andrew Macphail in Orwell, PEI
1880　Entrance to Prince of Wales College, Charlottetown
1882　First teaching position, in Melville, PEI
1883　Becomes principal of Malpeque grammar school
1885　Enters McGill University, Montreal
1888　Graduates in arts
1891　Wins international essay contest on vivisection
　　　Graduates in medicine
　　　Embarks on round-the-world trip as a journalist
1892　Further medical training in England
1893　Appointed professor in the University of Bishop's College Faculty of
　　　Medicine, Montreal
　　　Marries Georgina Burland
1894　Andrew and Georgina move to 216 Peel Street
　　　Birth of son
1896　Conducts research on canned lobster industry in PEI
1897　Joins Pen and Pencil Club of Montreal
　　　Birth of daughter
1902　Death of Georgina
1903　Becomes managing editor of the *Montreal Medical Journal*
1905　Commences spending his summers in Orwell
　　　Publishes first book, *Essays in Purtitanism*
　　　Death of his father
1906　Publishes novel, *The Vine of Sibmah: A Relation of the Puritans*
1907　Founds the *University Magazine*, which he edits and publishes from 216
　　　Peel Street
　　　Appointed McGill's first professor of the history of medicine
1908　(*ca.*) Commences agricultural experiments in Orwell
1909　Publishes *Essays in Politics*
1910　Publishes *Essays in Fallacy*

1911 Becomes founding editor of the *Canadian Medical Association Journal*
      His eyesight is seriously damaged in domestic accident
1914 Publishes *The Land: A Play of Character*
      Enlists for active military service
1915 Arrives in France
1916 Transferred from the front to a staff position
      Publishes *The Book of Sorrow*
1917 Transferred to London
1918 Knighted
1919 Returns to Canada
1920 Discontinues the *University Magazine*
      Death of his mother
1921 Publishes translation of *Maria Chapdelaine*
      Is wounded by gunshot in 216 Peel Street
1925 Publishes *Official History of the Canadian Forces in the Great War, 1914–19: The Medical Services*
1927 Publishes "American Methods in Medical Education"
1929 Publishes *Three Persons*
1930 Is vice-president of the Montreal Repertory Theatre at its founding
1931 Publishes *The Bible in Scotland*
1935 Travels to the Soviet Union
1937 Retirement from McGill
1938 Death in Montreal
1939 Publication of *The Master's Wife*
1961 Donation of his home to the province of Prince Edward Island

Bibliography

PRIMARY SOURCES

Sir Andrew Macphail's Writings

The following is a chronological list of Macphail's works. Within particular years, books are listed first, followed by articles arranged alphabetically by provenance, and untitled reviews. When a periodical carries more than one Macphail article in a single year, these are in chronological order. Some articles appear to have been widely reprinted; in such cases, a second provenance is noted only if the title was altered. Translations by Macphail have been clearly indicated as such.

Articles pseudonymously signed, unsigned, or signed "The Editor" are denoted as follows: ED, signed "The Editor"; PS, pseudonymously signed; US, unsigned.

1891
"Vivisection." In *Vivisection: Five Hundred Dollar Prize Essays*, compiled by George T. Angell, 27–43. Boston
1892
"Athletics in Japan." *Outing*, December
1893
"Bicycling in Japan." *Outing*, January
1894
"An Epidemic of Paralysis in Children." *Medical News* 65 (8 December): 619–25; also published in abridged form as "A Preliminary Note on an Epidemic of Paralysis in Children." *British Medical Journal*, 1 December, 1233–4
1896
"The Artificial Feeding of Children." *British Medical Journal*, 19 December, 1766–8
1897
Discoloration in Canned Lobsters: Report of an Inquiry into the Causes Leading to a Deterioration in the Quality of Canned Lobsters. Ottawa

1900

"The After-History of Applicants Rejected for Life Insurance." *British Medical Journal*, 15 December, 1697–1701

1902

"The Attainment of Consideration." *British Medical Journal*, 15 November, 1612–14

1905

Essays in Puritanism. Boston and New York

"Margaret Fuller." *McGill University Magazine* 4 (January): 52–81

"Sir William Dawson." *McGill University Magazine* 5 (December): 12–29

1906

The Vine of Sibmah: A Relation of the Puritans. New York

1907

"John Knox in the Church of England." *University Magazine* 6 (February): 15–23

"A Patent Anomaly." *University Magazine* 6 (February): 49–54 (PS as Angus Macfadyen)

"Loyalty – To What." *University Magazine* 6 (April): 142–51

"The Patience of England." *University Magazine* 6 (October): 281–90

"What Can Canada Do." *University Magazine* 6 (December): 387–411

1908

"The Authority of the Woman." *May Court Club Magazine* 1 (October): 14—18

"The 'American Woman,'" *Spectator* 101 (3 & 10 October): 497–8, 537–8

"The Dominion and the Spirit." *University Magazine* 7 (February): 10–24

"Protection and Politics." *University Magazine* 7 (April): 238–55

"Why the Conservatives Failed." *University Magazine* 7 (December): 529–45

1909

Essays in Politics. London

"How Canada Looks at American Tariff-Making." *American Review of Reviews* 39 (January): 85–7; partially reprinted as "The U.S. Tariff: A Canadian's View of Its Interest to the Two Countries." *Gazette* (Montreal), 19 January

"A Canadian View of Reciprocity and Imperialism." *Spectator* 102 (6 March): 372–3; reprinted as "Trade and Nationalism: Some Comments on Canada's Relations with Other Lands." *Gazette* (Montreal), 27 March

"New Lamps for Old." *University Magazine* 8 (February): 18–35

"British Diplomacy and Canada." *University Magazine* 8 (April): 188–214

"The Nine Prophets." *University Magazine* 8 (October): 398–406

Postscript note to Bram de Sola's "The Jewish School Question" (ED). In *University Magazine* 8 (December): 560

Review in *Montreal Medical Journal* 38 (October): 685–6 (US)

1910

Essays in Fallacy. London

"Medicine in Canada." *British Medical Journal*, 7 May, 1118–19

"An Imperial View of Education." *Cambridge Review*, 27 January, 217–18; reprinted as "Hints of the Progress of Knowledge: An Imperial View of Education." *World Wide* (Montreal), 26 March, 268–70

"Lord Grey in Canada." *Canadian Century* (Montreal), 2 July, 7–8

"The Psychology of the Suffragette." In *Empire Club Speeches: Being Addresses Delivered before the Empire Club of Canada during Its Session of 1909–1910*, 102–27. Toronto

"The Past Session." *Saturday Night*, 14 May

"The Poor Boy." *Saturday Night*, 21 May; reprinted as "The University's Work." *Gazette* (Montreal), 24 May

"Mark Twain's Successor." *Saturday Night*, 28 May

"Church and Politics." *Saturday Night*, 4 June

"Shall We Develop or Shall We Exploit?" *Saturday Night*, 11 June

"What Is the News." *Saturday Night*, 18 June

"Reciprocity." *Saturday Night*, 25 June

"The Manufacture of Opinion." *Saturday Night*, 9 July

"Canada's Loyalty." *Saturday Night*, 6 August

"Nation or Empire." *Saturday Night*, 20 August

"East and West." *Saturday Night*, 3 September

"British Diplomacy and Canada." *Saturday Night*, 17 September

"What Canada Owes to England." *Saturday Night*, 1 October

"Government by Party." *Saturday Night*, 15 October

"Self Defence." *Saturday Night*, 29 October

"The Businessman in Politics." *Saturday Night*, 5 November

"Canadian Writers and American Politics." *University Magazine* 9 (February): 3–17; (ED)

"Oxford and Working-Class Education." *University Magazine* 9 (February): 36–50

"As Others See Us." *University Magazine* 9 (April): 165–75 (ED)

"An Obverse View of Education." *University Magazine* 9 (April): 192–204

"A Voice from the East." *University Magazine* 9 (December): 517–23 (ED)

"The New Theology." *University Magazine* 9 (December): 683–97

1911

"Medicine in Canada." *British Medical Journal*, 1 July, 30–2

"Style in Medical Writing." *Canadian Medical Association Journal* 1 (January): 70–3 (US)

"The Degradation of Parliaments." *Halifax Chronicle*, 2 January

"Anglo-American Arbitration." *Brooklyn Eagle*, 10 April

"Government by Commission." *Guardian* (Charlottetown), 18 February

"Payment of Members." *Guardian* (Charlottetown), 25 February

"International Amity." *Saturday Night*, 1 July

"Canadian Citizenship." *Saturday Night*, 8 July

"Imperialism: The Problem." *Saturday Night*, 15 July

"Imperialism: The Solution." *Saturday Night*, 22 July

"The Poisoning of the People." *Saturday Night*, 29 July

"The Peril to Democracy." *Saturday Night*, 5 August

"The Education of the People." *Saturday Night*, 12 August

"The Going of the Greys." *Saturday Night*, 30 September

"The Coming of the Connaughts." *Saturday Night*, 7 October

"Canada and the United States – The Real Danger." *Spectator* 106 (18 February): 243–4

"Certain Varieties of the Apples of Sodom." *University Magazine* 10 (February): 30–46

"The Cleaning of the Slate." *University Magazine* 10 (April): 183–91 (ED)

"Confiscatory Legislation." *University Magazine* 10 (April): 192–206

"Why the Liberals Failed." *University Magazine* 10 (December): 566–80

"The Fielding-Taft Reciprocity Agreement." *Montreal Witness*, 21 February

"Protection and the Empire." [*ca.* 1911] ·

1912

"Prince Edward Island." In *Addresses Delivered before the Canadian Club of Toronto, Season of 1911–12*, 48–59. Toronto

"Conversion." *Proceedings of the American Medico-Psychological Association*, 68th annual meeting, 239–44

"The Tariff Commission." *Saturday Night*, 10 February

"The Interlude in Politics." *Saturday Night*, 17 February

"The Appeasement of the Farmer." *Saturday Night*, 24 February

"The Force of Attraction." *Saturday Night*, 2 March

"Bigotry in Parliament." *Saturday Night*, 9 March

"Our Chief End." *Saturday Night*, 16 March

"Town and Country." *Saturday Night*, 23 March

"The Church and the Theatre." *Saturday Night*, 30 March

"The End." *Saturday Night*, 6 April

"The Montreal 'Witness.'" *Spectator* 109 (16 November): 808

"The Tariff Commission." *University Magazine* 11 (February): 27–40

"The Cost of Living." *University Magazine* 11 (December): 526–43

Postscript note to N.A. Belcourt's "French in Ontario" (ED). In *University Magazine* 11 (December): 561

"Prince Edward Island." (a PEI newspaper), October

1913

"The Navy and Politics" *University Magazine* 12 (February): 1–22

"Unto the Church." *University Magazine* 12 (April): 348–64

"Theory and Practice." *University Magazine* 12 (October): 380–95

"The Hill of Error." *University Magazine* 12 (December): 533–9; (ED)

"The Dominion and the Provinces." *University Magazine* 12 (December): 550–67

"Stephen Leacock." *The Year Book of Canadian Art, 1913*, compiled by the Arts and Letters Club of Toronto, 3–7. Toronto

1914

The Land: A Play of Character, in One Act with Five Scenes. Montreal

"The Atlantic Provinces in the Dominion: Introduction." In *Canada and Its Provinces*, edited by Adam Shortt and Arthur Doughty, 13: 3–12. Toronto

"The History of Prince Edward Island." In *Canada and Its Provinces*, edited by Adam Shortt and Arthur Doughty, 13: 305–75. Toronto

"On Certain Aspects of Feminism." *Saturday Night*, 29 April

"Patriotism and Politics." *University Magazine* 13 (February): I–II (ED)

"On Certain Aspects of Feminism." *University Magazine* 13 (February): 79–91

"Consequences and Penalties." *University Magazine* 13 (April): 167–77 (ED)

"The Land." *University Magazine* 13 (April): 275–91

"The Day of Wrath." *University Magazine* 13 (October): 344–59 (ED)

"Val Cartier Camp." *University Magazine* 13 (October): 360–72

1915

"Lessons Proper for 1914–15." *University Magazine* 14 (February): I–9

1916

The Book of Sorrow. London

1917

"The Mind of the Soldier." *British Medical Journal*, II August, 188–9 (US)

"A Day's Work." *Lancet*, 30 June, 979–84

"An Ambulance in Rest." *University Magazine* 16 (October): 330–7

"In This Our Necessity." *University Magazine* 16 (December): 476–83

1918

"War and Business." In *Addresses Delivered before the Canadian Club of Toronto,
     Season of 1917–18*, 98–105. Toronto

"The War: A Wet Night." *British Medical Journal*, 7 December, 636–8

1919

"The Bridge-head." *British Medical Journal*, 15 February, 189–91

"The Education of Graduates." In *Contributions to Medical and Biological Research
     Dedicated to Sir William Osler Bart., M.D., F.R.S. in Honour of his Seventieth
     Birthday, July 12, 1919, by His Pupils and Co-Workers*. 1: 122–36. New York

"John McCrae: An Essay in Character." In John McCrae, *In Flanders Fields and
     Other Poems*, 47–141. Toronto

"Article Nineteen." *University Magazine* 18 (October): 311–26 (ED)

"The Last Days." *University Magazine* 18 (October): 327–43 (PS as "Staff Officer")

"The Conservative." *University Magazine* 18 (December): 419–44

1920

"The Immigrant." In *Addresses Delivered before the Canadian Club of Ottawa,
     1919–20*, 169–77. Ottawa

"Women in Democracy." *University Magazine* 19 (February): I–15

"The Peace and Its Consequence." *University Magazine* 19 (April): 119–32 (ED)

"The Immigrant." *University Magazine* 19 (April): 133–62

"Kismet and the Forests." *Saturday Night*, 20 March

1921

Maria Chapdelaine: A Romance of French Canada. Translated by Macphail. Montreal

"Sir William Van Horne." *Canadian Bookman*, new series, 3 (June): 30–2

"The Farmer." In *Empire Club of Canada: Addresses Delivered to the Members during
     the Year 1920*, 109–25. Toronto

"Introduction" to John Crichton, *A Vista: An Anthology of Verse*. Montreal

1922
"The American Novel." *Gazette* (Montreal), 17 November
1923
"In Memoriam: William E. Marshall." *Dalhousie Review* 3 (July): 152–4
1924
"Art in Democracy." *Dalhousie Review* 4 (July): 172–80
"Doctor John Andrew MacDonald." *McGill News* 5 (June): 5–6
1925
Official History of the Canadian Forces in the Great War, 1914–19: The Medical Services. Preface by A.F. Duguid. Ottawa
"A History of the Idea of Evolution." *Dalhousie Review* 5 (April): 22–32; also published slightly revised as "Evolution and Life." *Annals of Medical History*, new series, 1 (September 1929): 553–61
1926
"The Hand or the Book." *Dalhousie Review* 6 (July): 218–20
1927
"American Methods in Medical Education." *British Medical Journal*, 3 September, 373–80
"Robert Stanley Weir." *Transactions of the Royal Society of Canada*, 3rd series, 21: 8–9
1928
"Sir Henry Wilson." *Quarterly Review* 251 (July): 18–54
1929
Three Persons. New York
"Pierre Rocques." Translated by Macphail. In Supplement to *McGill News* 11 (December): 22–3
"Johnson's Life of Boswell." *Quarterly Review* 253 (July): 42–73
"Sir Sandford Fleming." *Queen's Quarterly* 36 (Spring): 185–204
"Child of Celt and Indian." *Saturday Night*, 30 November, Literary Supplement
1930
"The Burden of the Stuarts." *Quarterly Review* 254 (April): 218–29
"The Freedom of England." *Quarterly Review*, 255 (July): 1–16
"The Last Rising: A Melodrama." *Queen's Quarterly* 37 (Spring): 246–58
"News-Value in Literature." *Montreal Star*, 1 November
1931
The Bible in Scotland. London
"The Bible in Scotland." *Quarterly Review* 257 (July): 15–36
1932
"Our Canadian Speech." *McGill News* 14 (December): 27–8, 48
"The Graduate." *Queen's Quarterly* 39 (August): 377–91
"To the Reader." In Ethel McKenzie, *Secret Snow*. Philadelphia
Review in *Canadian Defence Quarterly* 9 (January): 282–3
1933
"The Source of Modern Medicine." *Canadian Medical Association Journal* 28 (March): 239–46

"The Reading of History." *Canadian Medical Association Journal* 29 (December): 664–71

"Armistice Day 1933." *McGill News* 15 (December): 39–42

"William Templeton Waugh." *Transactions of the Royal Society of Canada*, 3rd series, 27: 4–5

Review in *Canadian Medical Association Journal* 29 (September): 317

Review in *Canadian Medical Association Journal* 29 (November): 558–9

1934

"My Philosophy of Life." *Montreal Herald*, 10 December

"The Healing of a Wound." *Quarterly Review* 262 (January): 111–23

"The Short Story." *Quarterly Review* 263 (July): 16–28

"Sir Arthur Currie: The Value of a Degree." *Queen's Quarterly* 41 (Spring): 1–19

"Hindenburg." *Queen's Quarterly* 41 (Winter 1934–35): 433–52

"Sir Arthur Currie." *Transactions of the Royal Society of Canada*, 3rd series, 28: 12–14

"Conservative – Liberal – Socialist." *University of Toronto Quarterly* 3 (April): 263–85

1935

"The Goat and the Vine." In *Empire Club of Canada: Addresses Delivered to the Members during the Year 1934–35*, 161–72. Toronto

"Origins." *Quarterly Review* 265 (October): 189–98

"Woman of Danzig." *Saturday Night*, 17 August

"Woman of Leningrad." *Saturday Night*, 24 August

"Woman of Moscow." *Saturday Night*, 5 October

"A Pair of Brogues." *Saturday Night*, 21 December

"To the Reader." In A.S. Bourinot, *Selected Poems, 1915–1935*. Toronto

"Personal Tribute" [to John Redpath Dougall]. *Montreal Witness*, [ca. 18 September]

1936

"Medicine." In W.S. Wallace, ed., *Encyclopedia of Canada* 4: 257–67. Toronto

"The Royal Canadian Regiment: A Book Review." *McGill News* 18 (Winter): 34–5

"Greek Medicine." *Queen's Quarterly* 43 (Spring): 25–37

"The Four Musicians." *Saturday Night*, 1 February

"Company: A Play." *Saturday Night*, 9 May

1937

"The New *Scottish National Dictionary*." *Christian Science Monitor*, 10 March

"The Old School." *Patriot* (Charlottetown), 28 December

"Family and Society." *Quarterly Review* 268 (April): 214–24

"Design." *Queen's Quarterly* 44 (Spring): 28–35

"In Greek Soil." *Saturday Night*, 23 January

"The New House." *Saturday Night*, 12 June

"The Prince: A Memory." *Saturday Night*, 23 October

"The Shyness of Letters." *Montreal Star*, 30 November

1938
"The Old University." *McGill News* 21 (Spring): 27–9, 67
"The Old College." *Patriot* (Charlottetown), 3 January
"Robert Edward Lee." *Queen's Quarterly* 45 (Spring): 1–10
1939
The Master's Wife. Montreal
"Sir Gilbert Parker: An Appraisal." *Transactions of the Royal Society of Canada*, 3rd
    series, 33, Section 2, 123–35
1977
The Master's Wife. Toronto, New Canadian Library edn., with an introduction by
    Ian Ross Robertson
"The Traveller." *Island Magazine* 3 (Fall–Winter 1977): 27–30, with an introduction
    by Ian Ross Robertson, 26–7
1994
The Master's Wife. Charlottetown, facsimile reprint of 1939 edition, with (i) an
    enlarged introduction, explanatory notes, and corrigenda by Ian Ross
    Robertson; (ii) a preface by Harry Baglole, and the addition of (iii) "The Spirit,"
    a poem in Macphail's honour composed by a grandson, Jeffrey Burland Lindsay

Archival Collections

Beaverbrook Library, London, UK (BL)
    Lord Beaverbrook Papers
    John St Loe Strachey Papers
Bishop's University Archives, Lennoxville, PQ (BUA)
    Elizabeth Hearn Milner Papers
    University of Bishop's College, Minutes of the Faculty of Medicine
Dalhousie University Archives, Halifax (DUA)
    Archibald MacMechan Papers
Library and Archives Canada, Ottawa (LAC)
    Sir Robert Borden Papers
    Charles H. Cahan Papers
    Canadian Authors Association Papers
    Canadian Medical Association Minute Book Annual Meetings
    Canadian Medical Association Minute Book General Meetings
    Canadian Medical Association Minutes of Executive Council
    Sir Arthur Currie Papers
    John W. Dafoe Papers
    Wilfrid Eggleston Papers
    Fourth Earl Grey Papers
    Sir Wilfrid Laurier Papers
    Stephen Leacock Papers
    Newton W. MacTavish Papers
    Sinclair Ross Papers

Duncan Campbell Scott Papers
Sir John Willison Papers
McCord Museum of Canadian History, Montreal (MMCH)
E.B. Greenshields Diaries
E.B. Greenshields Scrapbook
Pen and Pencil Club of Montreal Minute Books
Pen and Pencil Club Papers
McGill University Archives (MUA)
McGill Principals' Papers
McGill University Board of Governors Minute Books
McGill University Corporation Minute Books
McGill University Faculty of Arts Minute Books
McGill University Scrapbooks
Cyrus Macmillan Papers
Sir William Peterson Letterbooks
Sir William Peterson Papers
Sir William Van Horne Papers
McGill University Archives, Archives of the Faculty of Medicine (MUA[AFM])
McGill University Faculty of Medicine Minute Books
McGill University Rare Book Room, McLennan Library (MRB)
Stephen Leacock Papers
McGill University Newspaper clippings
Eileen B. Thompson Papers
Osler Library of the History of Medicine, McGill University (OL)
"Bethune Material, 1924–42"
W.W. Francis Papers
C.F. Martin Papers
Public Archives and Records Office, Charlottetown (PARO)
William Macphail Family Papers
John A. Mathieson Papers
Prince Edward Island, Land Title Documents, Lot 50
Queen's University Library (QUL)
Stephen Leacock Papers
Lorne Pierce Papers
B.K. Sandwell Papers
Adam Shortt Papers
University of Durham Department of Palaeography and Diplomatic, UK (UD)
Fourth Earl Grey Papers
University of King's College Library, Halifax (KCL)
William E. Marshall Papers
University of Pennsylvania Archives and Records Center, Philadelphia, USA (UPA)
R. Tait McKenzie Papers
University of Toronto Archives (UTA)
Sir Robert Falconer Papers

University of Toronto Rare Book Room (UTRB)
  Mazo De la Roche Papers
  James Mavor Papers
  Sir Edmund Walker Papers
  George M. Wrong Papers
Victoria University Archives, Toronto (VUA)
  Pelham Edgar Papers

Private Collections

Etta B. Ehrlich Papers, Toronto
Alexander Macphail Papers, Ottawa
Sir Andrew Macphail Papers, Montreal
William Macphail Sr (1802–52) Papers, Montreal
William Macphail Jr (1830–1905) Papers, Montreal
James Mavor Papers, Toronto
Sir John Murray (1884–1967) Papers, London, UK

Interviews and Conversations

Bensley, Prof. E.H., Montreal, 23 June 1971
Bishop, Rev. Harvey, Charlottetown, 27 August 2003
Blanchard, Prof. J.-Henri, Charlottetown, 13 January 1967
Campbell, Mrs Dora, and Mrs Helen Chauvin, Montreal, 30 September 1970
Campbell, Mrs John, Charlottetown, 18 August 1971
Campbell, Prof. Roy, Charlottetown, 31 December 1970
Desbarets, Mlle Cecille, Montreal, 17 May 1968
Dewar, Katherine. A series of audiotaped interviews undertaken on Prince
    Edward Island by Katherine Dewar in 1990 and made available to the author
    in August 2002; those interviewed were people who had interacted with
    Macphail. There is also an interview, 1994, with a person who had worked on
    the restoration of the Macphail Homestead.
Haley, Miss Anne, Montreal, 23 July 1970
Harrison, Prof. W.E.C. and Elizabeth Harrison, Garden Island, Ontario, 7 June 1973
Igoe, W.J., London, UK, 7 July 1971
Ings, Earl, Mt Herbert, PEI, 6 September 1968
Lewis, Dr Sclater, Montreal, 17 May 1968
Lindsay, Mrs Dorothy, in Montreal and in Orwell, PEI, on several occasions,
    1968–81
MacDermot, Dr H.E., Montreal, 22 June 1971
MacInnis, Miss Goldie, and Miss Mary Martin, Orwell, PEI, 6 September 1969
MacKinnon, Prof. Frank, Charlottetown, 27 December 1967, and Toronto, 11
    August 1973
MacKinnon, Mrs W.E., Uigg, PEI, 26 June 1970

MacLeod, Mr. and Mrs. Malcolm "Mackie," Uigg, PEI, 4 September 1969
MacLeod, Percy, Orwell, PEI, 4 September 1969
Macleod, Miss Rachel, Orwell, PEI, 30 August 1969 and 26 June 1970
Macphail family, several members, at the Sir Andrew Macphail Heritage Days
    held at the Macphail Homestead, Orwell, PEI, 29–30 July 2000 and 10
    August 2002
Macphail, Prof. and Mrs M.S. Macphail, Ottawa, 18 May 1968
Martin, Prof. C.P., Montreal, 15 May 1968
Martin, Prof. William Macphail, Montreal and Orwell, PEI, on several occasions,
    2000–02
Stevenson, John A., Ottawa, 19 May 1968
Stewart, Group Captain H.R., and Mrs Stewart, Ottawa, 18 May 1968 and 10
    December 1970
Weber, Jean Macphail and Katherine Dewar, Orwell, PEI, 28 August 2004

Government Documents

Canada. *Census of Canada, 1880–81.* Vol. 1. Ottawa, 1882
– *Census of Canada, 1890–91.* Vol. 2. Ottawa, 1893
Prince Edward Island. *Debates and Proceedings of the Legislative Assembly.*
    Charlottetown, 1914
– *Journals of the Legislative Assembly.* Charlottetown, 1911–16
– *Report of the Parliamentary Committee Appointed to Investigate and Report upon
    the Manner in which the Education Law Has Been and Is Being Carried on in the
    Public Educational Establishments of this Island.* (Pamphlet), 1876
– *School Visitors' Reports,* 1845–69, 1871–72 (usually published in the journals of the
    House of Assembly or the Legislative Council or both)

DOCUMENTS RE MACPHAIL'S PRINCE EDWARD ISLAND HOME AND STEPS TAKEN TO PRESERVE HIS MEMORY (PRIVATE COLLECTION)

Abegweit Research Group, "Historic Resources Study of Selected Sites on Prince
    Edward Island," March 1976
Deed of Conveyance, from Mrs Dorothy Lindsay to Her Majesty the Queen in
    the right of the Province of Prince Edward Island, 14 June 1961
Deed of Conveyance, from Executors of the Estate of Mrs Dorothy Lindsay, and
    four children of Mrs Lindsay (acting as one party), to the Government of
    Prince Edward Island, 15 August 1991
Grant from the Province of Prince Edward Island to the Estate of Mrs Dorothy
    Lindsay, 22 November 1990
Indenture of Lease between Government of Prince Edward Island as represented
    by the Minister of Transportation and Public Works, Lessor, and Sir Andrew
    Macphail (of Orwell, PEI) Foundation Inc., Lessee, 15 August 1991

Release Agreement between Executors of the Estate of Mrs Dorothy Lindsay, and
   four children of Mrs Lindsay (acting as one party), and the Government of
   Prince Edward Island, 15 August 1991
n.a., "The Intent of a Park Master Plan" [September 1976]
n.a., "Sir Andrew Macphail Heritage Property, Development Plan, Summary," n.d.
   [15 January 1991]

SECONDARY SOURCES

Allan, Martha. [Obituary article], *The Cue* 8 (October 1938): 2–3
Allen, Richard. *The Social Passion: Religion and Social Reform in Canada, 1914–28.*
   Toronto, 1971
Armstrong, Christopher, and H.V. Nelles. "Competition vs. Convenience: Federal
   Administration of Bow River Waterpowers, 1906–13." In *The Canadian West:
   Social Change and Economic Development*, edited by Henry C. Klassen, 163–80
   & 214–19. Calgary, 1977
Atlas of Province of Prince Edward Island, Canada, and the World. Toronto, [*ca.* 1925]
Bacchi, Carol Lee. *Liberation Deferred? The Ideas of the English-Canadian Suffragists,
   1877–1914.* Toronto, 1983
Baglole, Harry, and David Weale, eds. *Cornelius Howatt: Superstar!* [Summerside,
   PEI], 1974
Baker, Janet. "Archibald MacMechan." In *Encyclopedia of the Essay*, edited by Tracy
   Chevalier, 511–12. London, 1997
– *Archibald MacMechan: Canadian Man of Letters.* Lockeport, NS, 2000
Beck, J.M. *The Pendulum of Power: Canada's Federal Elections.* Scarborough, 1968
Bensley, E.H. "Bishop's Medical College." *Canadian Medical Association Journal*, 15
   March 1955, 463–5
Benson, Eugene, and William Toye, eds. *The Oxford Companion to Canadian
   Literature*, 2nd edn. Toronto, 1997
Berger, Carl. "The Other Mr. Leacock." *Canadian Literature* 55 (Winter 1973): 23–40
— *Science, God, and Nature in Victorian Canada.* Toronto, 1983
— *The Sense of Power: Studies in the Ideas of Canadian Imperialism, 1867–1914.*
   Toronto, 1970
Bernier, Jacques. *Disease, Medicine, and Society in Canada: A Historical Overview.*
   Canadian Historical Association Historical Booklet no. 63. Ottawa, 2003
Bittermann, Rusty. *Rural Protest on Prince Edward Island: From British Colonization
   to the Escheat Movement.* Toronto, 2006
Bittermann, Rusty, and Margaret E. McCallum. "Upholding the Land
   Legislation of a 'Communistic and Socialist Assembly': The Benefits of
   Confederation for Prince Edward Island." *Canadian Historical Review* 87
   (March 2006): 1–28
Borden, Henry, and H.N. Macquarrie, eds. *Robert Laird Borden: His Memoirs.* 2
   vols. Toronto, 1969
Bottomore, T.B. *Social Criticism in North America.* Toronto, 1966

Bourne, J.M. *Who's Who in World War One*. London, 2001

Bowker, Alan, ed. *On the Front Line of Life: Stephen Leacock: Memories and Reflections, 1935–1944*. Toronto, 2004

– "Truly Useful Men: Maurice Hutton, George Wrong, James Mavor, and the University of Toronto, 1880–1927." PHD thesis, University of Toronto, 1975

– ed. *The Social Criticism of Stephen Leacock: The Unsolved Riddle of Social Justice and Other Essays*. Toronto, 1973

Bradbury, Bettina. *Working Families: Age, Gender, and Daily Survival in Industrializing Montreal*. Toronto, 1993

Brooke, Janet M. *Henri Hébert, 1884–1950: un sculpteur moderne*. Quebec, 2000

Brown, Robert Craig. "The Political Ideas of Robert Borden." In *Les idées politiques des premiers ministres du Canada/The Political Ideas of the Prime Ministers of Canada*, edited by Marcel Hamelin, 87–106. Ottawa, 1969

Brown, Thomas E. "Shell Shock in the Canadian Expeditionary Force, 1914–1918: Canadian Psychiatry in the Great War." In *Health, Disease, and Medicine: Essays in Canadian History*, edited by C.G. Roland, 308–32. Hamilton, 1984

Bruce, H.A. *Politics and the Canadian Army Medical Corps*. Introduction by Hector Charlesworth. Toronto, 1919

– *Varied Operations: An Autobiography*. Toronto, 1958

Bruce, Marian. *A Century of Excellence: Prince of Wales College, 1860–1969*. Charlottetown, 2005

Brunet, Michel. *Le présence anglaise et les Canadiens*. Montreal, 1958

Buchanan, Meriel. "The Peregrinations of a Professor." *Saturday Review* (London), 10 August 1935, 9–10

Buechler, Ralph W. "Treatise." In *Encyclopedia of the Essay*, edited by Tracy Chevalier, 853–4. London, 1997

Bumsted, J.M. "Historical Writing in English." In *The Oxford Companion to Canadian Literature*, 1st edn, edited by William Toye, 350–6. Toronto, 1983

– *Land, Settlement, and Politics on Eighteenth-Century Prince Edward Island*. Montreal & Kingston, 1987

Byrne, Deirdre. "*The University Magazine*: An Inclusive 'Conservative' Periodical." Research paper in History c47Y, Scarborough College, University of Toronto, 2000–01

Campbell, David. "I Would Not Have Missed It for the World: Sir Andrew Macphail's War." *Island Magazine* 51 (Spring–Summer 2002): 2–10

– "I Would Not Have Missed It for the World: Sir Andrew Macphail's War, Part 2." *Island Magazine* 52 (Fall–Winter 2002): 2–9

– "Politics, Polemics, and the Boundaries of Personal Experience: Sir Andrew Macphail as Official Historian." Paper presented to the annual meeting of the Canadian Historical Association, 27 May 2002

[Campbell, Henry C., and Janice Tyrwhitt] *Bartlett's Canada: A Pre-Confederation Journey*. Toronto, 1968

Campbell, Maida, and Roy Campbell. "The Murder at Goblin Hollow." *Island Magazine* 2 (Spring–Summer 1977): 32–5

Chevalier, Tracy, ed. *Encylopedia of the Essay*. London, 1997

Clark, Andrew Hill. *Three Centuries and the Island: A Historical Geography of Settlement and Agriculture in Prince Edward Island, Canada*. Toronto, 1959

Cleverdon, Catherine L. *The Woman Suffrage Movement in Canada*. Toronto, 1974 edn

Collard, Edgar Andrew. "Sir William Peterson's Principalship, 1895–1919." In *McGill: The Story of a University*, edited by Hugh MacLennan, 73–97. London, 1960

– "Voices from the Past." *McGill News* 53 (November 1972): 25

– ed. *The McGill You Knew: An Anthology of Memories 1920–1960*. Don Mills, 1975

Connor, William. "Canadian Essay (English)." In *Encyclopedia of the Essay*, edited by Tracy Chevalier, 143–7. London, 1997

Conron, Brandon. "Essays (1880–1920)." In *Literary History of Canada: Canadian Literature in English*, edited by Carl F. Klinck, et al., 340–6. Toronto, 1970 edn

Cook, G. Ramsay. *Canada and the French-Canadian Question*. Toronto, 1966

– "Stephen Leacock and the Age of Plutocracy, 1903–1921." In *Character and Circumstance: Essays in Honour of Donald Grant Creighton*, edited by John S. Moir, 163–81. Toronto, 1970

Cook, Tim. *Clio's Warriors: Canadian Historians and the Writing of the World Wars*. Vancouver, 2006

– "'Literary Memorials': The Great War Regimental Histories, 1919–1939." *Journal of the Canadian Historical Association*, new series, 13 (2002): 167–90

– "The Madman and the Butcher: Sir Sam Hughes, Sir Arthur Currie, and Their War of Reputations." *Canadian Historical Review* 85 (December 2004): 693–719

Cooper, John Irwin. *Montreal: A Brief History*. Montreal & London, 1969

Copp, Terry. *The Anatomy of Poverty: The Condition of the Working Class in Montreal, 1897–1929*. Toronto, 1974

Cox, Leo. *Fifty Years of Brush and Pen: An Historical Sketch of the Pen and Pencil Club of Montreal*. N.p., 1939

– *Portrait of a Club*. Montreal, 1962

Crichton, John. *A Vista: An Anthology of Verse*. Introduction by Sir Andrew Macphail. Montreal, 1921

Croteau, John T. *Cradled in the Waves: The Story of a People's Cooperative Achievement in Economic Betterment in Prince Edward Island, Canada*. Toronto, 1951

Davies, Gwendolyn. "Maritimes, Writing in the: 4." In *The Oxford Companion to Canadian Literature*, 2nd edn, edited by Eugene Benson and William Toye, 736–8. Toronto, 1997

Dickinson, G. Lowes. *Appearances: Being Notes of Travel*. London and Toronto, [1914]

Dickinson, John A., and Brian Young. *A History of Quebec*, 2nd edn. Toronto, 1993

Dictionary of Canadian Biography. Vols. 8 (1985), 9 (1976), 11 (1982), 12 (1990), 13 (1994), 14 (1998), 15 (2005). Toronto.

Drake Carolyn, "The Business of Anne" and "Protecting Anne's Image." *Guardian* (Charlottetown), 24 August 2004

Dyonnet, Edmond. *Mémoires d'un artiste canadien*. Preface by Jean Ménard. Ottawa, 1968

Edgar, Pelham. "Sir Andrew Macphail." *Queen's Quarterly* 54 (Spring 1947): 8–22

– "Sir Andrew Macphail (1864–1938)." *Transactions of the Royal Society of Canada*, 3rd series, 33 (1939): 147–9

– "Sir Andrew Macphail: An Appraisal." *Canadian Author* 16 (Autumn 1938): 7, 21

– "Stephen Leacock." *Queen's Quarterly* 53(Summer 1946): 173–84

Ensor, R.C.K. *England 1870–1914*. Oxford, 1936

Fabrius Cassius Funny Fellow [Keir, William]. *An Address to Prince Edward Island, by a Native*. [PEI], 1862

Ferns, H.S. "The Ideas of Mackenzie King." *Manitoba Arts Review* 6 (Winter 1948–49): 4–11

Ferns, H.S. and Bernard Ostry. *The Age of Mackenzie King: The Rise of the Leader*. London, 1955

Fingard, Judith. "The 1880s: Paradoxes of Progress." In *The Atlantic Provinces in Confederation*, edited by E.R. Forbes and D.A. Muise, 82–116. Toronto & Fredericton, 1993 .

Fong, William. *Sir William C. Macdonald: A Biography*. Montreal & Kingston, 2007

Forsey, Eugene A. *A Life on the Fringe: The Memoirs of Eugene Forsey*. Toronto, 1990

Francis, W.W. "Sir Andrew Macphail." *Bulletin of the History of Medicine* 7 (July 1939): 799–800

Friedland, Martin L. *The University of Toronto: A History*. Toronto, 2002

Frost, Stanley B. *McGill University: For the Advancement of Learning. Vol.I: 1801–1895*. Montreal, 1980

– *McGill University: For the Advancement of Learning. Vol. 2: 1895–1971*. Montreal, 1984

Fulton, Richard D. "*The Spectator*." *Encyclopedia of the Essay*, edited by Tracy Chevalier, 807–8. London, 1997

Gentilcore, R. Louis, and Geoffrey J. Matthews, eds. *Historical Atlas of Canada*. Vol. 2: *The Land Transformed*. Toronto, 1993 .

Gersovitz, Julia. "Sir Andrew Thomas Taylor." *The Canadian Encyclopedia*, 2nd edn. Edmonton, 1988

– "The Square Mile, Montreal 1860–1914." MSC (Architecture) thesis, Columbia University, 1980

Gillett, Margaret. *We Walked Very Warily: A History of Women at McGill*. Montreal, 1981

Gillis, Eliza, Viola Gillis, and Linda Jean Nicholson. *Leap Over Time: History and Recollections of One-Room Schools in the Belfast Area, 1803–1968*. N.p., 2004

Gordon, C.W. "The New State and the New Church." In Social Service Council of Canada, *The Social Service Congress of Canada, Proceedings*, 192–8. Toronto, 1914

Gorveatt, Nancy. "'Polluted with Factories': Lobster Canning on Prince Edward Island." *Island Magazine* 57 (Spring–Summer 2005): 10–21

Gournay, Isabelle. "Gigantism in Downtown Montreal." In *Montreal Metropolis, 1880–1930*, edited by Isabelle Gournay and France Vanlaethem, 153–82. Toronto, 1998

Graham, Jean. "A Man of Mark." *Saturday Night*, 4 October 1933

Grant, George Parkin. "An Ethic of Community." In *Social Purpose for Canada*, edited by Michael Oliver, 3–26. Toronto, 1961

Grant, J.W. [John Webster]. "Population Shifts in the Maritime Provinces." *Dalhousie Review* 17 (1937–38), 282–94

Grant, Judith Skelton. "Charles William Gordon." In *The Oxford Companion to Canadian Literature*, 2nd edn., edited by Eugene Benson and William Toye, 474–6. Toronto, 1997

Griffiths, N.E.S. *The Splendid Vision: Centennial History of the National Council of Women of Canada, 1893–1993*. Ottawa, 1993

Gross, John. *The Rise and Fall of the Man of Letters: Aspects of English Literary Life since 1800*. London, 1969

Hadley, Michael L., and Roger Sarty. *Tin-Pots and Pirate Ships: Canadian Naval Forces and German Sea Raiders, 1880–1918*. Montreal & Kingston, 1991

Hallowell, Gerald, ed. *The Oxford Companion to Canadian History*. Toronto, 2004

Hamer, Kathryn. "William Hume Blake." In *The Oxford Companion to Canadian Literature*, 2nd edn., edited by Eugene Benson and William Toye, 127. Toronto, 1997

Harris, Robin S. *English Studies at Toronto: A History*. Toronto, 1988

Harte, Walter Blackburn. "Canadian Journalists and Journalism." *New England Magazine*, new series, 5 (December 1891): 411–41

Harvey, D.C. *The French Régime in Prince Edward Island*. New Haven, 1926

Hathorn, Ramon. "Samuel Morgan-Powell." In *The Oxford Companion to Canadian Theatre*, edited by Eugene Benson and L.W. Conolly, 348–9. Toronto, 1989

Hatvany, Matthew G. "Tenant, Landlord, and Historian: A Thematic Review of the 'Polarization' Process in the Writing of Nineteenth-Century Prince Edward Island History." *Acadiensis* 27 (Autumn 1997), 109–32

Hay, Peter. *Vandiemonian Essays*. North Hobart, Tasmania, 2002

Heggie, Grace F., and Anne McGaughey, comps. *The University Magazine, 1901–1920: An Annotated Index*. Teeswater, Ont., 1997

Hesse, Douglas. "British Essay." In *Encyclopedia of the Essay*, edited by Tracy Chevalier, 103–13. London, 1997

Higham, Robin, ed. *Official Histories: Essays and Bibliographies from Around the World*. Manhattan, Kans., 1970

Hill, Charles C. *The Group of Seven: Art for a Nation*. Toronto, 1995

Hinds, Margery. "A Governor-General Goes North." *Beaver*, 303 (Winter 1972): 48–53

Hirschfeld, Magnus. *The Sexual History of the World War*. [Revd. edn, translated from German.] New York, 1946

Hobsbawm, Eric J. *Industry and Empire*. Vol. 3 of *The Pelican Economic History of Britain*. Harmondsworth, UK, 1969

Hodgins, Thomas. *The Alaska Boundary Dispute*. Toronto, 1903

– *British and American Diplomacy Affecting Canada*. Toronto, 1900

Hornby, Susan, ed. *Belfast People: An Oral History of Belfast, Prince Edward Island*. Charlottetown, 1992

Horowitz, David, ed. *Containment and Revolution*. Preface by Bertrand Russell. Boston, 1968 edn

Horowitz, Gad. "Conservatism, Liberalism, and Socialism in Canada: An Interpretation." *Canadian Journal of Economics and Political Science* 32 (May 1966): 143–71

– "Tories, Socialists, and the Demise of Canada." *Canadian Dimension* 2 (May–June 1965): 12–15

Houghton, Walter E. *The Victorian Frame of Mind, 1830–1870*. New Haven & London, 1957

Humphries, Mark Osborne. "The Horror at Home: The Canadian Military and the 'Great' Influenza Pandemic of 1918." *Journal of the Canadian Historical Association*, new series, 16 (2005): 235–60

Hyatt, A.M.J. "Official History in Canada." In *Official Histories: Essays and Bibliographies from Around the World*, edited by Robin Higham. Manhattan, Kans., 1970

Illustrated Historical Atlas of the Province of Prince Edward Island. [1880]; Belleville, Ont., 1972

Jeffery, Keith. *Field Marshal Sir Henry Wilson: A Political Soldier*. Oxford, 2006

Jones, Kim. "A Content Guide and Index to *The University Magazine*, Vols. IX–XIX, 1910–1920." MA thesis, Queen's University, 1954

Kerr, Donald, and Deryck W. Holdsworth, eds. *Historical Atlas of Canada*. Vol. 3: *Addressing the Twentieth Century*. Toronto, 1990

King, William Lyon Mackenzie. *Industry and Humanity: A Study in the Principles Underlying Industrial Reconstruction*. Introduction by David Jay Bercuson. Toronto, 1973 edn

Kulyk Keefer, Janice. *Under Eastern Eyes: A Critical Reading of Maritime Fiction*. Toronto, 1987

Lake, D.J. *Topographical Map of Prince Edward Island in the Gulf of St. Lawrence. From Actual Surveys and the Late Coast Survey of Capt. H.W. Bayfield*. Saint John, 1863

Lambert, Phyllis. "Foreword." In *Montreal Metropolis, 1880–1930*, edited by Isabelle Gournay and France Vanlaethem, 6–7. Toronto, 1998

Laqueur, Walter. *The Fate of the Revolution: Interpretations of Soviet History*. London, 1967

Lavigne, Suzanne, and Nicole Rodrigue. *Les rues de Montréal: répertoire historique*. Montreal, 1995

Leacock, Stephen. "Andrew Macphail." *Queen's Quarterly* 45 (Winter 1938): 445–52

– *Montreal: Seaport and City*. Garden City, NY, 1942

– *Sunshine Sketches of a Little Town*. Introduction by Malcolm Ross. New
   Canadian Library edn. Toronto, 1961
– *The Unsolved Riddle of Social Justice*. Plymouth, UK, 1920
Levitt, Joseph. *Henri Bourassa and the Golden Calf: The Social Program of the
   Nationalists of Quebec (1900–1914)*. Ottawa, 1969
– "Henri Bourassa and Modern Industrial Society, 1900–1914." *Canadian Historical
   Review* 50 (March 1969): 37–50
Lewis, Robert. *Manufacturing Montreal: The Making of an Industrial Landscape*.
   Baltimore & London, 2000
Lindsay, Mrs Dorothy. An address on weaving delivered to the Women's Institute
   in Orwell, PEI, *ca.* 1927
Linteau, Paul-André. "Factors in the Development of Montreal." In *Montreal
   Metropolis, 1880–1930*, edited by Isabelle Gournay and France Vanlaethem,
   25–33. Toronto, 1998
Lockerby, Earle. "The Deportation of the Acadians from Île St.-Jean." *Acadiensis* 27
   (Spring 1998): 45–94
– "Deportation of the Acadians from Île St.-Jean." *Island Magazine* 46 (Fall–Winter
   1999), 17–25
Lower, A.R.M. *Canadians in the Making*. Toronto, 1958
McAskill, J. Dan, and Kate MacQuarrie. *Nature Trails of Prince Edward Island*.
   [Charlottetown], 1996
McBrine, Ronald W. "The Development of the Familiar Essay in English
   Canadian Literature from 1900 to 1920." MA thesis, University of New
   Brunswick, 1967
McCrae, John. *In Flanders Fields and Other Poems*. Toronto, 1919
MacDermot, H.E. *One Hundred Years of Medicine in Canada*. Toronto, 1967
"H.E.M." [MacDermot, H.E.]. "Sir Andrew Macphail." *Canadian Medical
   Association Journal* 39 (November 1938): 482–3
– "Sir Andrew Macphail." *McGill News* 20 (Winter 1938): 16–17, 58
McDonagh, Josephine. "George Eliot." In *Encyclopedia of the Essay*, edited by Tracy
   Chevalier, 247-9. London, 1997
MacDonald, Colin S. *A Dictionary of Canadian Artists*. Vol 3. 3rd edn. Ottawa, 1991
MacDonald, G. Edward. *If You're Stronghearted: Prince Edward Island in the
   Twentieth Century*. Charlottetown, 2000
MacGillivray, S.R. "Marjorie Pickthall." In *The Oxford Companion to Canadian
   Literature*, 2nd edn., edited by Eugene Benson and William Toye, 918–20.
   Toronto, 1997
MacKay, Donald. *The Square Mile: Merchant Princes of Montreal*. Vancouver, 1987
MacKinnon, D.A., and A.B. Warburton, eds. *Past and Present in Prince Edward
   Island*. Charlottetown, [*ca.* 1906]
MacKinnon, Frank. *The Government of Prince Edward Island*. Toronto, 1951
MacKinnon, Kenneth. "Technique in *The Master's Wife*." *Essays on Canadian
   Writing* 31 (Summer 1985): 55–74

MacLaine, Brent. "Crooked Signs and Shining Things: The Magic of Books in the Literature of Atlantic Canadian Islands." In *Message in a Bottle: The Literature of Small Islands. Proceedings from an International Conference, Charlottetown, Prince Edward Island, Canada, June 28–30 [sic: June 26–28], 1998*, edited by Laurie Brinklow, Frank Ledwell, and Jane Ledwell, 37–50. Charlottetown, 2000

McLeod, Ellen Easton. *In Good Hands: The Women of the Canadian Handicrafts Guild*. Montreal & Kingston, 1999

MacLeod, Roderick. "Salubrious Settings and Fortunate Families: The Making of Montreal's Golden Square Mile, 1840–1895." PHD thesis, McGill University, 1997

MacLure, Millar. "Literary Scholarship." In *The Culture of Contemporary Canada*, edited by Julian Park, 222–41. Ithaca, 1957

MacMechan, Archibald. *Head-waters of Canadian Literature*. Toronto, 1924
– *Late Harvest*. Toronto, 1934

McMurray, Dorothy. *Four Principals of McGill: A Memoir, 1929–1963*. Montreal, 1974

McNally, Peter F. "Canadian Periodicals and Intellectual History: The Case of the *McGill University Magazine/University Magazine*, 1901–1920." *Papers of the Bibliographical Society of Canada* 19 (1980): 69–78
– "*The McGill University Magazine*, 1901–1906; An Evaluation and a Bio-bibliographical Analysis." MA Research paper, McGill University, 1976

Macpherson, C.B. *Democracy in Alberta: Social Credit and the Party System*. 2nd edn. Toronto, 1962
– *The Political Theory of Possessive Individualism: Hobbes to Locke*. London, 1964 edn

McQuaid, Sean. "Island Culture." In *Prince Edward Island: A Colour Guidebook*, edited by Laurie Brinklow, 64–8. Halifax, 1995

Mahoney, John L. "William Hazlitt." In *Encyclopedia of the Essay*, edited by Tracy Chevalier, 378–81. London, 1997

Malpeque Historical Society. *Malpeque and Its People 1700–1982*. Summerside, PEI, 1982

Marquis, T.G. "English-Canadian Literature." In *Canada and Its Provinces*, edited by Adam Shortt and Arthur Doughty, 12: 493–589. Toronto, 1914

Martin, C.F. "Sir Andrew Macphail." *Canadian Medical Association Journal* 39 (November 1938): 508–9

Masters, D.C. *Bishop's University: The First Hundred Years*. Foreword by A.R. Jewitt. Toronto, 1950

Mavor, James. *My Windows on the Street of the World*. 2 vols. London, 1923

Mellor, R.E.H. "Population." In *The Counties of Moray and Nairn*, edited by Henry Hamilton, 41–8. Glasgow, 1965

Milner, Elizabeth Hearn. *Bishop's Medical Faculty Montreal, 1871–1905, Including the Affiliated Dental College, 1896–1905*. Sherbrooke, 1985

Milner, W.S. "The Higher National Life." In *Canada and Its Provinces*, edited by Adam Shortt and Arthur Doughty, 12: 403–31. Toronto, 1914

Moir, John S. *Enduring Witness: A History of the Presbyterian Church in Canada*.
    N.p., 1987
Moore, Barrington, Jr. *Social Origins of Dictatorship and Democracy: Lord and
    Peasant in the Making of the Modern World*. Boston, 1967 edn
Moran, John. "Wittgenstein and Russia." *New Left Review* 73 (May–June 1972):
    85–96
Morgan, Henry J., comp. *Canadian Men and Women of the Time: A Handbook of
    Canadian Biography*. Toronto, 1898 & 1912 edns
Morgan-Powell, S. [Obituary article], *The Cue* 8 (October 1938): 2
– "Sir Andrew Macphail" (poem). *Montreal Star*, 26 September 1938
Moritz, Albert, and Theresa Moritz. *Stephen Leacock: His Remarkable Life*.
    Markham, 2002
Morton, Desmond. "The Supreme Penalty: Canadian Deaths by Firing Squad
    in the First World War." *Queen's Quarterly* 79 (Autumn 1972): 345–52
– *When Your Number's Up: The Canadian Soldier in the First World War*.
    Toronto, 1993
Mullin, Katherine. "Sir (John) Andrew Macphail." *Oxford Dictionary of National
    Biography*, 35: 977–8. Oxford, 2004
Munro, John A. "English-Canadianism and the Demand for Autonomy:
    Ontario's Response to the Alaska Boundary Decision." *Ontario History* 57
    (December 1965): 189–203
Murray, Heather. *Working in English: History, Institution, Resources*. Toronto, 1996
Neary, Peter. "Grey, Bryce, and the Settlement of Canadian-American Differences,
    1905–1911." *Canadian Historical Review* 49 (December 1968): 357–80
New, William H., ed. *Encyclopedia of Literature in Canada*. Toronto, 2002
Nicholl, Christopher. *Bishop's University, 1843–1970*. Montreal & Kingston, 1994
Noel, S.J.R. *Politics in Newfoundland*. Toronto, 1971
Noonan, Gerald. "William Henry Drummond." In *The Oxford Companion to
    Canadian Literature*, 2nd edn, edited by Eugene Benson and William Toye,
    333–4. Toronto, 1997
O'Brien, Charles F. *Sir William Dawson: A Life in Science and Religion*.
    Philadelphia, 1971
O'Connor, Ryan. "The Brothers and Sisters of Cornelius Howatt: Protest,
    'Progress,' and the Island Way of Life." In *Islands of the World*. Vol. 7: *New
    Horizons in Island Studies: University of Prince Edward Island, Charlottetown,
    Prince Edward Island, Canada, June 26 to 30, 2002*. Available online at
    http://bisd.hollandc.pe.ca/islands7
Orwell W.I. [Women's Institute]. *Orwell: Good Days in Orwell, History of Orwell,
    PEI*. N.p., 1985
Pacey, Desmond. "Literary Criticism in Canada." *University of Toronto Quarterly* 19
    (January 1950): 113–19
Parekh, B.C. "The Nature of Political Philosophy." In *Politics and Experience: Essays
    Presented to Professor Michael Oakeshott on the Occasion of His Retirement*, edited
    by Preston King and B.C. Parekh, 153–207. Cambridge, UK, 1968

Partridge, E.A. *A War on Poverty: The One War That Can End War*. Winnipeg,
   [1926]
Pen and Pencil Club, Montreal. *The Pen and Pencil Club, 1890–1959*. Montreal,
   1959
Perceval-Maxwell, Michael. "The History of History at McGill." Paper presented
   under the auspices of the James McGill Society, 2 April 1981
Pierce, Lorne. [obituary article], *Transactions of the Royal Society of Canada*, 3rd
   series, 33, section 2 (1939), 123
Pinney, Thomas, ed. *The Letters of Rudyard Kipling*. Vol. 4: *1911–19*. London, 1999
Porter, John, comp. *Canadian Social Structure: A Statistical Profile*. Toronto, 1967
Porter, Reg. "Architectural Treasures." In *Prince Edward Island: A Colour Guidebook*,
   edited by Laurie Brinklow, 89–95. Halifax, 1995
Rayburn, Alan. *Geographical Names of Prince Edward Island*. Ottawa, 1973
Read, Joseph. "Trade and Commerce." In *Past and Present in Prince Edward Island*,
   edited by D.A. MacKinnon and A.B. Warburton, 99–108. Charlottetown,
   [*ca.* 1906]
Reid, John G. *Six Crucial Decades: Times of Change in the History of the Maritimes*.
   Halifax, 1987
Rémillard, François, and Brian Merrett. *Demeures bourgeoises de Montréal: Le mille
   carré doré, 1850–1930*. Montreal, 1987
Reynolds, Mark. "The Campus That Never Was." *McGill News* 84 (Winter
   2004–05), 28–33
Richards, Eric. *A History of the Highland Clearances*, Vol. 1: *Agrarian Transformation
   and the Evictions, 1746–1886*. London, 1982
– *A History of the Highland Clearances*, Vol. 2: *Emigration, Protest, Reasons*.
   London, 1985
Rider, Peter E. "'A Blot Upon the Fair Fame of Our Island': The Scandal at the
   Charlottetown Lunatic Asylum, 1874." *Island Magazine* 39 (Spring–Summer
   1996): 3–9
Robertson, Ian Ross. "Andrew Macphail." In *Encyclopedia of the Essay*, edited by
   Tracy Chevalier, 512–13. London, 1997
– "Andrew Macphail: A Holistic Approach." *Canadian Literature* 107 (Winter
   1985): 179–86
– "The Historical Leacock." In *Stephen Leacock: A Reappraisal*, edited by David
   Staines, 33–49, 162–65. Ottawa, 1986
– "Maritimes 'Golden Age.'" In *The Oxford Companion to Canadian History*, edited
   by Gerald Hallowell, 391. Toronto, 2004
– "Recent Island History." *Acadiensis* 4 (Spring 1975): 111–18
– "Religion, Politics, and Education in Prince Edward Island, from 1856 to 1877."
   MA thesis, McGill University, 1968
– "Sir Andrew Macphail and Orwell." *Island Magazine* 1 (Fall–Winter 1976): 4–8
– "Sir Andrew Macphail and Prince Edward Island as a Way of Life." In *Message
   in a Bottle: The Literature of Small Islands, Proceedings from an International
   Conference, Charlottetown, Prince Edward Island, Canada, June 28–30 [sic: June*

26–28], 1998, edited by Laurie Brinklow, Frank Ledwell, and Jane Ledwell, 203–13. Charlottetown, 2000

– "Sir Andrew Macphail as a Social Critic." PHD thesis, University of Toronto, 1974

– *The Tenant League of Prince Edward Island, 1864–1867: Leasehold Tenure in the New World*. Toronto, 1996

– ed. *The Prince Edward Island Land Commission of 1860*. Fredericton, 1988

Robertson, Samuel N. "The Public School System." In *Past and Present in Prince Edward Island*, edited by D.A. MacKinnon and A.B. Warburton, 362a–72a. Charlottetown, [ca. 1906]

Rogers, John H. "V.S. Pritchett." In *Encyclopedia of the Essay*, edited by Tracy Chevalier, 676–7. London, 1997

Roland, Charles G. "Medical Schools." In *The Oxford Companion to Canadian History*, edited by Gerald Hallowell, 395–6. Toronto, 2004

Roper, Gordon. "New Forces: New Fiction (1880–1920)." In *Literary History of Canada: Canadian Literature in English*, edited by Carl F. Klinck, et al., 260–83. Toronto, 1970 edn

Ross, Aileen D. "The French and English Social Élites of Montreal: A Comparison of La Ligue de la Jeunesse Féminine with the Junior League." MA thesis, University of Chicago, 1941

Rubio, Mary, and Elizabeth Waterston, eds. *The Selected Journals of L.M. Montgomery*, Vol. 1: *1889–1910*. Toronto, 1985

– *The Selected Journals of L.M. Montgomery*. Vol. 2: *1910–1921*. Toronto 1987

St Pierre, Paul Matthew. "Andrew Macphail." In *Dictionary of Literary Biography*. Vol. 92: *Canadian Writers, 1890–1920*, edited by W.H. New, 225–8. Detroit, 1990

Sanderson, Heather. "Janice Kulyk Keefer." In *The Oxford Companion to Canadian Literature*, 2nd edn, edited by Eugene Benson and William Toye, 610–11. Toronto, 1997

Scriver, Jessie Boyd. "Slowly the Doors Opened." In *The McGill You Knew: An Anthology of Memories 1920–1960*, edited by Edgar Andrew Collard, 131–5. Don Mills, 1975

Sellar, Robert. *The Tragedy of Quebec: The Expulsion of its Protestant Farmers*. Introduction by Robert [Andrew] Hill. Toronto, 1974 edn

Shephard, David A.E. *Island Doctor: John Mackieson and Medicine in Nineteenth-Century Prince Edward Island*. Montreal & Kingston, 2003

– "An Island Doctor: The Life and Times of Dr. John Mackieson, 1795–1885." *Island Magazine* 38 (Fall–Winter 1995): 32–8

Shortt, Samuel E.D. "Essayist, Editor, and Physician: The Career of Sir Andrew Macphail, 1864–1938." *Canadian Literature* 96 (Spring 1983): 49–58

– *The Search for an Ideal: Six Canadian Intellectuals and Their Convictions in an Age of Transition, 1890–1930*. Toronto, 1976

– "Sir Andrew Macphail: Physician, Philosopher, Founding Editor of *CMAJ*." *Canadian Medical Association Journal*, 4 February 1978, 323–6

Sisler, Rebecca. *Passionate Spirits: A History of the Royal Canadian Academy of Arts, 1880–1980*. Toronto, 1980

Smith, W.I., ed. "Charles Tupper's Minutes of the Charlottetown Conference." *Canadian Historical Review* 48 (June 1967): 101–12

Spadoni, Carl. "The Publishers Press of Montreal." *Papers of the Bibliographical Society of Canada* 24 (1985): 38–50

Sperdakos, Paula. *Dora Mavor Moore: Pioneer of the Canadian Theatre*. Toronto, 1995

Squires, Bruce P. "Remembering Our First Editor." *Canadian Medical Association Journal*, 15 June 1992, 2127

Stacey, C.P. "From Meighen to King: The Reversal of Canadian External Policies, 1921–1923." *Transactions of the Royal Society of Canada*, 4th series, 8, section 2 (1969): 223–46

Stern, Fritz. *The Politics of Cultural Despair: A Study in the Rise of the Germanic Ideology*. Anchor edn. Garden City, NY, 1965

Stevenson, John A. "Sir Andrew Macphail." *Canadian Defence Quarterly* 16 (January 1939): 206–10

– "Sir (John) Andrew Macphail." *Dictionary of National Biography, 1931–1940*, 592–3. London, 1949

[Stevenson, John A.] Obituary article. *Times* (London), 24 September 1938

Stewart, H.R. "Address during the Unveiling of a Memorial to Sir Andrew Macphail." At Prince of Wales College, Charlottetown, 11 July 1955

Story, Norah. *The Oxford Companion to Canadian History and Literature*. Toronto, 1967

Strachey, J. St Loe. "The State and the Family." *National Review* (London), 50 (December 1907): 637–50

Strong-Boag, Veronica. "Independent Women, Problematic Men: First- and Second-Wave Anti-Feminism in Canada from Goldwin Smith to Betty Steele." *Histoire sociale/Social History* 29 (May 1996): 1–22

Stuart, H.A. "Sir Andrew Macphail (1864–1938)." *Calgary Associate Clinic Historical Bulletin* 9 (February 1945): 61–7

Surveyer, E.F. "Maria Chapdelaine." In *Addresses to the Canadian Club of Toronto, 1922–23*, 253–67. Toronto, 1923

Sutcliffe, Anthony. "Montreal Metropolis." In *Montreal Metropolis, 1880–1930*, edited by Isabelle Gournay and France Vanlaethem, 19–23. Toronto, 1998

Sweezy, Paul M. *The Theory of Capitalist Development: Principles of Marxian Political Economy*. Modern Reader edn. New York, 1968

Taylor, A.J.P. *Beaverbrook*. London, 1972

Taylor, Charles. "The Agony of Economic Man." In *Essays on the Left: Essays in Honour of T.C. Douglas*, edited by Laurier Lapierre, et al., 221–35. Toronto, 1971

Thomas, William Beach. *The Story of the Spectator, 1828–1928*. London, 1928

Thompson, Edward P. *William Morris, Romantic to Revolutionary*. London, 1977 edn

Thompson, I. MacLaren. "Sir Andrew Macphail (1864–1938)." *Canadian Medical Association Journal*, 6 January 1968, 40–4

Thomson, E.W. *Old Man Savarin Stories: Tales of Canada and Canadians.* Introduction by Linda Sheshko. Toronto, 1974 edn

Toker, Franklin. *The Church of Notre-Dame in Montreal: An Architectural History.* Montreal, 1970

Toye, William, ed. *The Oxford Companion to Canadian Literature.* Toronto, 1983

Trudeau, Pierre-Elliott. "La Province de Québec au moment de la grève." In *La grève de l'amiante*, edited by Pierre-Elliott Trudeau, 1–91. Montreal, 1970 edn

Try-Davies, John. *A Semi-Detached House and Other Stories.* Montreal, 1900

Tucker, Gilbert Norman. *The Canadian Naval Service: Its Official History.* Vol. I. Ottawa, 1952

Vance, Jonathan F. *Death So Noble: Memory, Meaning, and the First World War.* Vancouver, 1997

Wagg, Susan. *Percy Erskine Nobbs: Architecte, artiste, artisan/Architect, Artist, Craftsman.* Kingston & Montreal, 1982

Waite, Clifford F. "The Canadian Historical Novel." MA thesis, Acadia University, 1951

Waite, Peter B. *The Lives of Dalhousie University.* Vol. 1: *1818–1925, Lord Dalhousie's College.* Montreal & Kingston, 1994

– *The Lives of Dalhousie University.* Vol. 2: *1925–1980, The Old College Transformed.* Montreal & Kingston, 1998

Wallace, M.W., and A.S.P. Woodhouse. "In Memoriam: William John Alexander." *University of Toronto Quarterly* 14 (October 1944): 1–33

Wallace, W.S., ed. *The Macmillan Dictionary of Canadian Biography*, 3rd edn London & Toronto, 1963

Watt, F.W. "Critic or Entertainer: Leacock and the Growth of Materialism." *Canadian Literature* 5 (Summer 1960), 33-42

Waugh, Douglas. "Medical Education." *The Canadian Encyclopedia*, 3rd ed. Edmonton, 1999

Weale, David. "'The Minister': The Reverend Donald McDonald." *Island Magazine* no. 3 (Fall–Winter 1977): 1–6

– *A Stream Out of Lebanon: An Introduction to the Coming of Syrian/Lebanese Emigrants to Prince Edward Island.* Charlottetown, 1988

– "The Time Is Come! Millenarianism in Colonial Prince Edward Island." *Acadiensis* 7 (Autumn 1977): 35–48

Weale, David, and Harry Baglole. *The Island and Confederation: The End of an Era.* Summerside, PEI, 1973

Wells, Kennedy. *The Fishery of Prince Edward Island.* Charlottetown, 1986

Westley, Margaret W. *Remembrance of Grandeur: The Anglo-Protestant Elite of Montreal, 1900–1950.* Montreal, 1990

Whiteman, Bruce. "The Publication of *Maria Chapdelaine* in English." *Papers of the Bibliographical Society of Canada* 21 (1982): 52–9

Whittaker, Herbert. "Montreal Repertory Theatre." In *The Oxford Companion to Canadian Theatre*, edited by Eugene Benson and L.W. Conolly, 345–6.
   Toronto, 1989
– *Setting the Stage: Montreal Theatre, 1920–49*. Montreal & Kingston, 1999
Williams, Frances Fenwick. *A Soul on Fire*. Toronto, 1915
Williams, Raymond. *Culture and Society, 1780–1850*. Penguin edn.
   Harmondsworth, UK, 1963
Williamson, Moncrieff. *Robert Harris, 1849–1919: An Unconventional Biography*.
   Toronto, 1970
Vinyl recording incorporating readings from *The Master's Wife*: *"Island Scotch
   ...": A Medley from the Scottish Tradition in Prince Edward Island*. Produced by
   Wayne MacKinnon and Others for the Caledonian Club, Prince Edward
   Island, 1976

Illustration Credits

Connie Auld: Dr William Keir in his study in Malpeque
Confederation Centre Art Gallery, Charlottetown: Pen and Pencil Club 1908
menu card, front; Pen and Pencil Club 1908 menu card, signatures on the
back; Pen and Pencil Club menu card for 1913
Dalhousie University Archives and Special Collections: Archibald MacMechan,
University Photograph Collection PCI, box 10, folder 2, item 9
Fanning School Committee: Malpeque grammar school, 1942
Julia Gersovitz: Peel Street row house, 1894
Eleanor Lindsay Jarrett: Macphail's grandchildren, in Orwell
McCord Museum of Canadian History: Andrew Macphail, November 1886,
in Montreal, II-81719.1; Andrew Macphail in academic dress, 25 March 1891,
II-94859.1; the drawing room at 216 Peel Street at the time of Georgina's death,
1902, II-141731; Percy E. Nobbs, II-159967.1; Andrew Macphail, taken for the
Pen and Pencil Club, MP-1992.11.12; Frederick Parker Walton, MP-1992.11.22;
Stephen Leacock, II-141252; Paul T. Lafleur, MP-1978.129.14; advertising *Maria
Chapdelaine*, MP-1994.64.1.34
McGill University Archives: Sir William Peterson, PR008099
Musée national des beaux-arts du Québec (photographer Patrick Altman) and
Confederation Centre Art Gallery, Charlottetown, CAG 69.23 (64.3×59.8×34.2
cm.): bust of Macphail by Henri Hébert, 1927
Prince Edward Island Public Archives and Records Office: Prince of Wales
College, 1894, 3218/86, photo ID # P0000250
I.R. Robertson: Uigg grammar school; bell from Valleyfield church, Macphail
Homestead; the pillars, 1987; Macphail Homestead, 1988
Sir Andrew Macphail Foundation: frontispiece; Mary McPherson Macphail,
Andrew's grandmother; portrait of Andrew Macphail, 1897; portrait of
Georgina Burland Macphail, *ca.* 1900; Macphail Homestead, *ca.* 1912; Macphail
and friends at the pillars, Macphail Homestead; soldiers on horseback; Andrew
with his daughter Dorothy; Lisl; Macphail in rural setting, interwar years

Douglas Sobey: map of Prince Edward Island; map of southeastern Prince
   Edward Island; Macphail's bailiwick
Meg Lindsay Stanley: Macphail at his writing desk, interwar years
University of Prince Edward Island, University Archives: Alexander Anderson,
   principal of Prince of Wales College
University of Toronto, Cartography Office, Department of Geography: map of
   Andrew Macphail's Montreal
Victoria University Library (Toronto): Pelham Edgar; Marjorie Pickthall
Jean Macphail Weber: William and Catherine Macphail, Andrew's parents; the
   Macphail children, 1869; Andrew with son Jeffrey and brother Alexander; east
   side of the homestead, as restored

Index